KT-471-921

‖‖‖‖‖‖‖‖‖‖‖‖‖‖‖‖‖‖‖‖

# Philosophy and the Sciences of Exercise, Health and Sport

*Philosophy and the Sciences of Exercise, Health and Sport* answers these questions and more in a unique interdisciplinary study that calls on researchers working in sport, exercise and health to reflect critically on the nature and aims of scientific enquiry in these disciplines. The book addresses the underlying assumptions and development of both the very idea of science itself and what shape scientific enquiries ought to take in the fields of exercise, health and sport.

Written by a range of internationally respected philosophers, scientists and social scientists, each chapter addresses a key issue in research methodology. Questions asked by the authors include:

- Do natural and social scientists need to understand philosophy of science?
- Are statistics misused in sport and exercise science research?
- Is sport science research gender-biased?
- How do external and commercial interests skew professional guidelines in health and sport research?
- Should scientists focus their attention on confirmation of theories, or on attempts to falsify them?

*Philosophy and the Sciences of Exercise, Health and Sport* serves notice to sport and health researchers to think more philosophically about their subject and its scientific bases. It is essential reading for postgraduate researchers seeking to establish a sound theoretical foundation for their work.

**Mike McNamee** is Senior Lecturer in Philosophy at the Centre for Philosophy, Humanities and Law in Health Care at the University of Wales at Swansea, UK. He is also co-editor of the Routledge series, Ethics and Sport.

212  983

# Philosophy and the Sciences of Exercise, Health and Sport

## Critical perspectives on research methods

*Edited by*

## Mike McNamee

| NORWICH CITY COLLEGE LIBRARY | | |
|---|---|---|
| Stock No. | 212983 | |
| Class | 796.01 MAC | |
| Cat. | SSA | Proc. 3WKL |

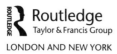

Routledge
Taylor & Francis Group

LONDON AND NEW YORK

First published 2005 by Routledge
2 Park Square,
Milton Park,
Abingdon,
Oxon OX14 4RN

Simultaneously published in the USA and Canada
by Taylor & Francis Inc
270 Madison Ave, New York, NY 10016

*Routledge is an imprint of the Taylor & Francis Group*

© 2005 Mike McNamee

Typeset in 10/12 Goudy by Keyword Typesetting Services
Printed and bound in Great Britain by TJ International Ltd, Padstow,
Cornwall

All rights reserved. No part of this book may be reprinted or reproduced or
utilised in any form or by any electronic, mechanical, or other means, now
known or hereafter invented, including photocopying and recording, or in
any information storage or retrieval system, without permission in writing
from the publishers.

Every effort has been made to ensure that the advice and information in this
book is true and accurate at the time of going to press. However, neither the
publisher nor the authors can accept any legal responsibility or liability for
any errors or omissions that may be mad.e In the case of drug administration, any medical procedure or the use of technical equipment mentioned
within this book, you are strongly advised to consult the manufacturer's
guidelines.

*British Library Cataloguing in Publication Data*
A catalogue record for this book is available from the British Library

*Library of Congress Cataloging in Publication Data*

ISBN 0-415-30016-9 (hbk)
ISBN 0-415-35340-8 (pbk)

For Cheryl, Megan and Ffion with love

# Contents

# Figures

# Tables

# Contributors

**Jacquelyn Allen Collinson** is a feminist sociologist at the University of Gloucestershire where she is a Research Fellow. Her previously published work includes research on occupational socialization and identities, while her current work is within the sociology of sport and coheres around the sporting body, the gendered body and the running body, and the use of auto/ethnographic approaches to examine these areas.

**Celia Brackenridge** runs her own research-based consultancy company, specializing in child protection and gender equity issues in sport and leisure. Celia previously worked at Sheffield Hallam and Gloucestershire Universities in the UK and is currently an honorary visiting Professor in the Centre for Applied Childhood Studies at Huddersfield University. She is an accredited BASES researcher, a World Class Adviser for the UK Sports Institute and was the first Chair of the UK Women's Sports Foundation. She is the author of *Spoilsports: Understanding and Preventing Sexual Exploitation in Sport* (Routledge, 2001).

**Precilla Choi** is Associate Professor at University, Australia. She has a background in health psychology and is internationally renowned for her ground-breaking research on gender and sport/physical exercise. She has conducted and published numerous research studies on psychological and sociocultural issues that influence physical exercise and health-related physical activity participation. She is author of *Femininity and the Physically Active Woman* (Routledge, 2000).

**Stephen-Mark Cooper** is Principal Lecturer in Biostatistics in the School of Sport, PE and Recreation at the University of Wales Institute, Cardiff, UK. He is an elected Fellow of the Royal Statistical Society and a member of the British Association of Sport and Exercise Sciences. His research interests are centered on the application of statistical methods in the sport and exercise sciences, and measurement issues relevant to performance in sport and exercise.

**John Hockey** is a Research Fellow at the University of Gloucestershire who has used ethnographic and authoethnographic approaches to study areas as diverse as the subculture of infantry, doctoral education and the sociology of sport. His current research within the sociology of sport focuses on "mundane" knowledge held by middle-distance and long-distance runners.

**Roger Homan** is Professor of Religious Studies at the University of Brighton, UK. His doctoral study and the thrust of much of his early work were in sociology. It was here that he got entangled in research ethics, to the study of which his principal contribution is *The Ethics of Social Research* (Longman, 1992).

**Graham McFee** is Professor of Philosophy in the University of Brighton, UK, and Vice President of the British Society of Aesthetics. He has written and presented extensively, both nationally and internationally, on many areas within philosophy, especially philosophical aesthetics and the philosophy of Wittgenstein. His recent publications include *Understanding Dance* (Routledge, 1992), *Free Will* (Acumen, 2000), *The Concept of Dance Education* [Expanded Edition] (Pageantry Press, 2004), and *Sport, Rules and Values* (Routledge, 2004).

**Mike McNamee** is Senior Lecturer in Philosophy at the Centre for Philosophy, Humanities and Law in Health Care at the University of Wales, Swansea, UK. His research interests are in the philosophies of education, leisure, science, sports, and in research ethics. His co-edited works include *Ethics and Sport* (Routledge, 1998), *Just Lesiure* (LSA, 2000) and *Ethics and Educational Research* (Blackwell, 2002), and he is series co-editor of *Ethics and Sport* (Routledge). He is a Past President of the International Association for the Philosophy of Sport. He is currently an Executive Member of the European College of Sport Science, the International Council for Sports Science and Physical Education, and is the inaugural Chair of the British Philosophy of Sport Association.

**Nanette Mutrie** is Professor of Exercise Psychology at the University of Strathclyde, Glasgow. She is a visiting Professor in the MRC Social and Public Health Sciences Unit in Glasgow University. Her main research interests are related to exercise and health with the theme of increasing activity in general and clinical populations.

**Alan Nevill** is the research Professor in the School of Sport, Performing Arts and Leisure, as well as a core member of the Research Institute of Healthcare Sciences at the University of Wolverhampton, UK. He is currently Editor-in-Chief of the *Journal of Sports Sciences*. Previously, he has served as Treasurer of BASES (1995–97) and Chairman of the Birmingham and District local group of the Royal Statistical Society (1994–96). He was also consultant statistician to the Allied Dunbar national fitness survey (1991–93).

**Tim Noakes** is the Discovery Health Chair of Exercise and Sports Science and is Director of the University of Cape Town/Medical Research Council Research Unit for Exercise Science and Sports Medicine at the University of Cape Town, South Africa. He has run more than 70 footraces of 42 km or longer and is the author of the definitive text, *The Lore of Running*. In 1985, he was the first to describe the condition of voluntary water intoxication in ultra-marathon runners and has spent the last 20 years trying to understand why over-consumption of any fluid during exercise can be fatal, and is also responsible for a novel interpretation of the factors that regulate exercise performance.

**Jim Parry** is Senior Lecturer in Philosophy at the University of Leeds, UK. He was formerly Head of the Department of Philosophy and of the School of Humanities, and held the International Chair in Olympic Studies at the Autonomous University of Barcelona for 2003. He is series co-editor of *Ethics and Sport* (Routledge), and co-author (with V. Girginov) of *The Olympic Games Explained.*

**Neil Spurway** is Emeritus Professor of Exercise Physiology at the University of Glasgow, UK. He taught and researched physiology – mainly that of vertebrate muscle and of human exercise – from 1960 to 2001. He is a former Chair, British Association of Sport and Exercise Sciences, and Vice-Chair, Physiology Steering Group of British Olympic Association and is currently President of the Royal Philosophical Society of Glasgow. He has a life-long interest in philosophy, especially that of science and a comparable enthusiasm for natural theology. He was the first elected Chair, Glasgow Gifford Lectureships Committee, and currently edits the *ESSAT News*, Journal of European Society for the Study of Science and Theology.

**John Sugden** is Professor in the Sociology of Sport at the University of Brighton's Chelsea School (UK). He has researched and written widely on a variety of themes around the relationship between sport and society. He is particularly well known for his work on sport in divided societies and his critical analysis of world football's governing body, FIFA. He is equally regarded for his ethnographic and investigative approach to research.

**Rhys Williams** is Professor of Clinical Epidemiology at the Clinical School, University of Wales, Swansea. He has a long-standing interest in diabetes – its epidemiology, economic consequences and the delivery of health services to those with diabetes and those at risk of developing it. He has been a visiting consultant at the World Health Organization in Geneva and has long been involved in the development of diabetes-related health policy at national and international levels.

**Simon Williams** is Principal Lecturer in Health and Exercise Science at the University of Glamorgan. His primary research interests focus on the physiology of obesity and type 2 diabetes, the epidemiology of these conditions and their prevention and treatment with nutritional and exercise interventions.

**M.R. (Fred) Yeadon** began life as a mathematics undergraduate where he was first coached in gymnastics by Nik Stuart. Subsequently he applied his mathematical background to the analysis of twisting somersaults for which he won awards from the International Society of Biomechanics and the American Society of Biomechanics. Currently he is Professor of Computer Simulation in Sport at Loughborough University, UK, where he uses both experimental and theoretical approaches to sports biomechanics to investigate technique in athletics, gymnastics, trampolining, springboard diving, freestyle skiing and ski jumping.

# Preface and acknowledgements

In these days of research selectivity, the reader will probably be aware that edited collections do not add much to one's professional CV. Writing chapters for such books then might appear to have even less prestige. The only currency in the market (it is said) is articles in internationally respected peer-reviewed journals. These are of course key indices of quality research output. They are not, however, the exclusive homes for 'real' scholarship that some believe. Something of importance must have driven the authors here to accept my invitation to contribute to this collection. Can they all be mistaken? I think not (well, I would say that, wouldn't I?!). Collections such as these, I believe, are highly important in this regard: if people are to teach courses in new areas, or new ones in old areas, they need resources. It is my hope that this book augments the research methods texts that proliferate in exercise, health and sports sciences and that it at least begins to open a space for more considered discussion of issues pertaining to the nature and methods of scientific enquiries, and the professional socialization of would-be scientists in these fields.

I thank the authors wholeheartedly for the wisdom they have shared in these pages and not least of all for their tolerance of my editorial interferences. Finally, my thanks go to Andrew Bloodworth for his diligent proof reading, to Simon Whitmore (formerly of Routledge) for his early encouragement of the text, and to Samantha Grant of Routledge (Taylor and Francis) for her patience and support.

# 1  Positivism, Popper and Paradigms: an introductory essay in the philosophy of science

*Mike McNamee*

## Philosophical questions in natural and social scientific research

That we need science to understand matters of disease, exercise, fitness, health, illness and so on is undisputed. Whether any empirical or scientific enterprise could properly proceed without philosophical reflection is not universally agreed. A simple thought, however, should arrest any potential dispute. How, we might well ask, could scientists investigate exercise, measure fitness, or evaluate health and illness without first clarifying the very concepts that they sought to research? Are exercise benefits objective or subjective? What type of fitness do we wish to measure? Shall we use broad or narrow conceptions of health? What are the logical relations between disease and illness? All these simple questions are essential to scientists and other professionals in the sphere of exercise, health and sport. And they are, of course, all philosophical ones pertaining to the concepts we employ, whether as students, or lecturers, or researchers, in our professional lives.

What is less obvious, perhaps, is the array of questions that are assumed in the very nature of the methods, reasonings or theories that underlie the activities of scientists. Why ought we to consider philosophical aspects of the production of knowledge in science? For researchers, and well-published ones at that, the kinds of reflections on fundamental questions seem a mere annoyance: Are there are any absolute truths? Is relativism the only alternative to absolute truth? Can science be interest-driven and objective? Are theories incommensurable? Is there a unity of method in science? Is and ought scientific enquiry to be viewed as amoral? These are questions that certainly get in the way for some. To what extent are they an obstacle to be overcome in the production of knowledge? Are they merely of antiquarian interest to the modern researcher? In short, is there a need for a Philosophy of Science in exercise, health and sport research?

It is my contention that philosophical reflections on the natures and methods of sciences is simultaneously critical *and*, sadly, marginalized. In the course of 20 years of lecturing I have found, in the various universities where I have taught, conditions favourable and unfavourable to philosophical reflection. Every year, in research methods courses, I have been called upon to perform two apparently valued tasks. I am sure my experience is not an isolated one. First, typically in

Lecture 1, the resident philosopher, if one's department is still lucky enough to employ one, will need to romp through the entire history of the philosophy of science. In this vein, I well remember a colleague complaining in a course planning meeting for a postgraduate research methods module, that they could not possibly fit into 3 hours an introduction to a certain software package. Is it not remarkable then, that one should be required to traverse – at speeds that the term 'breakneck' hardly begins to describe – the entire terrain of philosophy of science to students equally in/experienced in both science and philosophy. My colleague was impervious to the irony. Second, and increasingly these days, the philosopher is wheeled in to speak about research ethics in the conduct of scientific enquiries and to interrogate issues such as anonymity, confidentiality, privacy, the ab/uses of 'gatekeepers', voluntary informed consent and so on. These two functions are critical to the *education* of researchers and not merely their training. The cultivation of broader concerns to inform their knowledge and understanding of scientific research is critical to their becoming reflective practitioners as opposed to mere scientific technicians. Nevertheless, these two contributions aside, the remainder of such courses, typically, is a mixture of methods and techniques of data gathering and analysing, dissecting and disseminating. (And all shall worship at the wonders of scientific method and its techniques.) Yet, is this not proper? Ought one really to expect anything else in courses typically called 'Research Methods'?

Over the time of teaching such material, I have come increasingly to believe that most of the students, from doctoral to undergraduate programmes, could not give a coherent account of the distinctions between research methods and research methodologies. And their dissertations and theses often bear testimony to this assertion. Perhaps it is the fault of the supervisors, who may well stand in similar ignorance. Yet the ability to articulate one's methods is one thing; to justify them is another. To show how this problem may or may not have been conducted otherwise, and to show that the manner in which it was conducted was appropriate or even optimal, to show how observation is theory-laden, to appreciate how data can be a hostage to method, is crucial and all too often ignored. Even where it is not overlooked it is not taken seriously. This is a strong claim. Let me say a little more then about how I think this happens.

The processes whereby scientists typically become technicians is a complex one and I am not fit to tell the story especially well. I will therefore restrict myself to a few observations that will yield at least part of the context for the justification of this text as well as the provision more widely of philosophical reflection across the range of scientific domains.

The idea of the lonely scholar conducting experiments may find its romantic home in Galileo's tower, but it scarcely comes near the modern reality of scientific research in exercise, health and sports as elsewhere. Researchers typically hunt in packs. At the postgraduate level generally, but especially at doctoral level, research teams in and out of laboratories focus on specific issues and techniques. Those teams and laboratories become reputed for certain types of research: department X is brilliant with certain biochemical assays, department Y is more focused on epidemiological work; research unit Z is excellent on survey work; team F focus on high performance, department A on individualized qualitative work (or post-structuralist feminist critique, or figurational analysis, and so on). Their funding is generated by key publications which then secure private or governmental monies in order to produce more research, and so the cycle goes on. The mix can be either methodological and/or theoretical. And 'paradigmatically', as I shall note below, this all operates at a level below conscious consideration or reflection.

Scientific labour has necessarily become specialized. Teams divide their labour from the mundane blood collection techniques, the assays, or the questionnaires or interviews, the drafting of data tables and so on. The statistical analyses will typically be done by a specialist. Other critical tasks, whether writing the funding proposal, the review papers (state of the art [science] summaries), final versions of international journal articles, or the keynote lectures, will be assigned. That fragmentation of the process is now essential to much modern science. And, lest it be thought that I am biased, while this has been the norm in natural sciences for a long time now, it is increasingly becoming the norm in the social sciences too. Departments are rated more highly where their research themes are tightly focused and where their colleagues collaborate in shared ends and agreed methods. The benefits of such managed research are too obvious to recount, the drawbacks more subtle. I have often met PhD students who have already completed one or more experiments but performed no literature review. When asked how they decided upon the methodological approach they simply said – without a whiff of disquiet or even unease – that all that had been set out by the lab director or principal researcher or that the method was so obvious that no serious reflection was required on it. Equally, I have met funded PhD students in the social sciences who had failed to appreciate that their funding was predicated upon particular theoretical approaches that, mid-way through, they had come to challenge with great discomfort. Perhaps most pernicious of all, and increasingly prevalent in the days of 'publish or perish', is the attribution of authorship: whose name gets on to the published research – and often in what order – reveals hierarchies of power that seem ineradicable in much modern science. Yet the inputs to the research are often so varied in quality and quantity that there are real and pressing questions to be asked about the researcher's names on papers no less than the appearance of signatures on the originality clause at the front of every thesis. We can also ask questions of scientific integrity and the im/proper socialization processes of future generations into a particularly cynical conception of science. Such are the prices of modern, managed research and the efficient production of knowledge.

These sketchy scenarios raise questions about the relations between values, theory, method and data, about research funding, and about editorial biases in certain forms of research or historically privileged conceptions of scientific questions and solutions. They are every bit as important for researchers as the selection of case study or survey, or of invasive versus non-invasive techniques for the measurement of aerobic and anaerobic metabolism. These are the types of questions that I have asked the authors of this text to address. In the process of the book's history, I set out to find authors who had genuine authority in their fields and to offer them a question that was of some scientific and professional moment. I did not want a chapter written merely on a fascinating philosophical puzzle within a scientific context. I wanted to display the urgency and privilege of philosophical reflection *in* answering scientific questions. Very often, in the process of drafting and redrafting, that question became revised and refined; some authors fell by the wayside, others joined in. Equally it was my contention that the type of reflection we called 'philosophical' in scientific matters was not the exclusive province of philosophers. Every good scientist in their activities needs to address conceptual questions just as much as they must address epistemological ones. Ought not every scientist to consider the alternative conceptions of the phenomenon they are researching before they operationalize their definitions of the subject they propose to investigate? Ought not every scientist to reflect on the relations of theory, method and data? My contention that they should is carried into the choice of authors for the text. Only three are professional philosophers. Yet each of the natural or social scientists that have contributed to the text has, as is demonstrated here, thought deeply and philosophically about the nature and methods of their enquiries. I also confess to a deeper, political, motive. Were a philosophy of science text to be written merely by a philosopher or philosophers, I sceptically assume that it would not be received as well by the multiple audiences whom I have targeted. Indeed, it may not even be read by them nor reviewed in the natural and social scientific journals of exercise, health and sport. External criticism can often be dismissed as impractical and/or irrelevant, outdated, uninformed, and these are the most polite of the disavowals. Criticism from within the quarters of scientific domains, from authoritative voices, cannot be dismissed *ad hominem* with a clear conscience: whether the proposition a person propounds is true or false, it will not be so merely *because* it is the view of this or that particular person. Were mere philosophers to propound some of the views set out here, my intuition is that swift rejection might well follow.

The text is not an original one in the 'philosophy' of science. Nor is it even a typical one. And so for those who seek detailed discussions on the nature of causality, or of explanation, or of inference to the best explanation, realism and anti-realism in science, will be disappointed with the range of the material covered here. First, it is not intended that the authors especially challenge or add to the parent discipline. Rather the more modest aim is that they illustrate a range of philosophical questions that have grown in the fields of our professional endeavours. Second, the cut between natural and social scientific research makes these areas ripe for enquiry. In this way, the term 'fields' of enquiry takes on a more literal meaning. Typically, exercise, health and sport do not form single disciplinary contexts. They are properly to be understood within a matrix of disciplines from anatomy, biochemistry, biomechanics, philosophy, physiology, psychology, sociology and beyond. The book, I hope, instantiates the need for, and the benefits to be had from, a spirit of tolerance of the multidisciplinarity of contributions to our fields. What I shall do in the remainder is to further sketch out in a superficial way a selected portion of the philosophical terrain that provides little more than background notes to the chapters herein.

## Two cheers for positivism and *the* scientific method

'What are the objects of scientific enquiry?' we might ask. Recognizing that exercise, health and sports research have offered fruitful fields of scientific labour, could there be a science of anything or indeed everything? Well, of course, the idea that anything might be scientifically understood is a contestable claim. Not that long ago, however, it would have been clear that what designated a scientific enquiry was the method adopted. It is worth considering some historical aspects of this idea.

It is widely held that, until the seventeenth century, the term philosophy was used to refer to any systematic enquiry of any subject after which certain methods of enquiry, certain ways of arriving at knowledge, come to be privileged. A particular picture of rationality replaces the ancient tests of reasonableness (Toulmin: 2003). In the wake of the Copernican revolution, which dislodged the earth from the centre of the known universe while replacing it with the sun, came Galileo's use of a mathematical vocabulary to help to describe the physical world. Crucially, we witness the rise of the experiment to support careful observation and develop generalizations, hypotheses and theories for scientific explanations. Whether we are to label Bacon an inductivist[1] or not, there are clearly the seeds here of the patient accumulation of facts that are tested against experience in a controlled manner so as to become more certain of the order of the natural world. It is in the seeds of these loosely collected ideas that the term 'positivism' is typically situated.

It is something of a surprise then, that the term 'positivism' is not a hostage to the history of natural science itself. The term 'positivist philosophy' was first coined by the French sociologist Auguste Comte in the early nineteenth century. In the wake of the success of experimental methods, scholars typically cite the earlier empiricist influence of David Hume in his *An enquiry concerning human understanding* (1739) who rejects the reasoning from 'first' principles. He writes:

> When we run over libraries, persuaded of these principles, what havoc must we make. If we take in our hand any volume; of divine or school metaphysics, for instance, let us ask: *Does it contain any abstract reasoning concerning quantity or number?* No. *Does it contain any experimental reasoning concerning matter of fact and existence?* No. Commit it then to the flames: for it can contain nothing but sophistry and illusion. (Cited in Hacking 1983: 44.)

Among the things that Hacking notes from this quote is the positivistic penchant for slogans. That spirit survives today in those who assert blindly that unless problems have some quantificationist or experimental basis, they cannot claim scientific status. That which is not wrought from *the* scientific method must therefore surrender all pretence to science (thereby to proper objectivity). Of course a whole host of unscientific biases are in operation here (see Parry, Chapter 2, on the ideological elements of positivistic thinking). What we can retain here is the positivist's strong sense of antipathy to metaphysics, on which I shall comment below.

Of the term 'positivism' specifically, Halfpenny (1982: 15) notes not one but three senses or conceptions of the term in Comte's writing. First, positivism refers to a theory of historical development in which the growth of knowledge contributes to the development of progress and social stability. This conception of positivistic philosophy sounds very much a product of its age, while the second and third conceptions have a more modern ring.[2] Second, positivism refers to a claim that only a certain kind of knowledge counts as scientific and that it must be based upon observation of publicly available entities. Finally, positivism entails the claim that all science proper can be integrated into a unified system.

Even if academics were faithful to Comte's original work, confusion might arise in the applications of a term that slid between the three different senses. Yet modern natural and social scientific research methods talk in exercise, health and sport research is sometimes so loose that the term itself falls into disrepute. Nowhere is this more the case than with the all-pervasive term 'paradigm' (discussed below), which is typically cited without any precise meaning in mind. Likewise, calling a researcher or research design 'positivistic' often indicates little more than mild and unspecific abuse. When content seems to attach to the ascription, it might mean little more than a predilection for statistics, or a privileging of experimental method, or a dependence on hypothesis testing as a *sine qua non* of a proper researcher.

Comte's positivist philosophy owed a debt to Condorcet's *Essay on the development of the human mind* (Hacking 1983). In this development, which was in sympathy with Hume's empiricism, there were three phrases: (i) the theological stage; (ii) the metaphysical stage in which divinities were replaced by metaphysical entities; and (iii) the final stage of positive science. For Comte, positive science rested on the ability to determine the truth and/or falsity of propositions. Hacking (1983: 45) writes 'Propositions cannot have "positivity" – be candidates for truth-or-falsehood – unless there is some style of reasoning which bears on their truth value and can at least in principle determine the truth value'.[3]

Despite the heterogeneity of scientists and commitments that are often grouped (or merely thrown) together, Hacking (1983: 42–3) discerns six positivistic ideas which I summarize here:

1  an emphasis upon *verification* (or some variant such as *falsificationism*) to settle truth claims;
2  a commitment to *observation* as the content or foundation of all our non-mathematical knowledge;
3  a *rejection of innate causes* and instead an acceptance of the constancy with which events of one kind are followed by others;

4　a *downplaying of explanations* which should be used to organize phenomena but do not provide deeper answers to the 'why?' questions over and above the noting of their regular occurrence;

5　a restriction of reality to the observable and a *disavowal of theoretical entities*;

6　a summation of ideas 1–5 in the phrase *against metaphysics*.

Hacking concludes thus: 'Untestable propositions, unobservable entities, causes, deep explanation – these, say the positivists, are the stuff of metaphysics and must be put behind us' (1983: 42). A further point might be added to this list. Typically, in the first half of the twentieth century the philosophical branch of positivism (logical positivism as it came to be known) held specifically that our interrogation of language allowed us to set up discrete categories such as those between fact and value, and propositions that could be known to be true analytically (by definition of the words as in the closed concepts of mathematics or logic) or synthetically (by experience – for which substitute here: experiment). I shall refer specifically to the problems of the fact–value distinction in the final section below.

Despite the fact, then, that the term 'positivist' has fallen into disrepute, it still shares many ideas that natural and social scientists feel at home with, however much they might baulk at the term. Most scientists are still anti-metaphysical; many consider verification appropriate in certain circumstances. Even those committed to falsificationism, after Popper's radical ideas (see Spurway and Noakes, Chapters 3 and 4, for physiological applications of his ideas) there is still a positivistic element in the idea of a single criterion to demarcate science from non-science and a commitment to the unity of scientific method. So, if positivism is dead (I shall avoid a temptation to remark, after Twain, that reports to that effect might be a little precipitous), at least some of the spirit of positivism remains in logical empiricism, to which I shall briefly turn.

## (Logical) positivism, empiricism and Popper

Those who will not confess (in public anyway) to being positivists, or positivistic, might well own up to being fully paid up empiricists. The two are often slid together casually in research methods discussions. Clarifying their relations may be helpful if only to make sense of some of the important reactions to them in the work of philosophers such as Popper, Lakatos and Kuhn.[4]

Salmon (2001) claims that the fundamental tenet of logical empiricism is that empirical evidence in conjunction with logic as well as mathematics and formal logic underwrites all scientific knowledge. Importantly he notes that the form of reasoning that the logic takes may include either induction or confirmation. He goes on to issue a warning against the too casual use of labelling communities of scientists under specific commitments:

> Contemporary logical empiricists disagree, however, about such basic issues as the nature of empirical evidence, the status and structure of confirmation

or inductive inference, the nature of scientific explanation, and the character of scientific theories, to name but a few examples. (Salmon 2001: 233.)

In the early part of the twentieth century the logical positivists held very much to the view that meaningful (scientific) propositions had to be verified. Rudolf Carnap, one of its chief architects, stood continuous with the tradition that was committed to a bottom-up picture of science. Careful observation, systematic recording and controlled experimentation gave us data that accumulated to describe, predict and prosecute the regularity of the world.

Despite the reputation Karl Popper now enjoys, he was, during his early academic life, something of an outsider. The intellectual dominance of the 'Vienna Circle', which drove the logical positivist movement, was a group to which he neither belonged nor identified with.[5] Yet, as I have already remarked, he shares many of the commitments of the positivists such as the distinction between observation and theory, the movement toward the one true theory of the universe, the structure of reasoning and the unity of science (Hacking 1983); this is why Hacking still refers to him as a positivist. Among Popper's great contributions to the philosophy of science, however, is his effective reversal of the bottom-up procedure. Instead of making the spirit of confirmation drive scientists, he insists that it is falsification, not verification, that scientists ought properly to aim at in order to better understand the world (see Parry, Spurway and Noakes, Chapters 2–4 respectively[6]). What seems now obvious is a great leap forward in our understanding of science. Inductivism is based upon an inference from a great number of observations of the relations of phenomena (i.e. the sun has come up dutifully every morning – to use the crudest of examples) to a general conclusion – ideally a law-like formulation – that the sun will always rise in the morning. But, as Hume argued long before, this does not guarantee that the event will happen the next time. No proof is established, *viz.* the truth of the claim that the sun will come up tomorrow *because* it has with unfailing regularity come up in the past. By contrast, one observation to the contrary will falsify the generalization that the sun always comes up in the morning. As Magee puts it: 'The entire conception of science that had prevailed for getting on for three hundred years cannot be right. The rug is pulled out from under what had been the very basis of Western thought for centuries' (1997: 50). Perhaps, the nub of Popper's claim here is that scientific laws always go beyond experimental data and experience. Having challenged successfully the traditional method he proposed his own model of scientific method as a form of problem solving where one sought to reject weaker theories for stronger theories but always with the idea that the best knowledge we have is always provisional, never finally provable. Science at its best was an interplay of conjecture and refutation: a dialectic between opposing scientific theories and speculations that worked off the friction each gave the other in the processes of opposition. This idea, coupled with the belief in the unity of scientific method, drove him to demarcate science from what he called pseudo-sciences, such as Freudian psychology or Marxist sociology, both of which claimed to be scientific in the traditional sense. He found in Hume's original here the idea that if one could not *in principle* falsify propositions within a purported science – as was true of both Freudian and Marxist theory – then the claim to scientific status was bogus. The aftermath of this rejection, along with the dominance of an alternative paradigm in psychology, is still felt by Freudian scholars (see McFee for a critique of the often misguided rejection based frequently on misconceptions of his work in the context of sports psychology in Chapter 5).

Whatever revolution Popper sparked, perhaps the most notable aspect of continuity between his thinking and positivists' is the idea of the unity of science. However different verification and falsification are, they are both an attempt to provide a criterion of demarcation between science and non-science and as such they presuppose the idea of the unity of scientific method. In both cases, the positivistic conception of the science predicated on observation, hypothesis and experimental affirmation came under increasing attack.

In one clear way, the humility that attends Popperian science and the faith that we place in its spectacularly successful findings is supported or supplanted (depending on the statisticians involved) by ideas of probability. Given the impossibly heavy burden of truth, scientists of all persuasions typically trade in probabilities. Gower exemplifies this move in Bertrand Russell: 'In the induction chapter of *The Problems of Philosophy*, Russell makes it clear that the aim of inductive arguments is, given the truth of their premises, to make their conclusion *probably* true' (1997: 189, emphasis added.).

Russell's principle of induction runs something like this: given that we have a sufficient number of positive observations and no negative ones, then we can be nearly certain that a given law is true. As we have seen, this confidence is later shattered by Popper. But this does not render impotent the uses of probability. And the confidence of our probabilities can be put to good practical use – a point not lost in the public appreciation of science. Put at its most simple level, scientists and everyday folk want to assign a numerical quality to the relations between events, and they express these as ratios. This gives tremendous power to the idea that science can predict – with greater or lesser confidence – the likelihood of given occurrences. What ratios cannot do – but what many social and natural science undergraduates naïvely believe they do in fact do – is establish anything with absolute certainty: they prove nothing. Indeed it is argued by Reichenbach that an appreciation of the ramifications of this point rent asunder the positivists from the empiricists:

> An analysis of meaning [according to positivists] which any proposition of science contains nothing but a repetition of "report propositions." Since every report consists of statements about the *immediate present*, science states nothing but relations existing between present phenomena. This conclusion, however, is in sharp contrast to the actual practice of science, for scientific propositions make assertions about the *future*. Indeed, there is no scientific law which does not involve a prediction about the occurrence of future

events; for it is the very essence of a scientific law to assure us that under given conditions, certain phenomena will occur. (Cited in Salmon 2001: 235.)

Examples of precisely how statistical techniques are used in science are many and various and this is not the place to list them. But it is worth noting that one early view in empiricist thought was that they might be used not merely in the experiments themselves, but actually in preferring certain theories above others. Moreover, the force of tradition in statistics is not without its problems. Just as a community of scientists tends to approach problems and agree upon solutions in similar ways, so certain techniques and models come to dominate thinking in statistics (see Cooper and Nevill, Chapter 6, for a particular malaise in exercise and sport sciences) without critical reflection and in biomechanics, which itself cannot be undertaken without the support of statistical modelling (see Yeadon, Chapter 7).

The weight of a whole range of criticisms from the middle of the twentieth century onwards, from philosophers, historians and social scientists alike, culminates in an increasing attack on the scientific method. Bogen captures the reality of the scientific mindset as opposed to the naïve conception of science and scientific progress:

> People once believed a fabulous engine called the Scientific Method harvests empirical evidence through observation and experimentation, discards subjective, error ridden chaff, and delivers objective, veridical residues from which to spin threads of knowledge. Unfortunately, the engine is literally fabulous. Lacking a single method whose proper application always yields epistemically decisive results, real-world scientists make do with messy, quirky techniques and devices for producing and interpreting empirical data which proliferates as investigators improvise fixes for practical and theoretical problems which bedevil their research. (2001: 128.)

He goes on to observe that after the demise of positivism:

> Decades would pass before philosophers of science began to appreciate how much the epistemic value of empirical data as evidence for or against a scientific claim depends upon the way it was produced, and the degree to which some features of scientific practice can be illuminated by considering facts about data production instead of logical relations between theoretical claims and descriptions of empirical results. (2001: 132.)

Some of those features relate to the effects of technology and laboratory equipment, the salience of patterns of socialization for scientists and other cultural factors that affect observation and the perception of significance (see McFee, Chapter 5, Noakes, Chapter 8, Brackenridge *et al.*, Chapter 9, and Williams and Williams, Chapter 13, for a variety of instances of these problems).

There were of course other key contributions to the philosophical debate. Hansen's notion of the theory-ladenness of observation has long been well taken in the social sciences. Here the impossibility of theory neutrality is acknowledged by all and for a long time (the theory selection is at times bewildering: functionalism, structural-functionalism, Marxism, neo-Marxism, critical theory, figurationalism, the many forms of feminism, and so on are taught from the very beginning as the lenses through which we observe the social world). Yet in natural science, the shared backgrounds of researchers are often so tight that theoretical disagreement arises with much less frequency or is itself acknowledged with much less damaging implications. Equally, Lakatos' critique of Popper's oversimplified account of scientific progress and rejection (see Parry, Chapter 2) gave further reason for philosophers of science to sharpen their teeth on more realistic descriptions of the actual workings of natural scientists. The literature that developed further amplified the climate of scepticism towards the scientific project traditionally conceived. Yet it was Kuhn's historicized account of scientific methods and theory that contributed to what has been called the death of empiricism. Indeed, so strong was the tide of criticism launched by the book, that one author was moved to title an article 'Did Kuhn kill logical empiricism?' (Reisch 1991). I shall therefore consider a key feature of Kuhn's thinking, the paradigmatic nature of science, which is commonly passed over in the non-philosophical literature on research methods and methodologies.

## The unbearable slipperiness of paradigms

Kuhn's contribution to our critical understanding of science must be situated in the context of a growing disenchantment with positivistic philosophy of science. How ironic it is then, as many commentators have observed, that Kuhn's famous text *The Structure of Scientific Revolutions* was produced in a series entitled 'The Encyclopedia of Unified Science'. Unsurprisingly, perhaps, it became the last in the series. Effectively, it ended the myth. Kuhn much later on remarked:

> I aim to deny all meaning to claims that successive scientific beliefs become more and more probable or better approximations to the truth and simultaneously to suggest that the subject of truth claims cannot be a relation between beliefs and a putatively mind-independent or 'external' world (1993: 330).

But the reach of Kuhn's work and its complex nature are not charted here. Critical commentaries are legion (e.g. Horwich 1993). My concerns here are limited to his use, and the widespread subsequent use, of his novel idea: paradigms.

One of the problems that has bedevilled methodological discussion in theses and research papers has been the all too casual use of the term 'paradigm'. Indeed so proliferous and so careless is its use, that even though it has seen to become a *sine qua non* in methods discussions, it has, at the same time, been rendered almost meaningless because of a lack of precision in its use. The problem is twofold. In the first instance one wonders just how many of the authors who casually cite "paradigm" (Kuhn 1962) have even read the book. Before guilt is apportioned, expiation is in order. The fault lies partly with Kuhn himself, since in that first edition, as he later confesses:

> By and large I take great satisfaction from the interest it [*The Structure of Scientific Revolutions*] has aroused, including much of the criticism. One aspect of the response, however, does dismay me. Monitoring conversations, particularly among the book's enthusiasts, I have sometimes found it hard to believe that all parties to the discussion have been engaged with the same volume. Part of the reason for its success is, I regretfully conclude, that it can be nearly all things to all people.
>
> For that excessive plasticity, no aspect of the book is so much responsible as its introduction of the term 'paradigm,' a word that figures more often than any other, excepting the grammatical particles, in its pages (1977: 293–4.)

And even more starkly: '*Paradigm* was a perfectly good word until I messed it up' (Kuhn 2000: 298).

All this is more remarkable when set against the fact that the term does not appear in the index of the original 1962 edition of *Structure of Scientific Revolutions*. He then goes on to observe that were he now to insert the reference it would read 'paradigm' p. 172 *passim*. Masterman (1972: 61–5) went so far as to chart 21 different uses of the term. Given the tendency to refer without specification to the concept it is worth listing these senses here:[7]

1   a universally recognized scientific achievement (p. x);
2   a myth (p. 2);
3   a philosophy or constellation of questions (pp. 4–5);
4   a textbook, or classic work (p. 10);
5   a whole tradition, and in some sense, a model (pp. 10–11);
6   a scientific achievement (p. 11);
7   an analogy (p. 14);
8   a successful metaphysical speculation (pp. 17–18);
9   an accepted device in common law (p. 23);
10   a source of tools (p. 37);
11   a standard illustration (p. 43);
12   a device, or type of instrumentation (pp. 59–60);
13   an anomalous pack of cards (pp. 62–3);
14   a machine tool factory (p. 76);
15   a Gestalt figure which can be seen two ways (p. 85);
16   a political institution (p. 92);
17   a standard applied to quasi-metaphysics (p. 102);
18   an organizing principle which can govern perception itself (p. 112);
19   a general epistemological viewpoint (p. 120);

20   a new way of seeing (p. 121);
21   something which defines a broad sweep of reality (p. 128).

When, then, authors cite 'paradigm' and refer to Kuhn, one is left wondering which sense precisely they are adopting. Of course the items on the list are not entirely independent. Masterman classifies them into three broad categories which themselves are neither hermetically sealed nor exhaustive: (i) *metaphysical* or *metaparadigms* (senses 2, 3, 8, 17, 19, 21 and a potentially further sense: map (p. 108)); (ii) *sociological paradigms* (senses 1, 6, 9); and (iii) *artefact paradigms* or *construct paradigms* (senses 4, 9, 10, 12, 13, 15). Partly responding to Masterman, partly to a legion of other critics, Kuhn (1972, 1977) later responded that there were two general senses of paradigm:

> Whatever their number, the usages of "paradigm" in the book divide into two sets which require both different names and separate discussion. Our sense of "paradigm" is global, embracing all the shared commitments of a scientific group; the other isolates a particularly important sort of commitment and is thus a subset of the first. (1977: 294.)

A few observations are worth making here. First, working within paradigms in both senses allows scientists to get on with the business-as-normal of everyday scientific activities. As is well known, under this description of settled (if silent) agreement, scientists are operating in 'normal science'. Their activities are building upon received and – at that time, at least – unchallenged wisdom. What is less often observed is that the examples Kuhn persists with, and which inform and are informed by his famous analysis, are characteristic of natural science. In sharing the paradigm, therefore, these scientists have 'assimilated a time-tested and group-licensed way of seeing' (1970: 189). This is why, for them, questions regarding scientific method are not pressing. Second, it is far from clear then, how 'normal' science can pertain in the social sciences where the very idea of 'normal' science in his sense does not obtain. It might be argued that during the early periods of sociology, positivistic thought briefly held, but in modern times the situation was never so stable; agreement in theory and method was always elusive. And the prospects in postmodernity are certainly no better. His remarks bear this out directly: 'the practice of astronomy, physics, chemistry, or biology normally fails to evoke the controversies over fundamentals that today often seem endemic among, say, psychologists or sociologists' (1977: viii).

The precise nature of these 'controversies over fundamentals' begs questions regarding their relative status in the social and natural sciences as well as to their causes and effects. So it could be argued that either social scientists should either (i) reject the use of Kuhnian 'paradigms' altogether; or (ii) make it clear that when they use that term they have a particular meaning in mind other than simple theoretical and methodological diversity and conflict (in which case they should desist from referencing him!). If the latter is meant – and it is surely applicable – then perhaps the least confusion would arise in ignoring the term except for analogous reference.

Third, in his articulation of this simpler divide between the two senses of 'paradigm', Kuhn also attempted to put clear water between himself and Popper. One of the chief ways of doing this, and borne out by his later elaboration of paradigm-talk, was the relations between language and nature as they affected the initiation or apprenticeship of scientists into their respective scientific communities. In this regard, Kuhn was developing a central idea of the work of Michael Polanyi (1958) that we know more than we can tell; what in scientific contexts this implied was that scientists come to understand and order the world in special ways that are not as volitional or as deliberate as the theory-choice that Popper sets out. This idea, even as loosely hinted at as this, cuts across categories (i) and (iii) of Masterman's senses. Kuhn (1972) argues that it would have been better not to confuse matters by grouping the constellation of ideas that surround this one with the label 'paradigm' or 'paradigmatic'. He suggests that what enables scientists to agree upon and solve puzzles with such a uniform approach would be better captured in the phrase 'disciplinary matrix' (1972: 271; 1977: 297). His use of that term is justified by arguing that the disciplinary identity of scientists rests in part upon the shared possession of a matrix or ordered body of symbolic generalizations, models and exemplars of concrete problem-solutions (see for examples here: Chapter 5, McFee; Chapter 7, Yeadon; Chapter 8, Noakes; Chapter 9, Brackenridge *et al.*).

## Relativism and absolutism in research

In the trail of Kuhn's seminal book came a catalogue of others both more and less critical and supportive. One of the key elements of critical discussion related to the purported relativism of his idea that paradigms were themselves incommensurable. They were effectively competing and therefore not combinable intellectual currencies. Others (notably social scientists) have taken the idea much more strongly to argue that paradigms effectively locate scientists in different worlds. All knowledge becomes essentially located within competing paradigms. These stances betray a strong and a weak sense of incommensurability.

Harré and Krausz justify a weaker reading of the incommensurability thesis. They argue that the kind of wholesale upheaval that relativists latched onto in Kuhn's writings is not typical of western intellectual traditions. Of the authors cursorily cited here, I have at least gestured to the fact that their views stand on the shoulders of others, which is more or less true *mutatis mutandis*. Kuhn is not to be read in the radical fashion of someone such as Feyerabend, who discerns no historical rules that are universally applied in scientific reasoning and method. Of course some revolutions are of greater significance than others. But Kuhn can be understood as arguing that, for example, no scientist could be completely committed to both Aristotle and Newton in their approach to mechanics. Harré and Krausz write:

If paradigm shifts necessitated complete shifts in subject matter there would be no possibility for hunting for rational choice among paradigms. Paradigm shifts within the framework of that Western scientific tradition which had its origins in the ancient Greek traditions of enquiry, have never involved root and branch transformations of their generic ontologies. The deep, generic ontologies of individual substances and their attributes, located in the manifolds of space and time, has persisted however radically versions of this ontology have differed from one another. Incommensurability between paradigms has never been so radical and deep that it has not been possible to recognise this generic ontology embedded in every successive world view. (1996: 79.)

Related however, recent social scientists have certainly tested out the categories that are typically used to organize knowledge. Poststructuralists and postmodernists deny the givenness of boundary-setting disciplines. What they offer in return, however, is typically labelled relativistic. What does such a claim amount to? Harré and Krausz helpfully distinguish two sorts of relativism: sceptical and permissive.

It cannot be denied that these epistemological currents have scarcely dented the traditional topography of our universities and governmental institutions for research funding. Nor should it go without comment that their critique, in whatever clever clothes they are fashioned and in whatever language they are shrouded, is scarcely new. The idea of relativism goes back at least as far as Democritus and the ancient Greeks, whereas the idea of disciplines has a slightly more modern turn – but even then it reaches back to the 1600s. Toulmin remarks:

> The invention of disciplines, a change that began in the seventeenth century, involved both intellectual and institutional factors. Intellectually, Descartes's use of geometry as the model for knowledge provided its slogans; institutionally, the division of labour into professions and disciplines gave it wings. But the change did not happen quickly, and it has reached its peak only in the twentieth century. (2003: 29.)

Discussion of the non-givenness of disciplines, while having historical foundation, can easily be overblown. It is scarcely accidental. The challenge of relativism, founded in the power of the boundaries and the boundary-setters, often conflates a malign and a benign sense of the term respectively: as Harré and Krausz observe, the sceptical and the permissive.

1 *Skepticism*: no point of view is privileged, no description is true, and no assessment of value is valid.
2 *Permissive*: all points of view are equally privileged, all descriptions are true and all assessments of value are equally valid. (Harré and Krausz 1996: 3.)

The idea that there is one truth or none is a stark choice indeed. But it is no more pernicious than the idea that there is no route to true knowledge: the scientific method. The very idea of a dichotomy – one standard or none – is scarcely helpful. It has not been uncommon in multidisciplinary research seminars I have attended, organized or spoken at, to find natural and social scientists alike who polarize around these extremes. It is not merely that their languages, models and techniques differ, but that the very criteria that might make rational for preference or aversion appears to be contested. Is the reliability eschewed by social scientists using focus groups justified? Is validity invalidated in the recent trend for autoethnographic/autobiographical research (see Chapter 10, Allen Collinson and Hockey)? Is parsimony always criterial in theory-preference? Can narratives be treated as data in the same way that particles or propositions are? Is there no more to investigative sociology than journalism (see Chapter 11, Sugden)? Does the serious entertaining of these questions entertain the demise of science in which we can trust? The triumph of scientists and philosophy of science alike was in part due to the development and refinement of the scientific method. And in most social science and certain natural science its place at the head of the high table is now questioned with more or less promiscuity. Of course a more subtle analysis of relativisms is needed, as is a more patient explication of the kinds of absolutism that they kick out against.

Finally, we might ask, are there not merely epistemic but also ethical criteria that can help us to clarify where scientific endeavours overlap with other professional concerns to do with bytes, data, information? I shall turn to two final remarks on the relations between values and science in the context of traditional, positivistic, science.

## Science as value free (or: two-and-a-half cheers for Popper)

Putnam (1993) remarks that both philosophers and scientists have at different times wanted to cleave apart fact and values. Yet in many enquiries and experiments into exercise, health and sport *inter alia* the entanglement is unavoidable. And still many scientists claim to uphold the values of autonomy, neutrality and impartiality in their scientific labours (Lacey 1999). Others, such as critical feminists, insist on a stronger thesis that the social practices of science are inherently political and that notions such as these must be given up as hangovers from a precritical phase to be replaced by partiality and commitment in a more or less explicit way. Again, the picture that is being either supplanted or exculpated is the positivistic one. Putnam writes that positivism was 'fundamentally a denial of entanglement, an insistence on sharp dichotomies: science-ethics, science-metaphysics, analytic-synthetic' (1993: 15).

Much critical work was done in the beginnings of the philosophy of science that demonstrated – from a range of different directions and indeed disciplines – that values entered scientific processes. We can see how showing what now seems obvious to so many, was then so powerful. In their defence, positivists stressed the contexts of discovery were to be set aside from the contexts of justification. Very roughly put, while the latter were amenable to subjective influences (from cultural to psychological) the latter, it was claimed, assured scientific objectivity. The view is typically attributed to the empiricist Reichenbach (1938) but is also shared by Popper and other positivists, though some philosophers are sceptical of this claim (Shapere 2001). Ladyman (2002: 75) quotes Popper, however, in precisely such a vein:

> The act of conceiving or inventing a theory seems to me neither to call of logical analysis nor to be susceptible to it ... the question of how it happens that a new idea occurs ... may be of great interest to empirical psychology; but it is irrelevant to the logical analysis of knowledge (Popper 1934: 27).

While, therefore, anti-positivists all of persuasions have tended to celebrate the moves that were made by Popper in destabilizing logical positivism, we should be wary too of lionizing him. He too is a product of his age even if, unlike most of us, he was able to lift his head that much higher than most and gain a more critical perspective of the philosophical prejudices of his day. In general philosophical terms, merely to argue that the source of an argument is good/bad is inadequate. We may cite great authors who have been bad authorities in given topics or otherwise despicable writers whose views are soundly argued. In a sense Popper is right; from whom theories arise is not something that should enter the evaluation of their ideas. In another sense, and with an increasingly sophisticated awareness of the economic (see Chapter 8, Noakes), political, social and gender-driven biases (see Chapter 9, Brackenridge *et al.*) that enter into the processes of the production of scientific knowledge, the distinction loses some of its sharpness (see Shapere 2001: 416–17).

A final manner in which values have entered discussions of research is in what is termed 'research ethics'. In recent years, with the professionalization of research and the economically driven agendas of efficiency and effectiveness of research production and dissemination, the thought that science is an activity beyond morals – that is to say, amoral – is heard with less frequency. Both the processes of research and the products are increasingly open to ethical scrutiny. Despite, however, the emergence of various institutionalized responses to the wrongdoings of researchers, there is in inherent difficulty in the application of general ethical considerations to particular persons, practices and policies (see Chapter 12, Homan). What appears to be driving these agendas is a mix of the threat of legal redress and a genuine attempt to professionalize research (see Chapter 11, Sugden) in a manner that will at least in principle secure minimal standards of conduct and character, even if their application will always be a thorny affair.

At a more fundamental epistemic level, the traditional juxtaposition of fact and values is, as Putnam notes, due to an improper contrast between, for example, ethics and cultural knowledge generally and science in discussion of absolutism and relativism. In the contexts of health and well-being the effects of this contrast are at the centre of contemporary debates in philosophy as much as in politics. He notes that the contrast is often made in the following way: first one sets out highly generalized examples on the one hand (whether this culture or moral practice is good or bad as a whole – an eminently disputable affair) and then one opposes them with a specific and uncontested fact (whether this is green or that is hot – the truth of which is denied by no-one). The kind of absoluteness *assumed* in the latter case embodies the positivistic 'view of the world from nowhere in particular within it' (to use Nagel's celebrated phrase) and is wholly illusory. In making judgements in both cases we stand within traditions of thought and action: the conceptual frameworks are just so taken for granted in the latter case. Neither scepticism about knowledge, nor the scientistic or positivistic conception of science as the only method to secure knowledge, is satisfactory. Rather, he writes:

> The third possibility is to accept the position we are fated to occupy in any case, the position being who cannot have a view of the world that does not reflect our interest and values, but who are, for all that, committed to regarding some views of the world – and for, that matter, some interests and values – as better than others. This may be giving up a certain picture of objectivity, but it is not giving up the idea that there are what Dewey called 'objective resolutions to problematical situations' – objective resolutions to problems which are *situated*, that is, in a place, at a time, as opposed to an 'absolute' answer to 'perspective-independent' questions. And that is objectivity enough. (Putnam 1993:156.)

## Concluding remarks: an introduction to philosophical issues in science

The volume does not aim at comprehensiveness. Nor is it an introduction to the standard fare of philosophy of science texts. Though there is discussion of theories of science, of tolerance and ignorance thereof, and of the benefits and biases that attend positivistic science and philosophy, there is no space for more fundamental discussions of the nature of causality, determinism, explanation, realism and anti-realism and so on. What has driven my selection of the material is from my own professional experiences of topics that have caused fruitful professional frictions – in the various departments that I have worked in across the fields of exercise, health and sport sciences. This is one of the reasons why each chapter is in the form of a question – whether they are obvious or obscure is up to the reader to decide ultimately. I hope that the range of issues addressed here is not dismissed as mere philosophical intrusion – that much should be ensured by the standing of the authors and the quality of what they have written. *Ad hominem* argumentation is typically unacceptable, but academics of all persuasions still go in for it.

The aim of the book then is twofold. It is first to demonstrate the need for philosophical enquiry in the sciences of exercise, health and sport, whether that be undertaken by philosophers and/or philosophically minded scientists. Second, a certain hegemony is enjoyed by the natural sciences in these fields. I have often been struck by (some friends might add 'and struck back at') the hubris of the naïve natural scientist who believed uncritically in the deserved dominance of natural *science* and *the* scientific method. Such scientists too readily pour scorn on the alleged relativistic promiscuity of humanities scholars and social scientists in their attempts to embrace 'mere' scholarship or 'soft – qualitative' research. I prefer some rapprochement not least through dialogue in and between philosophers and other disciplinarians – irrespective of whether they identify themselves with that professional designation or not. Scientists have no choice but to engage in conceptual clarification and the coherence and justification of their data, methods, theories and, yes, paradigms too.

Finally, I hope this book will serve as an introduction for undergraduate or postgraduate students, teachers or researchers alike, in the sense of 'introducing' that is perhaps peculiar to philosophical work. For while the work introduces it should also offer some friction to those more experienced in the subject. Possibly the first philosophy text I purchased, A.D. Woozley's *Theory of Knowledge*, includes the following in its introductory remarks: 'controversy is desirable, only unreflective and passive acquiescence are to be avoided' (1949: 11). It is fitting that the book might be a minor 'Amen' to that.[8]

## Bibliography

Bogen, J. (2001) 'Experiment and Observation', in P. Machamer and M. Silberstein (eds) *The Blackwell Companion to the Philosophy of Science*, Oxford: Blackwell, 128–48.

Chalmers, A.F. (1999) *What Is This Thing Called Science*, Milton Keynes: Open University Press, 3rd edn.

Gower, B. (1997) *Scientific Method. An Historical and Philosophical Introduction*, London: Routledge.

Hacking, I. (1983) *Representing and Intervening: Introductory Topics in the Philosophy of Natural Science*, Cambridge: Cambridge University Press.

Halfpenny, P. (1982) *Positivism and Sociology: Explaining Social Life*, London: George, Allen and Unwin.

Harré, R. and Krausz, M. (1988) *Varieties of Relativism*, Oxford: Blackwell.

Kuhn, T.S. (1962) *The Structure of Scientific Revolutions*, Chicago: University of Chicago Press.

Kuhn, T.S. (1970) *The Structure of Scientific Revolutions*, 2nd edn, Chicago: University of Chicago Press.

Kuhn, T.S. (1977) *The Essential Tension: Studies in Scientific Tradition and Change*, Chicago: University of Chicago Press.

Kuhn, T.S. (1995) 'Afterwords', In P. Horwich (ed.) *World Changes*, Cambridge; MIT Press, 311–41.

Lacey, H. (1999) *Is Science Value Free? Values and Scientific Understanding*, London: Routledge.

Ladyman, J. (2002) *Understanding Philosophy of Science*, London: Routledge.

Lakatos, I. and Musgrave, A. (eds) (1972) *Criticism and the Growth of Knowledge*, Cambridge: Cambridge University Press.

Magee, B (1997) *Confessions of a Philosopher*, London: Weidenfield and Nicholson.

Masterman, M. (1972) 'The nature of a paradigm', in Lakatos and Musgrave op. cit., 59–89.

Nagel, T. (1980) *The View from Nowhere*, Oxford: Oxford University Press.

Polanyi, M. (1958) *Personal Knowledge*, London: Routledge and Kegan Paul.

Polanyi, M. (1966) *The Tacit Dimension*, New York: Anchor Books.

Popper, K. (1934) *The Logic of Scientific Discovery*, London: Hutchinson.

Putnam, H. (1993) 'Objectivity and the science-ethics distinction', in M. Nussbaum and A. Sen (eds) *The Quality of Life*, Oxford: Clarendon Press, 143–57.

Reichenbach, H. (1938) *Experience and Prediction*, Chicago: University of Chicago Press.

Reisch, G.A. (1991) 'Did Kuhn kill logical empiricism?' *Philosophy of Science*, 58, 264–77.

Salmon, W. (2001) 'Logical Empiricism', in W.W. Newton Smith (ed.) *A Companion to the Philosophy of Science*, Oxford: Blackwell, 233–42.

Shapere, D. (2001) 'Scientific change', in W.W. Newton Smith (ed.) *A Companion to the Philosophy of Science*, Oxford: Blackwell, 413–22.

Toulmin, S. (2003) *Return to Reason*, Harvard: Harvard University Press.

Woozley, A.D. (1949) *Theory of Knowledge*, London: Hutchinson.

## Notes

1 Hacking (1993: 246–51) for one certainly objects to such a label, even though it would appear commonplace in some introductory texts.

2 Of course, historians would remind me here that modernity is in part characterized by the rational disavowal of religious hegemony and the rise of science, which is consistent with the claim that the first sense of positivism here is modern. I merely mean that the latter are more contemporary.

3 For those interested, Hacking observes four epochs of positivism. After Hume (1739) and Comte (1830–42) come logical positivism (1920–40 – of which A.J. Ayer's classic 'Language, Truth and Logic' was the bible); and the contemporary philosopher Bas Van Fraasen (1980).

4 Whether Kuhn is properly to be thought of as a philosopher – his doctoral work was in physics, while he claims that his famous Structure of Scientific Revolutions is first and foremost a historical treatise on the development of science – is a point typically remarked upon in philosophical texts on science.

5 For a sympathetic account of this see Magee's autobiographical work, which weaves in a history of much modern-century philosophy in order to contextualize his own philosophical debts and commitments (Magee 1997: 46–55).

6 For further description and critique of Popper, see Chalmers' classic (1999: 59–86 and 87–103 respectively).

7 The original references Masterman cites are from the 1962 volume.

8 I am most grateful, and not for the first time, to my good friend Graham McFee for his insightful observations and critical comments on this chapter.

# 2 Must scientists think philosophically about science?

*Jim Parry*

## Introduction

What can a philosopher have to say about exercise, health or sport sciences? The scientists are those who have the experience, who make the observations, who know the facts. And as David Best has observed: 'People whose expertise is in a particular subject are often highly suspicious of a philosopher who takes a professional interest in that subject yet has nothing like a comparable level of practical expertise in it' (1978: 5).

But there are at least two possible defences against such a suspicion. First, philosophy is best seen not simply as a different subject from science, maths, history and the rest, but rather as in part constitutive of them and constituted with reference to them. Philosophy, as a subject, *includes* philosophy of science, philosophy of mathematics, philosophy of religion, and the rest; and each other subject is itself inadequately understood and explored without some attention to philosophical considerations.

Second, although the activity of applying philosophical procedures (of clarification, criticism, and the examination of presuppositions and justifications) is part of each subject, it may nevertheless be an interested outsider who gets the job, either because he has some philosophical expertise of an appropriate kind or because the scientists (in this case) are too busy getting on with their science. As an interested outsider, I hope I can open up some philosophical issues in the study of exercise, health and sport sciences through an examination of the very idea of science, the traditional notion of the scientific method and some key concepts in scientific enquiry.

## On science

In understanding the scientific components of the fields of study – exercise, health and sport – it might be thought that the best way forward is to offer a definition of science, so that we all know in advance what we are talking about. Fischer, in his undergraduate textbook, says 'it is important for us, at the outset of this book, to attempt to express a working definition of the word science, in order that the rest of the book will be meaningful' (1975: 4). I tested the hypothesis implicit in this statement by reading his last chapter before reading his working definition and found that: (a) the chapter was meaningful (I could read and understand it, at least) without the definition; (b) a subsequent reading of the definition made no further contribution to my understanding.

This is not surprising, really. Imagine my trying to begin to describe to you a visit by my vet: 'Daisy, that's my horse (you know, a solid-hoofed, graminivorous, perissodactyl quadruped) went down with colic (you know, severe paroxysmal griping pains in the belly) . . .' I need not go on to show how difficult communication would become if it were assumed that definitions were required to secure meaning. In practice, we are often at a loss to produce definitions of words of whose meaning we are well aware, and when we try to produce a definition, we often make matters worse (e.g. I have a fair grasp of what 'horse' and 'colic' mean, but I'm not sure that 'perissodactyl' and 'paroxysmal' give me any help at all – see Best 1978: 88–90).

I am not saying that there is never any point in providing definitions – only that there are dangers in assuming that one must be provided; and provided in *advance* of an investigation. Bambrough identifies one such danger:

> The question 'what is science?' has all too often been treated as if it were the question 'What is the definition of science?', and then answered in such a way as to deny the title of science to many of the sciences. (1973: 19.)

The same thing sometimes happens with the question 'What is knowledge?' which draws the answer: 'Scientific knowledge is the only *real* knowledge,' thus denying the title of knowledge to many areas of knowledge. Chalmers, whose classic book is called *What is This Thing Called Science?*, considers his title to have been misleading and presumptuous. In his concluding remarks he says 'It presumes that there is a single category 'science', and implies that various areas of knowledge, physics, biology history, sociology and so on, either come under that category or do not' (Chalmers 1982: 166).

One way of expressing this point is to say that any definition of science will generate a criterion of demarcation between what is and is not science. However, we can question whether we need such a 'hooray-category', or whether we should rather approach and accept each area of knowledge on its own terms, investigating its aims, its means and its degree of success in achieving its aims. But we are getting ahead of ourselves. We should begin not by offering a crisp once-and-for-all definition, but by exploring some of the many ways in which science is perceived and by examining some accounts of the nature of the scientific enterprise for their coherence.

## The traditional view

> Scientific knowledge is proven knowledge. Scientific theories are derived in some rigorous way from facts of experience acquired by observation and experiment. Science is based on what we can see, hear, touch, etc. Personal opinion or preferences and speculative imaginings have no place in science.

> Science is objective. Scientific knowledge is reliable knowledge because it is objectively proven knowledge. (Chalmers 1982: 1).

Chalmers begins the first edition of his book with this summary of 'a widely-held commonsense view of science'. It is not only the layperson, however, who may hold such a view. Until quite recently, at any rate, it was the preferred self-description of scientists:

> The image that the scientific community likes to project of itself … is that of rationality par excellence. The scientific community sees itself as the very paradigm of institutionalised rationality . . . . And in the noble … pursuit of (truth) the members of the community dispassionately and disinterestedly apply their tools, the scientific method, each application of which takes us a further step on the royal road to the much esteemed goal (Newton-Smith 1981: 1.)

What we might refer to as this Traditional View of scientific method may be described in terms of a series of stages (see Magee, 1973: 56):

1 observation and experiment
2 inductive generalization
3 hypothesis
4 attempted verification of hypothesis
5 proof or disproof
6 knowledge.

There are two main objections to the Traditional View, relating to stages 1 and 2, and if the objections hold then the remaining stages are deprived of their foundation.

### Stage 1: Observation

The Traditional View assumes that science begins with observation, and that this provides a firm foundation in brute fact for progress through later stages to proven knowledge.

> Perception alone gives us unvarnished news, in the form of brute, uninterpreted facts, and … without this foundation, we could know nothing of the world. The mind itself contributes nothing of substance. It is a tabula rasa or blank paper, on which experience writes the first knowledge. (Hollis 1994: 70).

So the traditional empiricist case against rationalism is that 'experimental' knowledge is pure and unmediated, whilst 'rational' knowledge depends on the constructions of the mind. But there are problems here. Imagine a particular observation (say, looking through a microscope at a bacterial culture) where you observe some blue blobs and black rods against a yellowish background. Now each such observation is undertaken by a *subject* – the *experience* of observation, pure and simple, is inescapably subjective. It looks as though this first stage of science, on which all else is based, is a subjective exercise. What could be more subjective than one's own personal sense-experiences?

However, we do not just *have* these experiences; we also report them to each other in statements which purport to describe what we observe. While my private experiences are not accessible to others, my public statements are – but this only suggests a symmetrical problem: while my private experiences are directly accessible to me, my public statements are *not*. Public observation-statements can only be made in a public language which furnishes me with the necessary conceptual apparatus with which to notice, identify, order, structure and describe the particular shapes and colours that are presented to my senses.

In this important way, our perceptual experiences are not innocent, and do not present us with brute facts. What we see and how we report it is dependent upon our previous experience, our knowledge and our expectations; and our observation-statements cannot even be made except in a public language which already incorporates theories of some kind.

Since our observations are theory-dependent, then it is to be expected that science cannot begin without those theories which precede observations. Moreover, our observation-statements are only as reliable as the theory within which they are articulated, and since the history of science is littered with discarded theories it is also littered with discarded observations. Whatever place observations do have in science, it is a mistake to see them as building blocks upon which the scientific edifice rests – their fallibility will not allow them to bear that weight.

### Stage 2: Induction

Even if science did start with observation, and observation did provide a secure foundation for scientific knowledge, there are still difficulties to face in the next stage of the Traditional View, which asserts that it is possible to arrive at scientific laws by inferring them from accumulated observations. This is the Principle of Induction, which seeks to link observations to theory by claiming that, as the observation-knowledge of workers in a certain area grows, so general features emerge from the data which can be systematized in law-like propositions. These hypotheses can later be tested and confirmed, if true, thus adding to our store of knowledge.

However, we should notice here that observations result in singular statements, whereas theories (or laws) are expressed as general statements. The crucial question is: how do we legitimately infer law-like generalizations from singular instances of observation (no matter how numerous)? The short answer is: we can't. No matter how many white swans we have observed, the generalization 'all swans are white' is never logically guaranteed, even though the generalization is a perfectly respectable example of induction. As Bertrand Russell points out: 'The man who has fed the chicken every day throughout its life at last wrings its neck instead, showing that more refined views as to the uniformity of nature would have been useful to the chicken' (1912: 63).

This example is uncomfortably applied to the human situation. In the literature on induction a common example used is that of the sun's rising tomorrow. If any of my beliefs is justified by induction, this one is, but the possibility of nuclear destruction of our planet puts even this induction in jeopardy. Possibly it is not only chickens who need to refine their views if they are to survive!

Since there is no strictly logical inference possible in inductive argument, it might be thought nevertheless that we could justify our belief in it by appealing to our experience of the success of inductions in the history of science. But this won't do either. The form of the argument is as follows (see Chalmers 1982: 15):

1   The principle of induction worked successfully on occasion T1.
2   The principle of induction worked successfully on occasion T2 etc.
3   The principle of induction always works.

But this is itself an argument that employs induction to demonstrate the validity of inductive argument, and this is clearly an illegitimate procedure, because it is circular.

If the criticisms of the Traditional View advanced in this section hold good, then what has been presented to us as objective, certain knowledge has been shown to be without the sort of 'objective' foundation which it has claimed for itself, and which it has conceived of itself as requiring.

Magee summarizes the quandary:

> The whole of our science assumes the regularity of nature … yet there is no way in which this assumption can be secured . . .. That the whole of science, of all things, should rest on foundations whose validity it is impossible to demonstrate has been found uniquely embarrassing … [I]nduction has presented an unsolved problem at the very foundations of human knowledge (1973: 20–2).

One attempt to defend inductivism against this sort of consideration lies in the retreat to probability (see Chalmers 1982: 17–18). Some scientists concede that we cannot be absolutely certain, on the basis of a number of observations, that the sun will rise tomorrow, or that a particular liquid will contract when cooled; but nevertheless they assert that the relevant generalizations are *probably* true, and the greater the number and variety of observations, the greater the probability.

Chalmers responds as follows: 'Given standard probability theory, it is very difficult to construct an account of induction that avoids the consequence that the probability of any universal statement making claims about the world is zero, whatever the observational evidence' (Chalmers 1982: 18). The reason for this is that observations are necessarily finite, whereas generalizations refer across an infinite number of situations.

With the degeneration of the inductivist programme, which fatally debilitates the Traditional View, we seem to be left with two possibilities: one is to accept that, at rock bottom, science cannot be rationally justified. The other is to deny that science is based on induction – to deny that the Traditional View is an adequate account of science.


## Karl Popper and falsificationism

The latter is the route taken by Karl Popper, whom some have considered the greatest philosopher of the twentieth century. He sidesteps the problem of induction by denying that the truth of a theory can be inferred from empirical evidence. His logical point is of the utmost simplicity: countless confirming instances can *never* conclusively verify a general proposition, but a single counter-example can conclusively falsify it. That is to say 'Only the falsity of the theory can be inferred from empirical evidence, and this inference is a purely deductive one' (Popper, 1963: 55).

Given the corrigibility of observation-statements, though, there would always be the possibility (and temptation) to evade the falsification of one's theory. Popper therefore insists that our methodology should force us to expose our theories to refutation. If a theory could not be wrong it could not be informative – and in order to be informative it must be potentially falsifiable.

As against the Traditional View, then, Popper's falsificationism proposes the following stages in the scientific method (see Magee 1973: 56):

1  problem (usually a rebuff to an existing theory or expectation);
2  proposed solution (in other words, a new theory);
3  deduction of testable propositions from the new theory;
4  tests (attempted refutations);
5  preference established between competing theories.

There are a number of things to notice about this account. The process begins not with the amassing of 'data' in the hope that something will emerge from them, but with problems and our attempted solutions of them. At the second stage, the scientist may make a bold imaginative conjecture which has more the character of a creative act than a logical inference from data. Science proceeds by a series of *Conjectures and Refutations* (the title of one of Popper's books). As Einstein writes in a letter to Popper:

> I really do not at all like the now fashionable 'positivistic' tendency of clinging to what is observable . . .. I think (like you, by the way) that theory

cannot be fabricated out of the results of observation, but that it can only be invented (in Popper 1968: 458).

The task of stages 3 and 4 is to deduce unknown consequences of a theory and to subject them to potentially falsifying tests, as a result of which we may learn which of our possible theories can cope most adequately with the results. As Lakatos puts it: 'Popper also indicated a further condition that a theory must satisfy in order to qualify as scientific: it must predict facts which are novel, that is, unexpected in the light of previous knowledge' (Lakatos 1981: 113).

The classic example of such a procedure occurred in 1919 when the Royal Society sent two expeditions to Brazil and West Africa, in order to attempt to photograph the field of stars in the Hyades group. A consequence of Einstein's General Theory was that light was attracted to heavy bodies and that therefore light rays should bend if passing close to the sun on their way to earth. Eddington calculated that during the eclipse of 29 May certain of these stars would become visible by day at a certain point in Africa, and the observations confirmed the General Theory. This procedure illustrates the way in which a scientific theory should seek to place itself at risk – to seek such falsification as would be informative. But it does not show that Einstein's theory is true. Popper says 'We cannot identify science with truth, for we think that both Newton's and Einstein's theories belong to science, but they cannot both be true, and they may well both be false' (Magee, 1973: 28).

Our readiness to accept Einsteinian physics indicates our belief that Newtonian theories have been falsified (as with the above experiment) even though they had been taught as truth for over 200 years. We should learn from this, says Popper, that what we call knowledge is necessarily provisional. We cannot prove the truth of our theories, although we can give reasons for our preference for one theory over another. We may assume the truth of our theories for working purposes, but should always remember that they may be shown to be false at any time. The challenge for modern physics is to falsify the theories of Einstein, an event which would mark a giant step in the progress of physics.

Popper's account of scientific method generates a demarcation criterion: properly scientific theories are those which are genuinely falsifiable, and so any theory which is unfalsifiable is not properly scientific. Examples of unfalsifiable theories advanced by Popper are those of Marxism, Freudian psychoanalysis, and Adlerian psychology. The latter theories do not generate falsifiable predictions; no possible observations could refute them; whatever happened in the world would be consistent with them and explicable by them. 'Popper saw that their ability to explain everything, which so convinced and excited their adherents, was precisely what was most wrong with them' (Magee 1973: 44).

Popper thought that, in the case of Marxism, falsifiable predictions *were* made, and in fact falsified – but Marxists defended themselves by producing reformulations of their theory, so that it remained intact. In this way, again, *whatever* happened in the world would be explicable by some version of the theory: either a revolution or no revolution; either a revolution in an advanced country or a backward one; either the polarization of the classes or the emergence of the petty-bourgeoisie; either the emiseration of the masses or the welfare state. So long as this remains the case, despite its claims and pretensions, Marxism cannot qualify as Popperian Science.

Typically, Marxists fail to see or consider any conditions under which they would give up their theories, and it is just this kind of commitment that Popper sees as unscientific. For him, everything in science is corrigible and provisional, a view known as 'fallibilism', and every theory (including one's own) should be approached with scepticism. This is what lies behind his famous critique (in *The Open Society and Its Enemies*, 1945) of social theories that proposed ideal societies.

## Lakatosian research programmes

In case we should now be thinking that Popper is *right*, I should remind us that, if Popper is to be regarded as a good Popperian, he will not regard his own theory as true or verifiable but at best tentatively preferable to its rivals and always corrigible. If it is to be seen as itself a scientific theory it must be open to falsification.

There are many objections to falsificationism (see Ladyman 2002: 81–90). However, I have only enough time and space here to record one way in which Popper's falsificationism has been challenged and developed in order to indicate the dynamic quality of the debate.

Imre Lakatos (Lakatos and Musgrave 1974) has taken Popper's theory to task on its own terms. Falsificationism says that a test is a contest between a theory and the world, the only interesting outcome of which is falsification of the theory. But the history of science does not square with this view, since scientists generally do not abandon their theories just because of experimental falsifications. To do so would be to introduce anarchy into scientific method. More commonly, scientists attempt to divert the force of anomalies by seeking explanations which do not threaten the central tenets of the theory, or by making modifications to the original theory to take account of anomalies. Normally, the *last* thing that scientists do is to give up their theories!

Lakatos proposes that we should rather regard scientific progress as a contest between rival theories in which the world acts as referee (see Newton-Smith 1981: 78–9) and that we should delay the assessment of the relative merits of competing theories until such time as modifications have been explored. This may take a considerable period of time, and will involve not just individual theories and falsifications, but a sequence of theories and modifications which we might call a scientific research programme: '[O]ne must treat budding programmes leniently; programmes may take decades before they get off the ground and become empirically progressive' (Lakatos, in Hacking 1981b: 131–2).

Lakatos sees these research programmes as containing a *hard core* of basic assumptions which are not open to modification. A rejection of part of the hard core entails a rejection of the programme (i.e. the scientist's commitment here motivates him to resist attempts at falsification). But in addition there is a *protective belt* of auxiliary hypotheses, initial conditions, observational hypotheses, etc., which *are* open to falsification and modification so as to conserve the hard core of defining characteristics of the theory (see Chalmers 1982: 80–1).

On this account we assess the relative merits of competing research programmes according to whether they are progressing or degenerating and this may take a long time to decide, which at least goes some way towards explaining the sort of theoretical disagreements we can observe in physics, psychology, sociology and the rest. Sometimes it is just very difficult to see which programme is progressive and which is not, and this accounts for fundamental (and irreconcilable) disagreements *within* science. If science were 'objective' in the required sense there would be no such disagreements possible, for it would be possible to demonstrate which view is wrong. Things are not quite as simple as that, which indicates that a vulgar objectivism is inadequate.

What I have tried to do in this section is to give some idea of the vigorous debate there has been within the philosophy of science on the question of the nature of science and its methodology – and it has not here been possible to allude to some of the more startling theories (e.g. of Kuhn and Feyerabend) which, in taking the line that science cannot be rationally justified, have presented relativist or anarchist threats to the self-image of science.

## The theory-dependence of practice

'Why bother with philosophy of science anyway?' you might be thinking. 'What has it to do with my concerns as a sport scientist?' The first thing that occurs to me is that every working scientist will adopt procedures and attitudes which are derived, consciously or not, from some basic beliefs about the scientific enterprise. What philosophy of science tries to do is to get these basic commitments out into the open so that they may be rationally examined. To find oneself to have been committed to an incoherent view of one's own activity might be the beginning of important changes in one's scientific practice and attitudes to knowledge. The Nobel Prize winner Sir John Eccles wrote: '[M]y scientific life owes so much to my conversion in 1954, if I may so call it, to Popper's teachings on the conduct of scientific investigations . . .' (in Magee 1973: 9). He advises others 'to read and meditate upon Popper's writings on the philosophy of science and to adopt them as the basis of operation of one's scientific life' (ibid.).

There can be no better testimonial than that, unless it is the following one by the astronomer Sir Herman Bondi: 'There is no more to science than its method, and there is no more to its method than Popper has said' (loc. cit.).

Whether or not their opinions regarding Popper are to be followed these days, it is nevertheless clear that they share the view that one's scientific practice (the methodology that one chooses to adopt) enshrines a view in the philosophy of science. There is an analogy here with teaching practice. Trainee teachers cannot escape the choice of *some* variety of methodology – but *whatever* they choose commits them to a view within the philosophy of education. In the practical endeavours of science and education there is no escape from philosophical presupposition. Of course, one can choose to avoid philosophical considerations altogether (Bertrand Russell once said: 'Most people would die sooner than think – and most do!') but this would be to choose to leap blindly into one's educational or scientific commitments, which can hardly square with any rational account of one's activity.

## Objectivity

The second reason for getting involved in philosophy of science has to do with coming to terms with prejudices regarding objectivity and certainty. Whether or not falsificationism is finally an acceptable theory choice, some acquaintance with the humility implicit in such an approach might decrease the degree of rather facile optimism and overconfidence which are to be discerned in some quarters amongst sport scientists, together with a certain regrettable arrogance towards other knowledge areas. A crash course in statistics and a bucketful of empirical methodology do not of themselves guarantee objectivity, or progress. Speaking of physics which, of all the sciences, has most reason to claim objective status, Bronowski says:

> One aim of the physical sciences has been to give an exact picture of the physical world – one achievement of physics in the twentieth century has been to prove that that aim is unattainable . . .. There is no absolute knowledge . . .. All information is imperfect. We have to treat it with humility. That is the human condition; and that is what quantum physics says. I mean that literally. (1973: 353.)

Scientists who have still not accepted this point are tempted to claim that science is 'more objective' than other areas of study, or that only if an object or process were being treated scientifically would it be treated objectively. As McFee has succinctly argued, this confuses two claims:

(A) All bits of X can be explained scientifically
(B) All (genuine) explanations of X are scientific. (McFee 1977: 23.)

(A) may be true, but (B) does not follow from (A). Take the classic example of this – dance. It may be possible to produce scientific explanations of all the movements of a dance, but this does not show that there is no *other* sort of explanation possible, nor that the scientific explanation actually tells us anything of interest about the dance. A biomechanical account of the movements of the limbs of the dancers would scientifically explain, in causal fashion, how movements were made and how one was able to follow on from another. But it would have nothing whatsoever to tell us about the meaning of the dance, for that relies upon an account relating to reasons, not causes. The idea that science will mature to a stage when it will be able to deal with such matters is the result of a simple category-mistake. As Best remarks, having granted the truth of (A):

> Dance, considered as an art form, is simply not the sort of activity to which the notion of empirical investigation is appropriate. It is like trying to measure ... my fear that rain will spoil the cricket season. (1973: xiii.)

Similarly in games: if you wish, you could measure the positions of all players on a football pitch when a certain variety of 'good pass' is made, the speed and direction of movement of players and ball, and so on. Let us say that this will be a scientific description of defence-splitting passes. Now, much may be learned from a scientific account, but one thing for certain will not be learned: and that is why it is a good pass. We already have to identify the good passes in order to know which ones to measure, so measurements of them do not constitute our knowledge of them but rather presuppose it. We know what counts as a good defence-splitting pass because we understand what football is and what reasons are operable within it. He who knows nothing of science may know more about football.

Nevertheless, it might be argued, what they know is not really scientific knowledge; it isn't exact, or measurable, or objective. Well, it is true that it isn't *scientifically* 'objective', but then it doesn't claim to be so, and we cannot require it to be so. The scientist appears to himself king only if he applies scientific criteria to all of our knowledge. Some of our knowledge, however, is not of the scientific variety, and so does not answer to such criteria – but this in no way invalidates it. Science does well (or badly) at scientific tasks, history at historical ones, philosophy at philosophical ones, and so on. Science cannot answer philosophical questions; it can't create or appreciate art, literature, humour or football; but I don't on that account despise it. Good science is good at what science is good at. We can't ask for more than that.

## Certainty and tolerance

Along with humility goes a certain degree of tolerance, an idea introduced by Bronowski in arguing against the claims to objectivity of science. All evidence, he says, is inherently inaccurate – we necessarily work within an area of tolerance. Exactness in our work does not require absolute accuracy (which is chimerical) but simply an honest recognition of the limitations of our methods and evidence.

However, he also proposes a Principle of Tolerance in a second sense, reminiscent of Popper's anti-authoritarian political critiques, which argues against those dogmas which are produced by people who are seduced by a conception of themselves as having access to knowledge that is certain (see Bronowski 1973: 356–74).

I can see him now, presenting his television series *The Ascent of Man*, an old man dressed formally in a dark suit standing by a pond at Auschwitz, saying, 'When people believe that they have absolute knowledge ... this is how they behave'. He quotes Cromwell at them: 'I beseech you, in the bowels of Christ, think it possible you may be mistaken' (1973: 374) and then he walks into the pond and grasps a handful of the grey mud created by the ashes of some four million of his people, as a symbol of human contact. His view of science and certainty is as follows: 'Science is a very human form of knowledge . . . .. Every judgement in science stands on the edge of error, and is personal. Science is a tribute to what we can know although we are fallible' (1973: 374).

## Ideology

What Bronowski was arguing against was an ideology of science, which we may call 'scientism', which seeks to use popular perceptions of science embodied in the Traditional View in order to endorse quite specific political positions. For example, a certain variety of psychology seeks to treat people as if they were machines and defends social policies based on IQ testing in the name of science. It is often, but by no means invariably, conservative positions which are defended by scientistic arguments. One thinks of arguments which seem ludicrous to us now but which were advanced for years by some in the medical profession in order to exclude women. 'Science' here was clearly used for ideological purposes, so as to preserve men's entrance to and control of the profession.

We should look carefully for signs of scientism in arguments about the space programme, or abortion law reform, or nuclear power, or the run-down of traditional industries, or the role of drugs in sport, or the effect of exercise on female physiology, and so on.

Of course, some radical positions are also prone to scientism, especially those forms of Marxism which claim to discern a pattern and sequence to human history through scientific analysis.

What we call our science is valued because (and to the extent that) it delivers the goods. It, and not other forms of prescientific activity such as witchcraft, herbalism, alchemy and ad hoc building methods, has survived and progressed and now dominates our thinking about the physical world of cause and effect and our interaction with it. Quite rightly so – it is the best source of such knowledge that we have, and to the extent that we value such knowledge, so shall we value the origin of it. But that should not blind us to two things:

- Science is not the only source of our knowledge.
- Science fetishism is an invitation to ideological intrusion.

I have suggested that every scientist necessarily occupies and employs a view within the philosophy of science, and that any such view has practical consequences for the conduct of scientific investigations. This is reason enough why every working scientist has an obligation to explore those philosophical considerations that bear not only on his immediate concerns, but also on the nature and value of the enterprise of science.

## Bibliography

Bambrough, R. (1973) *Reason, Truth & God*, London: Methuen.

Best, D. (1973) 'Empirical examination of dance – a reply', *British Journal of PE*, 4(3), 6 and 10.

Best, D. (1978) *Philosophy and Human Movement*, London: Allen & Unwin.

Bronowski, J. (1973) *The Ascent of Man*, London: BBC.

Chalmers, A.F. (1982) *What is This Thing Called Science?* 2nd edn, Milton Keynes: Open University Press.

Fischer, R.B. (1975) *Science, Man & Society*, 2nd edn, New York: W.B. Saunders.

Hacking, I. (ed.) (1981a) *Scientific Revolutions*, Oxford: Oxford University Press.

Hacking, I. (1981b) 'Lakatos's philosophy of science', in I. Hacking (ed.) *Scientific Revolutions*, Oxford: University Press, 128–43.

Harré, R. (1972) *The Philosophies of Science*, Oxford: Oxford University Press.

Hollis, M. (1994) *The Philosophy of Social Science*, Cambridge: Cambridge University Press.

Ladyman, J. (2002) *Understanding Philosophy of Science*, London: Routledge.

Lakatos, I. (1981) 'History of science and its rational reconstructions', in I. Hacking (ed.) *Scientific Revolutions*, Oxford: University Press, 107–27.

Lakatos, I. and Musgrave, A. (eds) (1974) *Criticism and the Growth of Knowledge*, Cambridge: Cambridge University Press.

Magee, B. (1973) *Popper*, London: Fontana.

McFee (1977) *Philosophy and Movement*, Chelsea Papers in Human Movement Studies, Brighton Polytechnic.

Newton-Smith, W.H. (1981) *The Rationality of Science*, London: Routledge.

Popper, K.R. (1945) *The Open Society and Its Enemies*, London: Routledge.

Popper. K.R. (1963) *Conjectures and Refutations*, London: Routledge.

Popper, K.R. (1968) *The Logic of Scientific Discovery*, rev. edn, London: Hutchinson.

Russell, B. (1912) *The Problems of Philosophy*, Oxford: Oxford University Press.

# 3 Can physiology be both Popperian and ethical?

*Neil Spurway*

## Conjectures and refutations

It is some time in the 1980s: the (UK) Physiological Society is in session. A dynamic young American visitor is conducting his audience through a sequential investigation. Three times in the allotted 10 minutes of his talk he says: 'So we challenged *that* hypothesis by . . .', and then describes his team's next experiment. To those who know a little philosophy of science, this is pure Karl Popper: conjectures, followed promptly by checks of what each conjecture would predict – i.e. by attempts at refutation.

Popper's most accessible statement of the view that this is how science ought to proceed – his 'demarcation criterion' between what was truly scientific and what, whether commendable or otherwise in itself, was not science – is in the title essay of his book, *Conjectures and Refutations* (Popper 1963: 33–65). Comparing the mounting of an astronomical expedition to test a prediction from Einstein's General Theory of Relativity with the way that Marxists, Freudians and Adlerians treated their theories, Popper became convinced that there was a crucial difference. For the latter groups, 'explanatory power' was the hallmark of a good theory, and their facility at fitting each and every new fact or observation into their respective preconceived frameworks was impressive. But, when predictions derived from their theory were not verified, the proponents would immediately adjust their interpretations, convinced not that the theory was wrong but that they had deployed it wrongly; with a little adjustment, incorporating the new knowledge into the theory itself or the way it was expressed, the theory would march on again, yet further enhanced (in their eyes) in its 'explanatory power'. By contrast, the attitude of the physicists to the astronomical expedition convinced Popper that, if the prediction of Einstein's theory had not been confirmed, they would have considered that the theory had itself been profoundly challenged, if not instantly refuted.

Popper (1963: 36–7, *my numbering*) concluded from this comparison that:

1 A theory which is not refutable by any conceivable event is non-scientific. Irrefutability is not a virtue of a theory . . . but a vice.
2 Every genuine test of a theory is an attempt to . . . refute it.

3 Confirming evidence should not count except when it is the result of a genuine test ... [which] ... can be presented as a serious but unsuccessful attempt to falsify the theory. Thus . . ..
4 The criterion of the scientific status of a theory is its ... refutability.

Even in the popular essay from which these sentences are quoted, the discussion of what constitutes the scientific approach to theory testing occupies only the first six of the 33 pages. Popper's overall output on the philosophy of science was immense and radical. Nevertheless, the criterion of in-principal refutability or 'falsifiability' remained a corner-stone, and was noticed with approval throughout the world of science at the time. It highlighted a core feature in the methodology, not only of experimental physics but of experimental chemistry, biochemistry, genetics, immunology, indeed of all sciences concerned with the way natural systems work – very much including physiology. The great and the good, during my early days in the profession, explicitly espoused the Popperian account. 'Popper is alright with me,' replied Sir Alan Hodgkin, the head of the group in which I was privileged to obtain a doctorate, to one of my tentative questions. His co-Nobel laureate, Sir John Eccles, advised young physiologists 'to read and meditate upon Popper's writings on the philosophy of science and to adopt them as the basis of operation of one's scientific life' (quoted by Magee 1973). And yet a third, knighted Nobelist, the immunologist Sir Peter Medawar, wrote repeatedly in Popperian terms (e.g. Medawar 1967).

In one important respect, the way Popper referred in this 1963 essay to the single astronomical expedition was unfortunate. It suggested that, when science was being done at its best, a single contrary observation should destroy the most major theory. I do not believe he ever thought this – there is a clear indication to the contrary within a few lines of the sentences I have quoted – yet he was widely assumed to do so. Chronologically, it is important to note that even the 1963 essay (originally given as a lecture in 1951) was sketching the development of Popper's thought as a young man in Vienna in the early 1920s. By 1963 such a simplistic view would have been doubly untenable, for the first edition of Thomas Kuhn's major work, *The Structure of Scientific Revolutions* (Kuhn 1962) had just appeared and made great impact. Kuhn's studies provided extensive evidence that substantial theories had never been withdrawn on the strength of a single contrary incident. A few years later, Imre Lakatos (1970) gave a much fuller account of what typically happens when a predicted result is not obtained.

At first, said Lakatos, the good experimenter will re-examine the 'auxiliary hypotheses' involved in interpreting the observations. These auxiliary hypotheses would include the specific assumptions underlying the design of the experiment; the principles and functioning of the equipment; and the success with which it was considered that the parameter being observed had been isolated from compounding factors, which may not all have been foreseen. (This last consideration is particularly imperative in biological experimentation, where the scope for the unplanned complication is especially large: any disturbance, from damage during dissection to the fact that the animal or human subject is incubating a virus, may confuse the best-designed experiment.) Usually such a critique will bring to the fore several possible reasons, well short of a failure in the fundamental theory, why the expected result had not been obtained. Yet even if this does not happen the scientific community will normally bide its time, suspecting that something has been overlooked in the analysis of the experiment, however assiduously this analysis has been undertaken. Kuhn's word, taken on by Lakatos, for a result neither predicted nor subsequently explained, was an 'anomaly'. The evidence from historical survey was that only when an unignorable number of anomalies have accumulated, has a substantial edifice of theory – the 'paradigm' (another Kuhn word) upon which the research has been modelled – ever been overthrown.

However, this is the way of the world with all ideals. The ideal of every experimental scientist remains Popperian: (s)he should seek, insofar as is humanly possible, to subject his/her hypotheses, and emergent theories to truly decisive tests. Popper's criterion of demarcation between science and non-science thus becomes an encapsulated challenge. In principle, if not in fact, we might consider it pinned on every laboratory wall, serving as, so to speak, a 'bench-side pulpit'.

Behind the interpretations of all three philosophers, Popper, Kuhn and Lakatos (and the great majority of those who have written more recently: see Chalmers 1999) is an acceptance that verbal accounts will be given and papers written to the end that other scientifically trained people, of broadly similar background, could repeat the experimental tests with a likelihood of similar results; and hence that, under the ambit of overall paradigms widely adhered to, something approaching objectivity will be claimable for the findings. There is no such thing as a theory-independent observation (Hanson 1958) or an absolutely objective conclusion (Lawson 2001) but, within cultures of commensurate development and linguistic background, close approaches to these ideals are attainable. The cultural aspect is readily evident: the endemic thought of aboriginal Australians, Kalahari Bushmen or Native Americans is so radically removed from the outlook of a modern, Western scientist that, unless one party or the other had taken exceptional pains to soak him/herself in the other's culture, discussion of an experiment would have no possibility of achieving comprehension. Ancient Chinese medicine may now have its adherents in the West, but the traditional explanations of how it works, however respectfully we may approach them, are no more comprehensible to us than gobbledygook. Even Russian or East European science, when I first began to read it around 1960, often had a strange feel, so that one was not quite certain whether the questions put or answers given meant precisely what the translations appeared to say; it is noticeable, however, that such an uncertainty is now infrequent, as political relaxation has allowed the cultures to converge. Both theory-dependence and objectivity are more technical concepts than the cultural one; in a book-length account each would have to be analysed at length, but here I hope it will suffice to say simply, in connection with both of them, that one is unlikely to see anything useful at all unless one has some idea of what one is looking for. Such perceptions as these, about culture, observation and objectivity are at the core of the received, philosophical viewpoint upon the mainstream sciences, and my underlying point at this stage is just that, in respect of its investigative intentions and the way it seeks to test its theories, experimental physiology *is* one of these sciences.

## Characteristics specific to physiological thought

When we come to consider the characteristics of the ideas that physiologists set out to test, we find many features more specific to the discipline.

First, it is assumed, until and unless substantial evidence to the contrary is generated, that every structure and every system has a function – a positive contribution to the life of the whole organism. Frequently this is expressed in the language of 'role' or even 'purpose', but the outsider must not take this language too literally. 'Purpose' talk is sometimes referred to as 'teleology', but it is *not* teleology in the Greek sense – an Aristotelian 'final cause'. It is simply a shorthand for 'contribution to survival'. Clearly, this in turn links to Darwinian evolution, and the more biologically sophisticated physiologists may, when they realize someone critical is listening, use a longer phrase such as 'confers adapt-ive advantage by . . .', instead of simply 'functions to . . .'. Whatever the form of words, however, this search for role or function is the essence of the physiologist's enterprise.

Yet it must be acknowledged that we are sometimes defeated in our attempts to find a current function. Then the likely conclusion is that the structure is vestigial – wholly so, as in the case of the 'vermiform' (intestinal) appendix, or of much diminished function, like the pineal gland. Or we may conclude that the form now seen has derived sub-optimally from some previous system – as upright stance derives from quadrupedal posture, and causes human beings almost certainly to suffer a great deal more backache than do cows. Yet it is worth noticing that this is an even more inescapably evolutionary position. It would be logically possible to study function physiologically if one believed in the separate (presumably divine?) design of every system; I just don't happen to know any physiologist who does. But to consider *past* functions is ineluctably evolutionary.

A more sophisticated challenge than simply to judge between present or past functions is to assess the *quantitative* adaptation to demand. This approach, which is largely a development of the last 20 or so years, brings together physiological and evolutionary thinking and so is termed 'evolutionary physiology'. It is accessibly described by Diamond (1993), in a book to which I shall shortly refer again for another chapter, by other authors. In most body systems there is about twice the provision we normally need; we can cope quite well, except in extreme circumstances, with one lung or one kidney, but not with half of one. Female mammals have twice as many nipples as an average litter for the species, and hardly ever produce more young than they have nipples. (Human triplets were vanishingly rare before modern fertility drugs.) Similar factors often apply at the molecular level, such as in the systems for adsorption of nutrients. Where the factor is much more than two, we must ask whether there is a reason. Cats, for instance, have ten times the capacity they might be considered to need for uptake of the nutrient arginine. However, arginine is vital for cats, and digestive processes may release it from different foodstuffs at different points down the length of the small intestine, so there has been adaptive benefit in providing considerable adsorptive capacity throughout that organ's length. This is not to claim that all adaptation is optimal: we have already seen that it is not. But we cannot even begin to identify many maladaptations, and to investigate the reasons for them, without precisely evaluating the degree of adaptation first.

There are deep philosophical questions aroused by evolutionary theory – such as the soundness of the concept of 'species', or whether the idea that the fittest survive is merely tautological (see, e.g. Mahner and Bunge 1997) – which do not affect physiology. Nor do the internal debates among evolutionists, about such questions as whether changes have accumulated at roughly similar rates over many millions of years or in intensive bursts punctuating long periods of virtual equilibrium. Physiological considerations of evolutionary history, even when the precision of adaptation is estimated quantitatively, are shallower than these subtleties.

If the investigation of function is physiology's first hallmark, the second is that the discipline confines itself to a certain range of scale. This is a matter partly of norm, of use and wont, but partly also of essence. At the upper end of the range, it is the essence of the discipline to be concerned with the individual organism. Most if not all practitioners would agree that there can be no true physiology of anything larger than a blue whale. If the 'physiology' of an ecosystem, or even the whole earth (Volk 1998), is spoken of, I am sure that every professional physiologist would consider that it is spoken of analogically, not formally. In practice, rough limits are accepted at the lower end of the size-range too. Physiological journals accept papers concerned with the behaviour and functions of cells, and certain extensive structures and systems within cells, such as their surface membranes or their contractile proteins, but when the scale is that of the individual molecule the work is more likely to be classified as biochemistry or molecular biophysics. Partly, these distinctions will be based on the techniques employed, and partly on the questions asked.[1]

Noble and Boyd (1993) give an excellent example of how the distinction between a biochemical and a physiological investigation might be drawn, at the bottom of the scale-range. I will rephrase it to avoid their more technical terms, but the idea is entirely theirs. They invite us to imagine two scientists, both of whom are manipulating the growth-processes of the same type of cell so that the same protein will be formed experimentally in its surface membrane. Perhaps they are even both interested in the effects of identical small changes in the protein's structure. To an outsider the two researchers' activities might appear indistinguishable. But one is concerned with the chemistry of the protein's conformation, and its consequent stability within the membrane; this investigation would therefore be categorized as biochemical. The other is concerned with the role of the protein as a channel for electrical current flow, and its consequences for the control of rhythm in the heart; this research is indisputably physiological, albeit at the smallest end of this discipline's scale.

A further feature of the Noble and Boyd example is that physiology has a characteristic style as well as a characteristic range of scales. The hallmark of the physiologist's mind is to be on the lookout for integrative mechanisms, whether at the cellular or the organismal level. A century ago, one body system was thought of as integrative above all others – the 'edifice' of the central nervous system (Sherrington 1906). Marginally ahead of Sherrington's consummate text, however, Bayliss and Starling (1902) – deviating from their own senior collaborator, Pavlov, who was as neurally focused as Sherrington – were proposing the new idea of chemical messengers which carried signals from one body-site to another via the blood stream, not by nerves. As this concept matured, its terminology developed: the messenger substances acquired the name 'hormones' and the principal structures producing them were termed 'endocrine' (internally secreting) glands – though Bayliss and Starling did not originally make this link. Nowadays the network of such endocrine control mechanisms, working in parallel or conjunction with the nervous system, is universally recognized, and the concept of endocrine control has become as powerful a paradigm as that of neural control. More elusive forms of integration, in which there is no identifiable master mechanism controlling the others, are also entering our range of understanding: interacting metabolic systems, or the mutual co-ordination of respiratory and cardiovascular systems under such challenges as exercise (Rowell and Shepherd 1996), exemplify this point.

An older idea, which the control systems just described subserve, is that of 'homeostasis' – staying the same (Cannon 1932). Bodily conditions do not, of course, stay *exactly* the same in the face of changes of food supply, physical activity or (in the case of warm-blooded animals) external temperature. The point of the term homeostasis is, however, that they deviate many times less than uncontrolled, non-homeostatic systems would; they seem to strive to stay, as nearly as possible, the same. And the capacity for such internal control is crucial to every animal's existence: 'Constancy of the internal environment is the condition of free, independent life' (Bernard 1878). As thus stated this comes close to dogma. It leads, however, to research programmes because it implies the existence of 'negative feedback', the principle that a deviation is first sensitively detected and thence strongly countered, so that the deviation actually occurring is many times less than if no such corrective mechanism existed (Machin 1964). Neural, endocrine and metabolic control systems all consist of complexly interacting negative feedback loops, each operating in this basic fashion, and a great deal of physiological research is concerned with identifying them and assessing their exact parameters (Windhorst 1996).

A number of comments suggest themselves at this point. The first is a historical one, drawn from Boyd and Noble: one of Bernard's original purposes in enunciating the insight just discussed was to counter the mid-nineteenth century optimism of organic chemists, principally in Germany, that in a few years they would have solved the problems of life. At the turn of the twenty-first century the same sense is present in the attitudes of many molecular biologists and workers on the genome, that they are unravelling the secrets of the living state. Their work is indeed exciting and hugely important, but it is not all that is required. The significance of a molecular feature can only be 'seen in the context of higher-order systems: whole cells, whole organs, whole organisms, even species and their environments' (Noble and Boyd 1993: 6). Yet Bernard's concept of the control required within several of these higher-order systems remains so strong that it has become a *leitmotif* of physiological understanding, independent of the philosophical challenge it was formulated to counter.

The second comment is that, if the word 'teleological' has a valid use in physiology, it is surely in describing such negative feedback systems, for there is a very real sense in which they can be considered purposive (though see Hull 1974). However, I suspect it is more constructive to call them 'cybernetic', remembering that the origin of that coinage in modern science was the governor, *kybernikos*, of a steam engine (Wiener 1961).

Third, physiologists aspire, almost as strongly as physicists, to represent their understanding of mechanisms in mathematical terms. A complete mathematical model is much harder to achieve in physiology, not so much because the measurements are insufficiently accurate (though that is sometimes the case), but more fundamentally because the systems studied are too complex. Nevertheless, the aspiration is there; and nowhere has it more frequently been demonstrated, to good effect, than in the analysis of control systems (Machin 1964; Windhorst 1996).

Non-biological control systems are the province of engineers; it follows that the mathematics of any control systems, biological or non-biological, is engineering mathematics. Strikingly, however, in almost every other branch of physiology to which mathematics has been productively applied – such as in the study of mechanical, electrical, chemical or hydraulic physiological systems – it is likewise the mathematics of engineering which has been found suitable. This is in contrast, for instance, to the probabilistic mathematics of much work in genetics and ecology. (Doucet and Sloep 1992, give instances of both approaches.)

Among the reasons for the frequency with which physiologists use engineering mathematics are one that is crude, another that is fundamental. The crude reason is that both engineers and physiologists are interested in mathematics that works, whether or not it is puristically rigorous. The more fundamental reason is that engineering systems also have clearly defined functions: they are designed to *do* specific things. In fact, physiology could well be characterized by the phrase of Dennett (1995), 'reverse engineering' – not designing new systems to work in a particular way, but analysing existing systems to find out how they work as they do. Whichever way round the analysis is done, the mathematics required will be the same.

## Metaphors and models

The philosophy of science, Anglo-Saxon style, rarely starts at the beginning: it emphasizes, as I have so far done, the way ideas are developed and tested, but not how they arise. The accepted way of summarizing this is to say that it operates in 'the context of justification' rather than 'the context of discovery'. Perhaps the Anglo-Saxon temperament has found discovery too personal to be a proper subject of enquiry? If so it is not surprising to find that the French have had no such inhibitions. They have considered the context of discovery at least as much as that of justification. From Henri Poincaré (c. 1900), through Gaston Bachelard to Michel Foucault (late 1960s) and beyond, they have explored the roles of irrational or pre-rational influences such as conceptual convention, metaphor and (more recently) social power, in the initiation of scientific ideas. Bachelard (1938) in particular has impressed me by the continuity of his treatment of metaphor in writings about both science and poetry.

The history of physiology provides many examples of metaphor in action – or, if not always metaphor in the sense which can also be applied to poetry, then certainly analogy or simile. Galileo to an extent, and markedly his pupil Borelli (in effect the earliest practitioners of biomechanics), saw the limb as a 'lever', and treated it that way in calculations of strength and load. Harvey, famously, perceived the heart as a 'pump'; he knew no more anatomy than the Greeks, yet the analogy which was the basis of his majestic insight was probably the lift pump, invented only a generation before him to get water into canals. Lavoisier, having studied chemical burning, and represented it in terms of reaction with oxygen rather than release of phlogiston, perceived that the respiration of a mouse in his calorimeter was essentially the same process as the burning of a candle there. Helmholtz modelled the tuning of the inner ear in terms of resonant physical cavities. Starling and Bayliss, as we have already seen, wrote of blood-borne signalling substances as chemical 'messengers'. Henderson perceived the sodium-rich fluids bathing our body cells as a 'sea' within us – not a modern sea either, but akin in its composition to the seas from which the first multicellular animals had emerged. Birds' feet can stay cold, yet their bodies hot, because the descending arteries and ascending veins in their long thin legs act as 'counter-current exchangers' of heat, as in engineering systems; and the solute-concentrating systems of the kidney work the same way. Nerve fibres are electrical 'cables'. Cell membranes are riddled with ion-conducting 'channels'.

I deliberately changed my language in those last three examples, because of course the analogy which provides the initial insight often survives as the model by which the system continues to be understood. The limb *is* a lever – a living lever. The heart *is* a pump – a living pump. Respiration may not be burning, *sensu strictu*, but at its cellular end-stage it is emphatically oxidation and it is the main source of body heat. The cochlea of the ear *is* a resonator (though more complex than Helmholtz could know). 'Messenger' and 'sea' remain more simply metaphorical, but the terms are still as vivid and pedagogically illuminating as when they were first deployed.

Notwithstanding widespread use, the word 'model' has many meanings even in academic discourses. Formal, mental models must precede mathematics. It is about the model, not the awful but probably irrelevant complexity of the real system, that one does one's calculations. The limb, the counter-current system and the nerve fibre are examples of systems analysed in terms of models which simplify both geometry and functional properties relative to the biological reality. A friend with whom I used to argue regarded such formal models as relating to the world in the same sense as that claimed for propositions (statements asserting facts) by the early Ludwig Wittgenstein: 'The proposition is a model of the reality as we think it is' (Wittgenstein 1922: 4.01). I am not persuaded that this is correct. The relation between a conceptual simplification of an experimental system and that system in its complex entirety is not convincingly the same as the relation between a linguistic proposition and the world. Of course there are (dare one say?) analogies between the two relationships, but the conceptual model used in scientific practice would, at a minimum, need many propositions to describe it. Indeed, one might question whether it could be embodied in a finite group of propositions at all, for a model selected by a perceptive scientist may be considered to embody tacit, non-verbal knowledge (cf. Polanyi 1958). Nevertheless, whether the model/world relation and the proposition/world relation are closely parallel or not, the fact that so influential a philosopher as Wittgenstein, in both his earlier and his later phases, spoke extensively of models has undoubtedly enhanced the currency of the word.

But by no means are all models merely formal. Lord Kelvin famously asserted that he could not fully understand any system of which he could not actually make a physical model – which, at his time, almost always meant a mechanical one. Mechanical models are rarely used at the research stage of a physiological problem, though studies of hearing, from Helmholtz to von Bekesy (1960) and beyond, have been exceptions. They are, however, frequently used in teaching – especially, but by no means solely, where access to the system in a living animal is inappropriate or even illegal. Models of the heart and blood vessels are particularly powerful in demonstrating the effects of interacting adjustments in different parts of the cardiovascular system. Yet other uses of the term 'model' refer to systems which are actually biological, not inanimate. Tissues in culture are studied as models of the same tissue *in situ*. Unfortunately (and too seldom recognized by the opponents of animal experiments), only after thorough checks on whole animals or human volunteers can we determine, in any given instance, whether the cultured tissue has provided a good or a misleading model. Most strikingly and gruesomely of all, however, a laboratory animal may these days be referred to as a 'model' – presumably, though this is never explicitly stated, a model of the human being. Phrases like, 'in the rat model' are now many times more common at meetings than direct references to the challenging of hypotheses, though tacitly the latter process continues unabated. Personally, I squirm at this linguistic turn as much as, I suspect, most readers of this volume will. But, in an appropriately detached account of physiological philosophy, the trend must not go unmentioned.

This rueful acknowledgement has taken us some distance from the examples, introduced three paragraphs ago, in which the accepted conceptual model has grown out of an original analogy or metaphor. Several of these can profitably be discussed further. First, let us look in a little more detail at Harvey's unsurpassable insight (1628). I have suggested that he could understand the heart as a pump because he had seen a pump, whereas Aristotle, Galen and even Leonardo (who had just the right sort of mechanism-oriented mind) had not. Prompted by this analogy, Harvey had shown that when a vein was compressed, it was on the peripheral not the central side that it swelled up, indicating that blood was reaching it from the tissues, not down the large veins from the heart. But he had to make an immense leap of faith nonetheless. To propose that the blood was pumped only in one direction through the heart, rather than flopping to and fro, so that it circulated from arteries to veins and thence back again to the heart, Harvey had to suggest that it permeated through the tissues from the last arterial-side vessels he could see to the first venous-side vessels he could see. He speculated that there must be interstices in the tissues, through which blood could pass from arteries to veins; yet, without the aid of a microscope, no such interstices could be seen. In this sense, Harvey's insight conflicted with existing evidence. It was not until 33 years later, when the very first microscope had been invented, that Malpighi saw capillaries – channels, just wide enough to accommodate one blood cell at a time – providing continuous passage from the arterial to the venous side of Harvey's postulated 'circulation'.

In terms of the theme with which I began, this was Popper deferred. If there really had been no interstitial channels, the blood could not have been circulating. Harvey dared a prediction, not knowing whether it could ever be checked. Malpighi acquired the technical means to perform a Popperian check of Harvey's concept, and in fact found elegantly *for* Harvey. It is impossible not to accept that, had he done the opposite – by which I mean not just that he had not seen through-channels of some sort (which would have been indecisive), but had positively seen channels which turned blood back from one artery to another, and one vein to another, with none continuing through – Harvey's grand postulate would have collapsed.

My second point comes from examination of the 'channel' concept. It started like the capillary, in that at the outset (e.g. Hodgkin and Huxley 1952) it was purely hypothetical; indeed it was not even quite explicit, in that the word 'channel' is not used in the great paper cited, yet in retrospect it is clear that all the key features of the idea were enunciated there (Hille 1984). In 1952 no one could see an ion-sized hole in a cell membrane, any more than in 1628 one could see capillaries in tissues. Unlike capillaries, however, normal channels can still not be seen, but features supporting that kind of concept can be. Specifically, a channel occupies, *ex hypothesi*, a particular location on the membrane's surface. The implied contrast is with diffusion through the bulk material making up the membrane, which is a 'lipid' (fatty) layer. The two respiratory gases, oxygen and carbon dioxide, can dissolve in fats and thus pass quite easily through the membrane, whereas ions – charge-carrying, water-dissolved particles – cannot; it is for them that molecular-width pores through the centres of proteins, normally filled with water but capable of allowing the passage of the ions, are postulated. Now such ordinary channels, proposed as conducting ions in large numbers, are too small to see, even by the latest techniques of electron microscopy. However, certain particularly large derivative forms, which transport the ions against concentration gradients or electrical fields with the aid of metabolic energy, can now be identified. So can another specialized form, in which the channels are open only when a neural 'transmitter' substance has so 'instructed' them (note two further metaphors!). Thus the idea of localized points at which ions can pass through membranes has gained some microscopical support, though the routes first proposed and most widely studied cannot themselves be seen and, on present understanding, never will be.

In addition to these structural indications in natural membranes, chemical models of such membranes can be made. Firstly, an ultra-thin film of lipid molecules is formed. When it has air on each side it looks black, like the thinnest parts of a soap bubble, yet when such a 'black membrane' is fabricated instead between two salt-containing (and so electrically conducting) solutions it presents an extremely high resistance to the flow of current from one to the other. But if a drop of liquid containing dissolved 'ionophores' is introduced into one of these volumes, the membrane's resistance falls by many orders of magnitude. Ionophores are fairly large molecules, of precisely known structures, which have circular or tubular form, and into whose central holes single ions of one or another chemical species fit almost precisely; by contrast, the outer surfaces of the ionophore molecules are highly tolerant, not of an ionic but of a lipid neighbourhood. So, when introduced into a salty solution in contact with a lipid film, they rapidly take up residence in the film and form ion-conducting routes. According to their size and shape these routes may be either fairly stationary channels constituting a permanent pore, or alternatively 'carriers' shuttling to and fro between the two surfaces of the lipid film; either way, they represent independent transmembrane routes for ion movement and therefore current flow. The idea that they are acting in a fashion closely analogous to that of natural channels would be powerfully suggested by this alone, but there is yet stronger evidence. If a system with very small numbers of ionophores (say one to five) is studied electrically, the current flows in finite steps, increasing and decreasing in a way which can only mean that the channels are opening and closing, forming and disappearing, according to their positions within the lipid layer. And when similar electrical studies are made, of small areas of natural cell membrane, similar upward and downward steps of conductivity are invariably seen. It has never been found possible to propose any interpretation for this observation on the natural systems other than the opening and closing of transmembrane channels. Yet further evidence (Hille 1984; Ashcroft 2000) has come from studies of molecular genetics: the genes which determine transmembrane conductivity do so by controlling the production of proteins which look like ionophores. The existence of ion-conducting channels is therefore regarded as confirmed, though indirectly.

In the philosophy of physics, one of the standard questions concerns the real existence of theoretical entities (Toulmin, 1953; McMullin, 1984). Electrons were once in this category, though only the most academic purist would contend that they still are; the Higgs boson[2] by contrast, emphatically still is. The development of ideas about electrons and those about ion channels have run very similar courses. Channels are still in a strict sense, theoretical entities, yet they are entities in which virtually every practitioner believes. Much the same might be said about several other classes of structure at the low end of the size-range dealt with by physiologists: the various 'receptor' molecules on cell-membrane surfaces at which drugs, neurotransmitters, and olfactory stimuli are considered to act, constitute a whole further family of instances.

A further example of small-scale conceptual model, which at first was interestingly ambivalent, is that of the 'independent force generators' proposed by Nobel Laureate Sir Andrew Huxley (1957) as the sites at which the fundamental property of muscle cells, the generation of contractile force, was located. A year or two earlier, in electron micrographs that Jean Hanson and Hugh Huxley (no relative of Andrew) had just produced, of the two kinds of parallel protein filament that fill the muscle cell, regularly spaced knobs could be seen on one type of filament, potentially or actually bridging the gaps to the other. These were obvious candidates to be the force generators, and almost certainly contributed to the concept in Andrew Huxley's mind. But he took care that his theory would not fall, if the knobs should be found to be artefacts of the microscopical preparation, until its own logical consequences had been thoroughly tested. Therefore, in the early years after the independent force generators were proposed, they were treated as entirely theoretical entities, though now no mainstream muscle biologist would doubt either that they exist, or that they are indeed the knobs on the filaments first seen in a few pinnacle-of-the-art electron micrographs half a century ago.

## Paradigms

I have argued that the concepts of function (or value for survival) and of homeostatic feedback, and the focusing of attention within a certain range of scales, are specific hallmarks of physiological thought. In many other respects, however, from the role of metaphor and analogy in the inception of ideas to the ways in which they are developed and tested by experiment, physiology has a logical structure and methodological approach closely concordant with that of other laboratory sciences.

A further respect in which the structure of physiological research activity is closely similar to that of the disciplines more often discussed by philosophers of science, but which has only been implied, not spelled out so far, is that key advances become paradigms for a whole new school of practice. I have already noted that, when Bayliss and Starling (1902) discovered their first hormone, they set in train a ramifying research programme; not only the *idea* of a hormone but the way they had looked for it were closely followed for some time. Such double-aspect emulation of the pioneer approach is the essence of what Kuhn (1962) sought to characterize when he coined the term 'paradigm', to designate an influence greater than that of any one concept, model or even fully formulated theory. (Early commentators insisted that he had embraced too many functions under the one word, 'paradigm', but the general idea has stuck, and the term is widely used.) Again when Hodgkin and colleagues first defined the properties of sodium and potassium channels in squid nerve fibres, their work was both conceptually and methodologically paradigmatic. In the following decade or so, the same two kinds of channel were identified in other cells. Gradually, after this phase, it became clear that calcium ions could carry brief bursts of current into cells just as sodium ions could, yet the effect was not to weaken the paradigm but to extend it in principle to other charged species capable of moving through lipid membranes.

As for the Huxley concept of localized force generators, the methods by which he and his colleagues pinned this concept down in skeletal muscle fibres have been less generally applicable, because other motile systems are very differently organized, but the concept of force-generating molecular sites, working independently, has found application in the understanding of phenomena as disparate as the beating of cilia in the bronchial tree, the flow of cytoplasm along nerve fibres, and even the energy-storing processes of intracellular organelles (Banting and Higgins 2000). In the breadth of its influence, therefore, if not as a methodological role model, Huxley's approach too has achieved paradigmatic status.

However, it would be seriously misleading to cite, as examples of physiological science, only instances where there is a single, dominating paradigm and its associated theoretical predictions have been extensively confirmed. So let us end this part of our discussion by considering a case, from the physiology of exercise, where two rival views are currently in contention.

Lactate accumulates in the blood when muscles are working hard. However, its concentration does not increase linearly with the intensity of effort: on the contrary, almost all lactate accumulation occurs in the upper half of the work-intensity range. One theory, which has existed in outline since about 1920, is that the muscles are being increasingly starved of oxygen, as the limits of the cardio-respiratory system's ability to supply it to them are approached (Wasserman *et al.* 1973). Another view, from the 1980s, notes that a single small muscle in a body otherwise at rest produces lactate, when working at 50 per cent or more of its own maximum – and there is no evidence of oxygen-lack in transverse slices of the muscle fibres (Connett *et al.* 1986). In my judgement (Spurway 1992) the latter evidence is convincing, but the disciples of the earlier standpoint yield only very slowly. The older theory is elegant, easily understood, and capable of explaining most observations. The few it does not explain, such as the experiment on the single active muscle, are widely overlooked or ignored. Such is the power of paradigmatic allegiance. The few upholders of the old view who have really taken the trouble to inform themselves about the newer one cast about for ways in which it is possible that the experimental results upon which it is founded could be misleading.

The situation falls convincingly into the area in which the writings of Kuhn and Lakatos prevail. The protective belt of auxiliary hypotheses, which must be accepted if the newer theory is to win the day, is what the aware defenders of the older view attack; they argue for non-obvious explanations of Connett's experiments. However, a-rationality and closed minds are common in this field, partly at least because the majority of participants are applied scientists rather than fundamental researchers, so that it is still the case that only a minority of exercise physiologists even know of the newer evidence. This is disappointing to one of its proponents! Yet I take comfort from the fact that it is also closely reminiscent of many past interactions within the scientific community. There has been a widespread pattern of intense investigative commitment at first, followed by a period of uncritical, perhaps even rather lazy orthodoxy (Kuhn 1962). The unity of science is yet again upheld, even if, in this case, perhaps not entirely edifyingly!

## The ethics of experimentation

I now turn to the aspect of physiological study which most disturbs many people – the inescapable consequence of its being the discipline concerned with how living bodies work. In this volume, investigations involving human subjects will probably be considered of even greater relevance than animal experimentation, but concern over this latter should first be acknowledged.

The overwhelming bulk of physiological knowledge has been acquired through experimentation on animals – from molluscs and worms to higher primates. Humankind has thus been, we might say, an intellectual carnivore. Every physiologist would contend that the benefit to humanity, through medical and health science – and, let it never be forgotten, to countless other animals through veterinary science – justifies the sacrifices of animal life involved. However, the stance that, in a civilized society, this should on principle never happen, is an absolutely fair one, provided it is upheld by vegetarians. My own view, indeed, is that the justification for the parsimonious and sensitive recourse to animal experimentation is much greater than that of eating meat, for there are excellent alternatives to meat eating and often no alternatives to the experiment other than continuing ignorance. One can thus be a vegetarian physiologist with perfect consistency, but not a meat-eating anti-vivisectionist.

What is absolutely unacceptable is the inflicting of substantial pain, whether physical or emotional. The images which the word 'vivisection' has been made to conjure up, of terror-stricken animals in agony, rightly horrify every civilized person. The invalidity of the propaganda which propagates these images is the suggestion that they apply to what goes on in modern laboratories. Society's defence against their ever nowadays being valid is that the licensing regulations of all advanced governments (e.g. those operated by the Home Office in the UK) absolutely oppose such practices, and are very rigorously enforced – the experimenter's entire career being at stake in cases of contravention. However, there is often an even stronger defence – the disposition of the scientist. Not only is a person who is driven by the sense of wonder and awe at the beauty of physiological mechanisms unlikely to be prepared to cause distress to the animals in whom (s)he studies them; an equally basic point, of which a good experimenter will be always conscious, is that the physiology of an animal in fear or pain is highly abnormal. Thus, while defending in principle the sacrifice of animal life under conditions of minimum pain, I would never defend the imposition of substantial distress, whether physical or emotional.

However, defence 'in principle' does not entail defence in every instance of practice. While research into cancer, conducted with restraint, sensitivity, and after serious consideration of alternatives, is for me desirable, research into cosmetics is not. The first is to be balanced against extensive human and animal agony, caused by cancers for which there is not adequate treatment. The second, however, is weighed only against the gratification of the well-to-do and self-admiring, and the profits of companies that pander to these people's self-esteem. To my mind the first balance justifies animal experiments, the second does not. If cosmetics are to be tried, let this be on human volunteers, not rabbits!

I acknowledged above that there are possible alternatives to certain animal experiments (FRAME 2002). Quite a lot can be done by computer simulations of physiological systems and, in the specific but commercially critical field of drug design, a great deal of initial work uses molecular modelling programs. These approaches can refine and focus experiments, and reduce their number, but will never mean they can be avoided entirely. Tissue cultures, obtained once from an animal or human being but often maintained over innumerable subsequent 'generations', can also give a lot of information. Both these alternatives to animal experiment are quicker and usually cheaper. Thus no scientist, under pressure to publish and having to justify every outlay to grant-giving bodies – even one who felt no other compunction – would consider opting for animal experiments which were not necessary. But the ultimate test of every computer prediction and tissue-culture result *must* be the response of the whole, integrated physiological system that is the living animal or person.

That remark brings us to the human subject. The philosophy of investigations on other human beings must be that of maintaining the greatest respect towards them, and continually recognizing the privilege embodied in being able to make the study. There can be few higher ethical demands than to interact in the most appreciative and respectful way with other people who have volunteered their time, and often agreed to undertake stressful and uncomfortable activity (and/or accept stressful and uncomfortable interventions) in the interests of a research project.

It used to be said that one could do much more severe things to human volunteers than to laboratory animals. In the past decade this has largely ceased to be true, not because animal legislation has been relaxed in the least degree but because more stringent conditions for research on people have come into operation. Ethics committees, operating in Britain and Europe under an EU directive, have become much more critical, often forbidding the volunteer to undertake things (s)he would have been perfectly prepared to do. The concerns usually are ethical in the strict sense – as where the committee must be sure not only that the fullest possible medical cover is in place wherever the proposed intervention carries finite risk, but also that no student could possibly have been led to volunteer by the belief that exam marks at the end of the year might otherwise be unfavourably influenced. Another purely ethical requirement is that enough subjects will be studied to ensure that the results will be statistically significant and therefore publishable. Concerns about adverse publicity or litigation are sometimes also raised by these committees, which are encouraged by the institution concerned to act as custodians of its name, whether or not the matter is one of ethics in the narrow sense. Where it is not, however, this is an incidental function, performed by such bodies because they are conveniently placed to do so; the strictly ethical aspect of their remit is their *raison d'être*.

In many of these respects the physiologist's situation is no different from that of the psychologist, sociologist or other human researcher. The majority of constraints – such as those on the numbers of subjects and the pools they are drawn from – are of identical form; and the risk of psychological damage to the person being experimented upon may be regarded as equivalent to that of physical injury. But the physiologist has bodily to touch his subjects – and I pointedly say 'his' here; where the subject is young, vulnerable or of the opposite sex, and very much more so when the experimenter is male than when she is female, suspicions of abuse are inevitably aroused in today's zero-trust society. On a small number of regrettable occasions the suspicions appear even to have been justified. A monitoring person has therefore to be present whenever procedures involving contact are undertaken.

The overt considerations of the last two paragraphs have been of social policy and law, rather than philosophy. Nevertheless, it is satisfactory to note that every one of the statutory requirements is consonant with our philosophical standpoint. For this reason, the researcher must strive to accept them, not merely with reluctant tolerance but with ready cooperation.

It is interesting, however, to note that the word still used, for the volunteers who have physiological measurements made upon them, *is* 'subject'; it is not, for instance, 'participant', more appealing though that term might at first sight seem. I have heard it suggested that the conscious or unconscious intention of those using the word 'subject' is to emphasize the power and status of the scientist, relative to the person whose physiology is being studied. It must adamantly be insisted that, whatever the interpretation put upon the usage, power relationship has nothing to do with its intention. The intention is that the person studied must be neutrally disposed towards the results obtained; by contrast, 'participant' rather suggests that willed effort in a particular direction is expected. That would, of course, vitiate the whole endeavour.

## Applications of research to sport

Obviously, animal results will be only indirectly applicable to the human athlete. Nonetheless, our understanding of almost every aspect of exercise physiology has been very considerably advanced by animal studies. This applies as much to the heart's almost instant responses to physical activity as it does to the responses of the endocrine system, which are on the scale of hours; it applies to our comprehension of every component of physical performance, from temperature regulation to the biology of training.

When we do turn to human studies, a limitation immediately arises. The great majority of available subjects are university students – for the purposes of this book, particularly sport and exercise science students, though the contributions of the long-suffering medical student over the years should not go unacknowledged! Physiologists are usually pretty confident that the first-class athlete differs only quantitatively, not qualitatively, from the average, fit sports science student; however, convincing coaches of this may be a long-term project. In rare cases, with which it is an especial privilege to work, the debate reaches its ultimate level, and the question becomes: 'Is the Gold Medal performer different again from the merely first class in qualitative, and not just quantitative respects?' Once more, the physiologist suspects not, but in this case proof is logically impossible, unless the medallist him/herself volunteers to become a subject.

Sometimes, where the investigation is non-invasive, this does happen: I am told that Steve Ovett once ran on the treadmill at the British Olympic Medical Centre, and had to be asked to run up a gradient because the equipment's maximum speed couldn't stretch him on the flat. A few muscle biopsies have also been obtained, but to my knowledge only from retired medallists – perfectly valid for genomic studies, but unable to give direct information about the condition they had attained during peak training. I know of no finding which has challenged the physiologist's assumption that the physiological differences between élite and non-élite are quantitative only. For working purposes this is certainly the right view to take, for one could in principle give no guidance to an individual who was, in significant respects, different in *kind* from those who have been studied. But, as Popper himself never failed to point out, absence of disproof falls far short of proof.

Some recent work including top-rank mountaineers has indicated three groups within the population in respect of two versions of a particular gene, labelled D and I. People can have two Ds, two Is, or one of each. Almost half the climbers, including the very best high-altitude performer, had the II pattern, and almost none had DD. Then a further study, among army recruits, found that the II recruits responded 11 times better to a weight-training programme than their DD billet-mates (Montgomery *et al.* 1998). The two challenges seem tenuously related, so this looks like a gene with considerable influence on physical performance. Nevertheless, there must be many others, whether with broad or specific influence. One could conceive that the ultra-élite performer in any field is one blessed with pairs of favourable genes for each of a large raft of properties. At the genomic level, this might be considered to imply that the performer was qualitatively unique – but so is every human being, in that formal, statistical, sense. And the performance differences in which each individual gene results will remain quantitative only – a matter of degree, not kind. The athlete may be at the extremes of many Gaussian curves, but is still on the curves.

## Physiological support for athletes

'Support' is the standard British term for work that is not research, but is aimed solely at assistance to the individual athlete. Where the assistance consists only in advice, it may be based entirely on the researches discussed under the preceding heading. Then the problems are simply those already acknowledged.

Frequently, however, physiological support involves performance testing. The runner performs on a treadmill, the oarsperson on a rowing ergometer, and in either case expired air is collected and capillary blood sampled for the analysis of lactate. The gymnast undergoes flexibility tests and the injured footballer has quadriceps/hamstring strength ratios measured on a costly dynamometer. Body fat may be assessed, or blood cholesterol, or urine concentration . . .. All the results will take the form of completely 'objective' figures, which, however, will be meaningless unless interpreted. And it is, sometimes, the case that lack of time, training or interpersonal skills may impede the physiologist's success in conveying that interpretation to the person concerned. Equivalent situations are, of course, all too common in clinical consulting rooms, and the same three insufficiencies – time, training, or interpersonal skill – are always at issue.

In my experience, the time problem is at least as likely to be on the part of the athlete or coach as that of the physiologist. A thorough exploration of the test-results and their likely significance, in the light of their changes over time, is almost certainly essential if proper benefit is to be had; yet the coach and athlete are often reluctant to come back for discussion. So a terse paper report is substituted, and only if the coach is unusually informed about physiology will anything like the proper benefit be derived.

I stress the point also about changes over time. The inter-individual variations, the Gaussian distributions, acknowledged above mean that absolute figures, obtained once, allow only rather weak comparisons between the individual subject and the mean. Substantial variations also exist between different pieces of equipment designed to measure the same variable (lactate concentration is a particular problem here) and between the techniques of different experimenters. Comparisons, not with published means but with the means obtained in the laboratory concerned, will considerably assist with the latter two problems, but the change in the individual subject's figures – obtained in the same laboratory, by the same hands – are many times more instructive still. So the performer must be prepared, not only to come back for discussion after any given test day, but to come for a series of test days as training or recuperation advances. Then it *is* up to the physiologist!

In this situation, one major difference obtains from that of fundamental research. When an athlete (which here means not only the track-and-field performer but any physical sportsperson) presents him/herself for test, statutory regulations still apply but many of the rules and procedures concerning research on the human person do not; nor is the Ethics Committee's opinion to be sought. The logic is that here the person being experimented on will be the beneficiary, whereas in fundamental research this is rarely the case – instead the likely benefit is to humankind in general, and the likely timing quite probably near if not into the next generation. The same respect must be afforded to the athlete, buying one's services, as to the subject in a research programme, contributing at best to the story line in the next generation's textbooks. Care for the athlete's health will, if anything, be even greater, since the least niggle impeding performance will not be countenanced by the subject or his/her coach. But the extent of the intervention will be decided between those individually involved, not by a remote committee.

## Reprise

This chapter has stressed the centrality of philosophical concerns, both Popperian and ethical, and whether voiced or tacit, to the practice of physiology. It has travelled from pure physiology and the guiding principles of its research to sports science support. The links, however, are not tenuous. The concepts of body function, built up over the centuries of disciplined research, in which biological vision has been honed by critical challenge, underlie each encounter between athlete and physiologist. Limb as lever, heart as pump, respiration and muscle action – no mechanisms could be more central than these to all physical sports. Hearing does not matter all the time, but it is essential often enough. Hormonal controls are crucial in the metabolic adjustment to exercise. Fluid balance and thermoregulation are the paramount concerns of physiologists looking after athletes in hot climates. Ion channels may seem a little more remote at present, yet it has been known for half a century that the whole function of the nervous system is founded upon them. Furthermore, evidence is accumulating that many diseases are attributable to slightly abnormal channels for one ion or another (Ashcroft 2000). What if some of the features which distinguish the élite athlete from the merely good are also genetically determined differences of channel function? This conjecture is entirely speculative, but the manner in which it would be refuted or reinforced can already in principle be sketched. The physiologists who perform such studies will probably not be the ones who pass on any consequent advice to athletes. But let us trust that the two groups have in common the driving vision that 'we are fearfully and wonderfully made' (Psalm 139), though some will undoubtedly be better at expressing this sense than others.

So let me end with one more word about the aesthetic driving force underlying all studies of the body's mechanisms. There is a temperament for which the use of that word 'mechanism' (and even worse its adjective, 'mechanistic') implies that the stance of the investigators towards the phenomena they address is detached and emotionless, if not indeed coldly derogatory: reductionist in the worse sense. There could scarcely be a less appropriate assumption. In asking questions about the mechanisms underlying and making possible a supernova, an oceanic wave formation or a particle interaction, the physicist in no way implies that these manifestations are not also beautiful, exciting, awesome. Much more probably (s)he is studying them precisely because that is exactly how (s)he *does* perceive them. Likewise, the physiologists: indeed, for Harvey, for Hodgkin, for Bayliss, for Huxley, and for every lesser but genuine researcher in their fields, the beauty, the excitement, the awe which is the archetypal response to confrontation with the living state are underlined and amplified by the elegance and essential simplicity of the mechanisms which turn out to be involved. Thus there can be no greater misunderstanding than that underlying Keats' anguished cry:

> There was an awful rainbow once in heaven:
> We know her woof, her texture; she is given
> In the dull catalogue of common things.

It is a strange view indeed, that there is more elegance and more romance in ignorance than in comprehension.

## Bibliography

Ashcroft, F.M. (2000) *Ion Channels and Disease*, San Diego, CA: Academic Press.

Bachelard, G. (1938) *La formation de l'esprit scientifique*, Paris: Corti. Translated as *The New Scientific Spirit*, Boston: Beacon Press, 1984.

Banting, G. and Higgins, S.J. (2000) *Molecular Motors*, London: Portland Press (Essays in Biochemistry series).

Bayliss, W.M. and Starling, E.H. (1902) 'The mechanism of pancreatic secretion', *Journal of Physiology*, 28, 325–53.

Bernard, C. (1878) *Leçons sur les phénomènes de la vie communs aux animaux et aux végétaux*. Paris: J.-B. Baillière et fils.

Cannon, W.B. (1932) *The Wisdom of the Body*, New York, NY: Norton.

Chalmers, A.F. (1999) *What Is This Thing Called Science*, 3rd edn, Buckingham: Open University Press.

Connett, R.J., Gayeski, T.E.J. and Honig, C.R. (1986) 'Lactate efflux is unrelated to intracellular $PO_2$ in a working red muscle in situ', *Journal of Applied Physiology*, 61, 402–8.

Dennett, D.C. (1995) *Darwin's Dangerous Idea*, London: Allen Lane (The Penguin Press).

Diamond, J.M. (1993) 'Evolutionary physiology' in C.A.R Boyd and D. Noble (eds) *The Logic of Life. The Challenge of Integrative Physiology*, Oxford: Oxford University Press, 89–111.

Doucet, P. and Sloep, P.B. (1992) *Mathematical Modelling in the Life Sciences*, New York, NY: Ellis Horwood.

FRAME (2002) *Researching Alternatives to Animal Testing: 21 Years of the FRAME Research Programme 1982–2002*, Nottingham: Fund for the Replacement of Animals in Medical Experiments.

Hanson, N.R. (1958) *Patterns of Discovery*, Cambridge: Cambridge University Press.

Harvey, W. (1628) *Exercitatio anatomica de motu cordis et sanguinis in animalibus*, Frankfurt: Guilielmi Fitzeri.

Hille, B. (1984) *Ionic Channels of Excitable Membranes,* Sunderland, MA: Sinauer Associates.

Hodgkin, A.L. and Huxley, A.F. (1952) 'A quantitative description of membrane current and its application to conduction and excitation in nerve', *Journal of Physiology,* 117, 500–44.

Hull, D. L. (1974) *Philosophy of Biological Science,* Eaglewood Cliffs, NJ: Prentice-Hall.

Huxley, A.F. (1957) 'Muscle structure and theories of contraction', *Progress in Biophysics and Biophysical Chemistry,* 7, 255–318.

Kuhn, T. (1962). *The Structure of Scientific Revolutions,* Chicago, IL: University of Chicago Press.

Lakatos, I. (1970) 'Falsification and the methodology of scientific research programmes', in J. Lakatos and A. Musgrave (eds) *Criticism and the Growth of Knowledge,* Cambridge: Cambridge University Press, 91–196.

Lawson, H. (2001) *Closure. A Story of Everything,* London: Routledge.

Machin, K.E. (1964) 'Feedback theory and its application to biological systems', in G.M. Hughes (ed.) *Homeostasis and Feedback Mechanisms. Symposia of the Society for Experimental Biology,* XVIII, Cambridge: Cambridge University Press.

Magee, B. (1973) *Popper,* London: Collins (Fontana Books).

Mahner, M. and Bunge, M. (1997). *Foundations of Biophilosophy,* Berlin: Springer.

McMullin, E. (1984) 'A case for scientific realism', in J. Leplin (ed.) *Scientific Realism,* Berkeley, CA: University of California Press. Reprinted in Y. Balshov and A. Rosenberg (eds) *Philosophy of Science: Contemporary Readings,* London: Routledge (2002).

Medawar, P.B. (1967) *The Art of the Soluble,* London: Methuen.

Montgomery, H.E., Marshall, R., Hemingway, H. *et al.* (1998) 'Human gene for physical performance', *Nature (London),* 393, 221–2.

Noble, D. and Boyd, C.A.R. (1993) 'The challenge of integrative physiology', in C.A.R. Boyd and D. Noble (eds) *The Logic of Life. The Challenge of Integrative Physiology,* Oxford: Oxford University Press, 1–13.

Polanyi, M. (1958) *Personal Knowledge. Towards a Post-Critical Philosophy,* London: Routledge and Kegan Paul.

Popper, K.R. (1963) *Conjectures and Refutations. The Growth of Scientific Knowledge,* London: Routledge and Kegan Paul.

Rowell L.B. and Shepherd, J.T. (1996) 'Exercise: regulation and integration of multiple systems', *Handbook of Physiology. Section 12,* New York, NY: Oxford University Press.

Sherrington, C.S. (1906) *The Integrative Action of the Nervous System,* New Haven, CO: Yale University Press.

Spurway, N.C. (1992) 'Aerobic exercise, anaerobic exercise and the lactate threshold', *British Medical Bulletin,* 48, 569–91.

Toulmin, S. (1953) *The Philosophy of Science. An Introduction,* London: Hutchinson (University Library).

Volk, T. (1998) *Gaia's Body. Toward a Physiology of Earth,* New York, NY: Springer (Copernicus Books).

Von Bekesy, G. (1960) *Experiments in Hearing,* New York, NY: McGraw-Hill.

Wasserman, K., Whipp, B.J., Koyal, S.N. and Beaver, W.L. (1973) 'Anaerobic threshold and respiratory gas exchange during exercise', *Journal of Applied Physiology,* 35, 236–43.

Wiener, N. (1961) *Cybernetics, or Control and Communication in the Animal and the Machine,* 2nd edn, New York, NY: MIT Press and John Wiley and Sons.

Windhorst, U. (1996) 'Regulatory principles in physiology', in *Comprehensive Human Physiology. From Cellular Mechanisms to Integration*, Berlin: Springer.

Wittgenstein, L. (1922) *Tractatus logico-philosophicus*, London: Routledge and Kegan Paul.

## Notes

1 However, the question/technique distinction is not always simple, for although among well-established techniques one chooses – as far as costs allow – the one which best suits the question, a new technological development often triggers a rush of questions framed, whether for noble or ignoble motives, simply to use it.

2 This is an 'elementary' particle, of particularly esoteric properties, postulated a generation ago by Peter Higgs, to resolve a number of other problems in particle theory. It has not yet been seen, and indeed – if I understand correctly – is itself expected to leave no track, but the hope is that its existence will be deducible from the tracks of particles produced by its decay in the coming generation of super-accelerators.

# 4 How does a foundational myth become sacred scientific dogma?

## The case of A.V. Hill and the anaerobiosis controversy

*Tim Noakes*[1]

### Introduction

The basis of the scientific method is the development of intellectual models, the predictions of which are then subjected to scientific evaluation. Indeed the real value of these models is the predictions they make. Whether or not these models are 'true' is not crucial since it is only through the testing of their predictions that their fraudulence can be exposed. As Nobel Laureate A.V. Hill wrote in 1965:

> I have long believed, and am still inclined to believe, that all theories of muscle contraction are wrong. But they have been very useful in stimulating new research. In fact, many of the best theories are self destructive, by provoking fresh inquiry and leading to new facts which they cannot explain. The only useless theories are those that cannot be tested and can explain everything (362–3).

Thus the crux of such models is the attempt to refute or falsify their predictions. Successful refutation forces revision of each model; the revised model persists as the 'truth' until its predictions are, in turn, refuted. Thus any scientific model should persist for only as long as it resists refutation. This form of science, however, is not always popular; we are usually rather too keen to confirm that the theories of our founding scientific heroes are, naturally, correct. This latter approach seems to be particularly prevalent in the exercise sciences. But when we adopt this deferential approach we risk becoming a tribe of scientific marionettes. Most certainly we betray the efforts of our scientific founders who would much prefer that we disprove and hence perfect their imperfect theories.

My special interest in the exercise sciences has focused on an understanding of the factors that limit exercise performance especially during high-intensity exercise of short duration. The most popular current explanation is that the cardiovascular system has a limited capacity to supply oxygen to the active muscles, especially during maximal exercise. As a result, skeletal muscle oxygen demand outstrips supply, causing the development of skeletal muscle hypoxia (reduced oxygen concentration) or even anaerobiosis (absence of oxygen) during vigorous exercise. This hypoxia stimulates the onset of lactic acid (lactate) production as the exercising muscles begin to produce an increasing proportion of their energy from those 'anaerobic' metabolic pathways, capable of producing energy even in the absence of oxygen. The most effective such pathway is the incomplete breakdown of the main skeletal muscle carbohydrate store, glycogen, to lactic acid (lactate). Accordingly this model predicts that the most important factor determining exercise performance is the body's capacity to transport and utilize oxygen and that fatigue results when the maximal capacity for oxygen transport is exceeded. As a consequence, it is argued that the most important effect of any intervention that alters exercise performance, be it exercise training, nutritional interventions, drug use or disease, is to change oxygen delivery to, and oxygen utilization by the active muscles during exercise. Thus it is believed that the common consequence of all the physiological, biochemical and functional adaptations that enhance exercise performance is to reduce skeletal muscle hypoxia or anaerobiosis during exercise.

The historical basis for this model is the original research of Nobel Laureate from the Universities of Manchester and London, Archibald Vivian Hill, which has survived in the classic theory that oxygen consumption 'plateaus' during progressive exercise to exhaustion, proving the development of skeletal muscle anaerobiosis (Hill 1925; Hill and Lupton 1923; Hill *et al.* 1924a, 1924b). But I contend that Hill's quite simple research methods failed to establish the existence of the 'plateau phenomenon' during exercise so that I argue that this core component of his historical model remains unproven (Noakes 1988, 1991, 1997, 1998, 2002; Noakes *et al.* 2001). Furthermore, definitive evidence that skeletal muscle anaerobiosis ever develops during exercise in humans and that this anaerobiosis initiates lactate production and its accumulation in blood, is not currently available (Mole *et al.* 1999; Richardson *et al.* 1998; Graham and Saltin 1989). As is appropriate, my contentions have been vigorously refuted (Bassett and Howley 1997, 2000; Bergh *et al.* 2000; Ekblom 2000; Wagner 2000).

In this process I realized that this historical physiological model has become what Waller terms a 'Foundation Myth' (Waller 2002) and, as a consequence, has escaped modern disinterested, intellectual scrutiny. The reasons for this serve as a warning of the fallibility of scientists and the current scientific methods under which we labour.

The writer Salman Rushdie, who spent many years in seclusion when his life was threatened because of his heretical views, has said: 'The journey creates us. We become the frontiers we cross'. My personal intellectual journey did not begin as a scientist but as a medical doctor training in a small city, far distant from the historical axis of academic excellence in Europe and North America, in a country that at that time was ruled by a repressive dictatorship that discouraged free thought. I was fortunate for the exposure to those frontiers. It is here that I begin the story.

## Lessons from a medical training

The first great lesson of medicine is to teach one's supreme level of personal stupidity. Indeed there is a collective level of medical ignorance, so brilliantly described by Dr Lewis Thomas (1985: 10):

> The greatest single achievement of science in this most scientifically productive of centuries is the discovery that we are profoundly ignorant. . .. I wish there were some formal courses in medical school on medical ignorance; textbooks as well, although they would have to be very heavy volumes. We have a long way to go.

Indeed, the beauty of the Textbooks of Ignorance would be their accuracy. I am reminded of these quotations whenever a scientist expounds the ignorance of absolute certainty. Regardless of any appearance of individual brilliance, we are each profoundly ignorant. And never more so than when we are absolutely certain of our most brilliant opinions.

This distinctive characteristic of modern medicine to challenge the truth (Le Fanu 1999), explains the intellectual paradox captured in the classic quotation attributed to a former Dean of Harvard, Dr Sydney Burwell by G.W. Pickering (1956: 14), himself formerly Professor of Medicine at the University of London and a protagonist in one of the classic medical arguments of the twentieth century (Swales 1985): 'My students are dismayed when I say to them, "Half of what you are taught as medical students will in 10 years have been shown to be wrong. And the trouble is, none of your teachers know which half"'.

The second great advantage of my medical education was that it included nothing about the exercise sciences, other than that which I taught myself. Learning in this way has important disadvantages, but one unique advantage is the avoidance of indoctrination, which is the tendency towards a stubborn, if subconscious, acceptance of a specific scientific mindset or prejudice that we acquire from our venerated tutors whom we assume to be intellectually infallible (Waller 2002). This could perhaps be termed the Tyranny of the Founder Effect. It is an effect for which the exercise sciences are especially susceptible since the profession is still very young and a relatively small band of famous founders including A.V. Hill in Britain, David Dill in the United States of America, Cyril Wyndham in South Africa, Wolder Hollman in Germany, Erling Asmussen, Erik Hohwu Christensen, Marius Nielsen and August Krogh in Copenhagen, P.O. Astrand and Bengt Saltin in Stockholm, and R. Margaria in Italy, have bequeathed an inordinately influential legacy. Indeed the second generation of scientists trained by those giants are only now approaching retirement age. Thus it is likely that the global teaching in the exercise sciences still reflects the powerful influence of those remarkable founding scientists.

My point is that a crucial outcome of our scientific training conditions us to accept only a limited sample of all the possible truths. Further we are more likely to accept those 'truths' that we learned from the giants who educated us and, in particular, their 'foundation myths' (Waller 2002). So ignorance of the historic precursors to that which is the presently considered 'truth' or received wisdom, can be a formidable attribute. For it allows the freedom to consider any intellectual possibility.

## Lessons from a scientific training

### *The concept of refutability and the burden of disproof*

Self-taught in science, I also learned some fundamental truths that are not always included in a more conventional scientific training. In his influential text, Viennese philosopher Karl Popper (1969) explains the pivotal importance of research that aims to disprove the currently considered 'truth'. He begins by posing the fundamental question: What identifies empirical science and therefore distinguishes it from pseudoscience? He concludes that: a statement (a theory, a conjecture) has the status of belonging to the empirical sciences if, and only if, it is falsifiable (Popper 1969). According to this criterion, a statement or theory is falsifiable, that is, able to be refuted, if and only if there exists at least one potential falsifier – at least one basic statement that conflicts with it logically. He continues that the falsifier does not itself have to be known to be true, only that it logically refutes the conjecture.

In Popper's view, an important aim of science is therefore to generate theories that are able to be refuted (falsified). Successful refutation (falsification) of successive conjectures leads to new and, occasionally, revolutionary theories, each of which is likely to be somewhat closer to the truth than all its predecessors. Victor Katch (1986) was one of the first to bring this to the attention of modern exercise scientists.

Popper also concludes that we will never know whether a specific conjecture is the final truth, for the reason that our scientific methods and our logic are too imprecise, ever to be certain that we have subjected a particular theory to every possible test of falsification. We must always presume that there is still one technique or technology, yet to be conceived, the application of which may yet allow the next experiment to disprove a long-favoured hypothesis. Thus, a theory that has yet to be refuted is the nearest we ever approach the truth. In this analysis, even Einstein's theory of relativity is simply a conjecture which has, for the most part, escaped refutation (Will 1986). Einstein understood this for he wrote: 'No amount of experimentation can ever prove me right; a single experiment may at any time prove me wrong'; and 'No fairer destiny could be allowed to any physical theory than that it should itself point out the way to introducing a more comprehensive theory in which it lives on as a limiting case' (Einstein, cited in Popper 1988:131).

Some would argue that too few scientists approach these lofty goals too infrequently. For the surprising nature of much scientific endeavour is a profound resistance to those new ideas which threaten to refute the favoured dogmas of the intellectual giants, our gods, at whose feet we have studied and on whose shoulders we are fortunate to stand (Waller 2002).

## The development of intellectual mindsets (paradigms)

A characteristic of the scientific mind is the development of intellectual mindsets or frameworks within which we interpret all new information (Hawking 1993). Popper (1988, 17) described this subconscious process accordingly:

> Thinking people tend to develop some framework into which they try to fit whatever new idea they may come across; as a rule, they even translate any new idea which they meet into a language appropriate to their own framework. One of the most characteristic tasks of philosophy is to attack, if necessary, the framework itself.

The value of these intellectual frameworks is that, when accepted by the entire community, they facilitate communication. The basis for this common understanding does not need endlessly to be reviewed or restated as all the experts in that specialist field accept that the prediction of that particular model have yet to be refuted so that, at that particular moment, it represents the yet-to-be-disproved 'truth'.

Thus frameworks or paradigms represent those scientific frontiers in which an intellectual truce has been declared; the intellectual battles have been fought, the arguments have been exhausted and a common consensus has been achieved, at least for the time being. There is a common acceptance that no further advantage can be gained by arguing the intellectual basis of the paradigm. Rather the accepted framework makes predictions which scientists are then eager to evaluate. Kuhn (1970) refers to this as 'normal' science.

As is elegantly described in the analogy of Friedman (1994), the danger of such frameworks is that, like clothes, these ideas can become too comfortable and are not easily discarded:

> Accepting a new paradigm is like acquiring a new wardrobe. Initially, the garments fit well, look stylish, and are suitable for almost all occasions. However, with the passage of time, the clothes become too loose or too tight, frayed and tattered, and the wearer begins to feel unsuitably dressed for certain events. At this point, he or she can either alter the outfits or purchase a new wardrobe. But the older clothes are not so easily cast aside. They are more comfortable in some ways, they served long and well, they are like old friends; a certain attachment has set in. Indeed the wearer may decide to keep the old wardrobe and restrict his or her activities accordingly, passing up occasions at which the clothes seem out of place. The activities that are dropped become defined as unimportant and eventually no longer belong to the wearer's 'real' world. Choosing a new wardrobe, on the other hand, is comparable to what Kuhn terms a paradigm revolution: the basic framework that defines activity is altered, and 'normal' science is replaced with a new range of possibilities. We may call this a new 'reality' (282–3).

### The dependence of reality on the specific model we choose to believe

The eminent mathematician Stephen Hawking has written a remarkably successful popular book on astrophysics (1989). His book describes models from which we can attempt to understand how the universe is (currently) believed to work. These models make predictions that can be tested, but there is no guarantee that they exist beyond the minds of their creators. As Hawking explains:

> We cannot distinguish what is real about the universe without a theory ... [But] ... it makes no sense to ask if a theory corresponds to reality, because we do not know what reality is independent of a theory. ... How can we know what is real, independent of a theory or model with which to interpret it? (1993: 38, 40.)

This is a perennial problem in philosophy; biological scientists can at least fashion experiments to disprove their models. Exercise scientists spend their academic lives developing models of how the body works. We need to remember that there is no guarantee that these models (Noakes 2000) are either real or the absolute truth. According to these ideas, we might propose that 'truth' implies only the absence of a significant refutation and that truth reveals itself through the refutation of the less true. As a consequence, scientific truth is subject to change, which often occurs with rude suddenness. Finally, all 'truth' is model-dependent; that is, the 'truth' predicted by one model may be the opposite of a 'truth' foretold by a different model.

### Novel ideas are not easily accepted by the scientific community

Hawking has described a phenomenon wherein scientists hold on to their scientific commitments even in the face of growing critique:

> The theory always came first, put forward from the desire to have an elegant and consistent mathematical model. The theory then makes predictions, which can be tested by observation. If the observations agree with the predictions, that doesn't prove the theory; but the theory survives to make further predictions, which again are tested against observation. If the observations don't agree with the predictions, one abandons the theory. Or rather, that is what is supposed to happen. In practice, people are very reluctant to give up a theory in which they have invested a lot of time and effort. They usually start by questioning the accuracy of the observations. If that fails, they try to modify the theory in an ad hoc manner. Eventually the theory becomes a creaking and ugly edifice. Then someone suggests a new theory in which all the awkward observations are explained in an elegant and natural manner (1993: 36).

Hawking also identifies a popular method which is employed to delay the acceptance of a new conjecture. In this technique labelled 'refutation by denigration', the scientific credibility of the person who questions the accepted model is brought into doubt and his or her professional standing is subtly undermined. It is the classic technique of shooting the messenger so that the message may be conveniently ignored. This method is unfortunately still very popular in many branches of science.

It would seem that even the intellectually brilliant are not immune from a reluctance to accept novel intellectual models. Both Newton and Einstein, two of the most revolutionary scientists, could not accept predictions of their own theories that were in conflict with a religious dogma. Newton refused to accept the impossibility of defining the absolute position of a large object in space as this conflicted with his belief in an absolute God. Similarly, Einstein would not believe that the position of the very small was also indeterminate (the Heissenberg Uncertainty Principle) because it also conflicted with his religious belief. 'God', Einstein wrote, 'does not play dice' (Hawking 1993: 91). His prediction of the existence of astronomical black holes led Hawking to suggest that: 'God not only plays dice but also sometimes throws them where they cannot be seen' (1993: 103).

Finally, there is the danger of the perpetuation of a 'foundation myth'. The greatest danger is the attempt to immunize a particular hypothesis from all attempts at refutation once it becomes the established mindset supported by all the influential scientists. As Miller (1983: 10) has exhorted: 'It is the perpetuation of errors that interferes with our understanding; and it is this, rather than their perpetration, that we must exert ourselves determinedly to avert'. Influential scientists can harm their discipline if they lose the desire to challenge the dogmas they have created.

During much of my scientific career I have considered two intellectual constructs in the exercise sciences that, in my opinion, have to a lesser or greater extent, become 'ugly and creaking edifices' (Noakes 1997). Here I review the history of the evolution of the construct that fatigue during high intensity exercise is caused by the development of anaerobiosis in the exercising skeletal muscles. I then present some of the evidence that conflicts with that interpretation and which, according to Popperian theory, should result in the replacement of that ugly edifice with a novel model that is better able to explain all the currently published information.

## The A.V. Hill cardiovascular/anaerobic/catastrophic model of exercise physiology

The work of Nobel Laureates Frederick Grover Hopkins (Fletcher and Hopkins 1907) and Archibald Vivian Hill and their colleagues (Hill 1925, 1965; Hill and Lupton 1923; Hill *et al.* 1924a, 1924b) forms the basis for the popular conjecture that an oxygen limitation develops during maximal exercise causing skeletal muscle hypoxia/anaerobiosis to terminate exercise. This model enjoys an almost complete acceptance in virtually all modern textbooks of exercise physiology and has survived, essentially without serious intellectual challenge, for almost 80 years (Bassett and Howley 1997, 2000; Bergh *et al.* 2000, Ekblom 2000; Wagner 2000; Bassett 2002).

This model holds that exercise performance is determined by the capacity of the athlete's large heart to pump unusually large volumes of blood and oxygen to the muscles. This allows the muscles to achieve higher work rates before they outstrip the available oxygen supply, developing skeletal muscle anaerobiosis (Figure 4.1). This model remains the most popular for explaining why fatigue develops during exercise; how the body adapts to training; how these adaptations enhance performance and health and, as a consequence, how effective exercise training programmes should be structured.

This model further predicts that training increases 'cardiovascular fitness' especially by increasing the body's maximum capacity to consume oxygen, measured as the maximum oxygen consumption ($VO_2$ max). This effect results from an increased maximum capacity of the heart to pump blood (the cardiac output) and an enhanced capacity of the muscles to consume that oxygen, the latter by increasing the number of blood vessels (capillaries) in the skeletal muscles and the number and size of those subcellular structures, the mitochondriae, which produce the energy for the exercising muscles. It is argued that these adaptations delay the onset of skeletal muscle anaerobiosis during vigorous

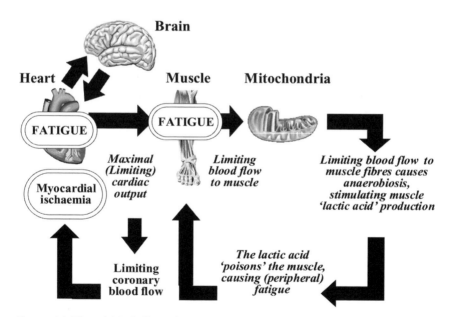

*Figure 4.1* The A.V. Hill cardiovascular/anaerobic/catastrophic model of exercise physiology. In this model, the development of myocardial ischaemia (reduced blood flow to the heart) leads to skeletal muscle anaerobiosis, lactic acidosis and muscle fatigue (poisoning).

exercise, thereby reducing blood lactate concentrations in muscle and blood at all exercise intensities above the so-called 'anaerobic threshold' – the threshold which apparently indicates the onset of skeletal muscle anaerobiosis and the sudden onset of high rates of lactic acid (lactate) production by the increasingly anaerobic muscles. The delayed onset of this blood lactate accumulation after training then allows the exercising muscles to continue contracting for longer at higher intensities before the onset of fatigue. An important but unrecognized prediction of this model is that increases in (coronary) blood flow to the heart must be an essential adaptation to training (Noakes 2000). The higher coronary blood flow allows a greater pumping capacity of the heart, producing a greater cardiac output to perfuse the exercising muscles, which can then achieve a higher exercise capacity.

This model finds strong support from the confirmation that these changes do indeed result from training, as fully documented in the literature. The key question is whether these changes are causally linked; that is, do these changes cause the change in exercise performance or do they occur *pari passu* with one or more other adaptations that are the real cause of changes in exercise performance. For there are important deficiencies in this model which have been fully argued (Noakes 1988, 1991 1997, 1998, 2000, 2002; Noakes *et al.* 2001; Noakes and St Clair Gibson 2004) and counter-argued (Bassett and Howley 1997, 2000; Bergh *et al.* 2000, Ekblom 2000; Wagner 2000) elsewhere and which do not need to be repeated here. But the fundamental contention of this model is the foundation belief that oxygen delivery determines the exercise performance; that is that oxygen delivery (A) *causes* the exercise performance (B) (Figure 4.2).

My special interest in this topic began when I read David Costill's classic textbook *A Scientific Approach to Distance Running* in which he wrote: 'Since the early work of Hill and Lupton (1923), exercise physiologists have associated the limits of human endurance with the ability to consume larger volumes of oxygen during exhaustive exercise' (1979: 25–6).

This quote clearly identified what the recently retired Costill, representing as he does the link to the previous generation of influential exercise physiologists in the United States, considered to be the key foundation on which this universally accepted theory rests. It was when reading those studies that I detected a critical flaw and an unexpected hypothesis, both of which had been ignored (or perhaps dismissed) for more than 50 years.

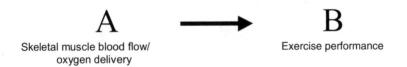

$$A \longrightarrow B$$

Skeletal muscle blood flow/          Exercise performance
oxygen delivery

*Figure 4.2* Cardiovascular/anaerobic/catastrophic model of factors determining maximal exercise performance.

The foundation of the classical Hill cardiovascular/anaerobic/catastrophic model (Noakes 2000; Noakes and St Clair Gibson 2004) can be traced to the pivotal influence that the original study of Fletcher and Hopkins (1907) at Cambridge University exerted on the thinking of Hill and his colleagues in Manchester. Fletcher and Hopkins wished to establish whether or not 'within a muscle itself, means exist for an oxidative control of its own acid formation, or for the alteration or destruction of acid which has been formed, either there or by muscular activity elsewhere in the body' (1907: 16). They were perplexed by the consistent finding at that time, that lactic acid (lactate) concentrations in excised skeletal muscle preparations were always high, regardless of the experimental conditions, for example whether the excised muscle came from rested, exercised, fresh or preserved tissue. They wondered whether this unexpected finding resulted not from 'the technical difficulties of lactic acid estimation, but that it is due to the difficulties inherent in the extractive treatment of an irritable muscle' (Needham and Baldwin 1949: 59).

By rapidly immersing the excised muscle in ice-cold alcohol, they were able to show that the freshly excised hind limb muscles of frogs had low initial lactic acid concentrations and released little lactic acid during the first 24 hours when incubated in air at room temperature. Even less lactate was produced when the muscles were stored in oxygen-enriched air also at room temperature. Lactic acid production was substantially increased when the muscles were stored in hydrogen; this effect was increased at higher temperatures. Next, they electrically stimulated the muscles in the excised hind limbs to contract until they no longer responded to stimulation. After prolonged stimulation, muscle lactic acid concentrations were elevated but were only about one-half the concentrations measured in muscles exposed acutely to chemical- or heat-induced damage. Finally, previously stimulated muscles were left to recover for 18 or more hours either in room air, or in nitrogen or oxygen at different temperatures. In all cases, lactic acid concentrations were lowest in muscles exposed to oxygen at any temperature. Accordingly Fletcher and Hopkins (1907) concluded that:

> The lactic acid content of muscle is profoundly affected by the nature of the treatment received before or during the extraction. . ... The increase of acid is most rapid under anaerobic conditions, is slower in air, and it is not to be observed in an atmosphere of pure oxygen (297–8).

Thus

> the excised but undamaged muscle when exposed to a sufficient tension of oxygen has in itself the power of dealing in some way with the lactic acid which has accumulated during fatigue and regaining irritability in an atmosphere of pure oxygen, their content of lactic acid is greatly reduced (ibid: 297).

They concluded that 'Lactic acid is spontaneously developed, under anaerobic conditions in excised muscle' and that 'fatigue due to contractions is accompanied by an increase of lactic acid' (ibid: 301).

Fletcher and Hopkins (1907) did not conclude either that anaerobiosis was the sole reason for increased lactic acid production by amphibian muscle or that the 'increase of lactic acid' caused fatigue. They merely described these separate phenomena whilst developing a novel technique (immediate immersion in ice-cold alcohol), to measure accurately muscle lactic acid concentrations. Historically, however, these studies have been interpreted somewhat differently. They have been seen to establish the classical interpretation that lactic acid production by skeletal muscle during exercise requires the absence of skeletal muscle aerobiosis (hence *a*naerobiosis) and that the increased production of lactic acid causes a peripherally located skeletal muscle fatigue, according to the mechanism shown in Figure 4.1.

As a result, when Hill and his colleagues measured increased blood lactate concentrations during exercise in humans (Hill *et al.* 1924b), they were bound to conclude that the muscles were contracting anaerobically since: 'Lactic acid does not accumulate so long as the oxygen supply remains adequate' (Hill *et al.* 1924a: 136). Thus arose the first pillar of the concept that oxygen deficiency limits maximum exercise performance (Noakes 1988, 1991, 1997, 1998, 2000, 2002; Noakes *et al.* 2001; Noakes and St Clair Gibson 2004) specifically as a result of skeletal muscle anaerobiosis and a resulting lactic acidosis.

The second pillar arose from a series of experiments in which Hill and his colleagues measured oxygen consumption ($VO_2$) every 30 seconds in subjects who ran for 3 minutes at different speeds on a circular grass track 85 m in circumference. Their relevant findings are reproduced in the main graph of Figure 4.3. The authors' interpretation of their data was the following (Hill and Lupton 1923):

> When muscular exercise is taken in man at a constant speed, the lactic content of his active muscles increases gradually from its resting minimum at the start. This rise in lactic acid content increases the rate of oxidation, so that finally, if the oxygen supply be adequate, a 'steady state' is reached in which the rate of lactic acid production is balanced by the rate of its oxidative removal, and its concentration remains constant in the muscle as long as exercise at that speed is maintained.... The lower three curves represent a genuine steady state, the uppermost curve only an apparent steady state in which the oxygen intake is at its maximum and the oxygen debt is rapidly increasing (148–9).

Hill and Lupton (1923) concluded that the constant $VO_2$ they measured at the fastest running speed (16 km.h$^{-1}$ in Figure 4.3) represented an apparent, not a true steady state. The basis for this conclusion was a circular argument based on Hill's subconsciously held model explaining fatigue during exercise (Figure 4.4). For Hill began with the subliminal premise that fatigue during exercise is caused

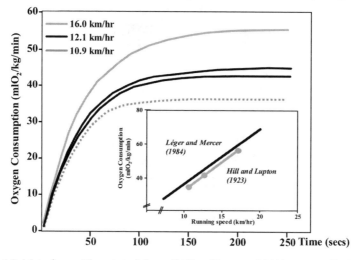

*Figure 4.3* Main figure: The original data of Hill and Lupton (1923) purportedly showing a 'plateau' in oxygen consumption during 'maximal exercise'. Insert: The data of Hill and Lupton (1923) fail to show any 'plateau' in oxygen consumption with increasing running speed.

by an oxygen deficiency; for reasons described in the introduction, he naturally interpreted his findings within that conceptual framework.

From the subjective feelings of the fatigue that he experienced when he ran at $16 \, \text{km.h}^{-1}$, Hill drew the equally subjective conclusion that this must have been caused by an oxygen deficiency, hence anaerobiosis, in his active muscles. As a result he concluded that his real $VO_2$ must have been higher than that which was objectively measured at $16 \, \text{km.h}^{-1}$ (top line in the main graph of Figure 4.3). On this basis, Hill and Lupton (1923) produced their classic speculation that defines their cardiovascular/anaerobic/catastrophic model: 'Considering the case of running... there is clearly some critical speed for each individual ... above which, the maximum oxygen intake is inadequate, lactic acid accumulating, a continuously increasing oxygen debt being incurred, fatigue and exhaustion setting in' (Hill and Lupton 1923: 151) and that 'However much the speed be increased beyond this limit, no further increase in oxygen intake can occur: the heart, lungs, circulation, and the diffusion of oxygen to the active muscle-fibres have attained their maximum capacity' (Hill and Lupton 1923: 156). Hill (1925: 93) further concluded that: 'The oxygen intake may attain its maximum and remain constant merely because it cannot go any higher owing to the limitations of the circulatory and respiratory systems'.

Not only did Hill and his colleagues fail to measure concurrently either the oxygen debt or muscle or blood lactate levels or cardio-respiratory function during these or subsequent studies, they also failed to subject their hypothesis to the accepted process of refutation. For the next logical study would have been to measure Hill's rate of oxygen consumption ($VO_2$) when he ran at a speed faster

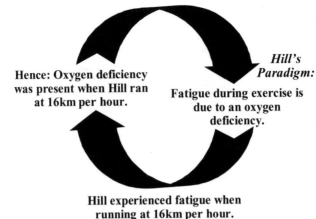

*Figure* 4.4 The circular logic that led Hill to believe he had developed an oxygen deficiency when running at 16 km per hour in Figure 4.3.

than $16 \text{ km.h}^{-1}$. Their hypothesis would have been supported if the $VO_2$ at that higher speed was either the same or lower than that measured at $16 \text{ km.h}^{-1}$. Given that that experiment was not performed, Hill and his colleagues could not conclude that Hill's $VO_2$ had 'plateaued' and was indeed maximal at $16 \text{ km.h}^{-1}$. Thus, their major conclusion that $VO_2$ reaches a plateau during exercise of progressively increasing intensity was not proven because this test of refutation was not conducted. I have since submitted their conclusions to such refutation, though some sixty-odd years later (Noakes 1988, 1997).

The data shown in the inset panel of Figure 4.3 confirm that Hill did not reach 'some critical speed ... above which, the maximum oxygen intake is inadequate.' For the data clearly show a linear relationship between Hill's mean $VO_2$ at three different speeds. This proves that his oxygen consumption rose appropriately without any evidence for a 'plateau' as Hill increased his speed from 10 to $16 \text{ km.h}^{-1}$. Hence those data do not provide any evidence for a 'plateau phenomenon' which Hill believed was the necessary proof that his exercise terminated as a direct consequence of skeletal muscle anaerobiosis. Nevertheless this is the interpretation that has survived in the popular model depicted in Figures 4.1 and 4.2.

The next significant event in this controversy was the publication in 1955 of a paper by Taylor *et al.* in which they attempted to define the criteria for the establishment of this oxygen 'plateau phenomenon'. They began the article thus:

> The classic work of Hill [Hill and Lupton 1923] has demonstrated that there is an upper limit to the capacity of the combined respiratory and cardiovascular systems to transport oxygen to the muscles. There is a linear relationship between oxygen intake and workload until the maximum oxygen intake is reached. Further increases in workload beyond this point

merely result in an increase in oxygen debt and a shortening of the time in which the work can be performed (78).

Yet it is clear from the inset panel in Figure 4.3 that Hill had failed to show any such 'increase in oxygen debt'.

Further support for this interpretation came in 1971 when a paper describing the meaning of the maximum oxygen consumption was published in the *New England Journal of Medicine* (Mitchell and Blomqvist 1971), arguably the most influential medical journal in the world. Next, was the development of one of the most popular teaching diagrams in the exercise sciences, shown in Figure 4.5 (Rowell 1993).

Under the heading 'What limits the ability to increase the oxygen uptake', this diagram suggests that such a limitation may occur in the respiration, the central or peripheral circulation, or in the muscle metabolism. Notably missing in the picture is the presence of the central (brain) and peripheral nervous systems.

Thus a central tenet of this model is the *belief* that the brain plays no role in exercise performance. Of course at the time he undertook his studies, Hill would not have had access to equipment to measure the brain's contribution to exercise performance; thus he would be expected to ignore that which he could not

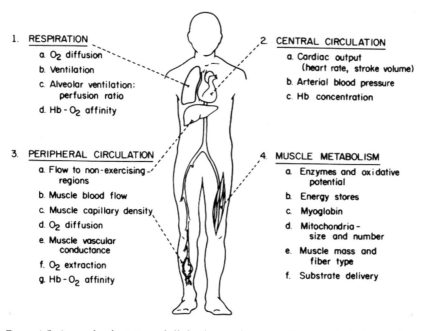

*Figure 4.5* A popular depiction of all the factors that are believed to limit the maximum oxygen consumption (VO$_2$max). Missing are the central (brain) and peripheral nervous systems.

measure. Yet it is a measure of the strength of a 'foundation myth' (Waller 2002) that even though scientists now have the capacity to measure the brain's potential contribution to exercise performance, yet so few do (Gandevia 2001; Kayser 2003; Nybo and Secher 2004).

Once I realized that Hill had failed to prove his hypothesis, I began to wonder how a system could fail even when there was no evidence that that failure was caused by 'anaerobiosis' (Graham and Saltin 1989; Mole *et al*. 1999; Richardson *et al*. 1998, 1999). Since my doctoral training was in cardiac physiology and metabolism (Resink *et al*. 1981a, 1981b; Van Der Werff *et al*. 1985) I was aware of the core teaching that the heart and skeletal muscles use quite different techniques to increase their total power output.

Although both heart and skeletal muscles are a collection of many individual muscle fibres (cells), the heart acts as if it comprises just one. Thus a single nerve impulse is all that is required to produce a simultaneous contraction of all the heart muscle fibres. Thus complete recruitment of all heart muscle fibres occurs each time the heart contracts; none remain quiescent and unrecruited. Thus for the heart to increase its power output, the strength of each of the molecular interactions (actin–myosin cross-bridges) that produce muscle contraction must increase. An increase in the power output of the individual actin–myosin cross-bridges is known as an increase in *contractility*.

In contrast, the *total* number of fibres in a particular skeletal muscle are innervated by many different nerve fibres, each of which therefore innervates only a portion of all the fibres making up a particular skeletal muscle. Thus the maximum power output of a particular skeletal muscle can only be achieved if there is a simultaneous contraction of all its multitude of muscle fibres. This requires that all the nerves innervating that muscle must be actively recruited by the (motor cortex in the) brain at the same time. This method for increasing skeletal muscle power output is known as an increase in skeletal muscle *recruitment*. Thus, unlike the case in the heart, the brain is the principal site regulating any increase in power output by the skeletal muscles; skeletal muscle power output rises as more fibres are recruited by the brain and falls when fewer fibres are recruited. This alternative model of exercise performance is depicted in Figure 4.6. Here the arrow of causality is reversed; the brain, not the heart, is the driver of performance. Thus to increase the power output of the skeletal muscles, the brain recruits more muscle fibres which then require an increased blood supply to cover their increased oxygen and energy requirements. In this way, the exercise performance causes the oxygen consumption, and not the reverse.

Hill's understanding of these concepts were of course limited by the knowledge of the day; thus he assumed that all available muscle fibres are recruited at exhaustion. Indeed he must have realized, even if only subconsciously, that the 'poisonous' lactic acid, that he considered to be the peripheral regulator of performance (Figure 4.1), could not regulate the function of those quiescent muscle fibres that have yet to be recruited. He supposed quite reasonably that, to avoid exhaustion, the brain would simply recruit more of those quiescent muscle fibres, thereby allowing the exercise to continue until all the

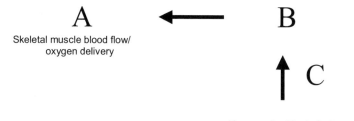

A &larr; B

↑ C

Skeletal muscle blood flow/
oxygen delivery

Unrecognized brain factor
(Skeletal muscle fibre recruitment by the CNS)

*Figure* 4.6 Alternative (neuromuscular recruitment) model of factors determining maximal exercise performance.

available muscle fibres had been recruited. Rather more culpably, all the exercise scientists who have subsequently embraced his cardiovascular/anaerobic/catastrophic model must also have made this assumption. This explains why the central and peripheral nervous systems are not included in Figure 4.5. The assumption has to be that there is complete skeletal muscle recruitment at exhaustion in all forms of exercise. Hence, according to this logic, any contribution of the central nervous systems to exercise performance can be ignored.

Yet this clearly conflicts with the most basic physiological truth, which is that the power output of skeletal muscle is determined by the number of muscle fibres that are recruited by the brain (Gordon *et al.* 2001; Katz 1992). The contrasting assumption of the alternative (muscle recruitment) model (Figure 4.6) is that, if the force output of skeletal muscle is less than maximal, then there must be a less-than-maximal skeletal muscle fibre recruitment. If this is the case then the exercise performance is clearly regulated by the brain through its control of the number of muscle fibres that are recruited in the exercising muscles.

Since, in the late 1980s, I too seem to have assumed that the recruitment of skeletal muscle fibres are always maximal at exhaustion in all forms of exercise, it was also natural that my first attempt to explain how a muscle could fatigue during maximal exercise included this subconscious assumption that all the available muscle fibres are simultaneously active at exhaustion. That is, my assumption was that, at exhaustion, the skeletal muscle acts as if it is a heart in which all available muscle fibres are simultaneously active. In which case, skeletal muscle failure, expressed as fatigue or exhaustion, can only occur if there is widespread failure of the *contractility* of the individual muscle fibres.

Thus I originally proposed that fatigue develops during maximum exercise because of a centrally (brain) initiated down-regulation of the contractility of all the muscle fibres in the maximally recruited muscles:

> [A] critical review of Hill and Lupton's results shows that they inferred but certainly did not prove that an oxygen limitation develops during maximal exercise . . . .. This review proposes that the factors limiting maximal exercise performance might be better explained in terms of a failure of muscle

contractility ('muscle power'), which may be independent of tissue oxygen deficiency. The implications for exercise testing and the prediction of athletic performance are discussed (Noakes 1988: 419).

What, in retrospect, is quite surprising is that I did not consider that the far more likely factor determining large changes in skeletal muscle power production is an alteration in the number of skeletal muscle fibres that are recruited by the central nervous system, as is the classical teaching (Gordon *et al.* 2001, Katz 1992). For even a simple calculation could have shown how much more probable is this alternative explanation. For example, the maximum power that an athletic human can produce for a few seconds with his legs is about 2000 W (Calbet *et al.* 2003c). But during a maximum exercise test lasting more than a few minutes, there are few humans who can achieve a power output of more than about 500 W. Similarly during an hour's exercise, few can exceed an average power output of about 400 W. This means that *if* all the available muscle fibres are recruited at all times, then the force output (contractility) of the multitude of individual molecular interactions that produce the total muscle power output would need to vary by a factor of 2000/400, that is five-fold. I am unaware of any known biological mechanism that could produce a five-fold increase in the contractility of individual skeletal muscle cross-bridges. Whilst mechanisms that can increase the contractility of heart (myocardial) cross-bridges are well understood (Gordon *et al.* 2001; Katz 1992; Resink *et al.* 1981a, 1981b), (i) these are unlikely to produce a five-fold increase in contractility and, more importantly (ii) such mechanisms are not known to exist in skeletal muscle (Gordon *et al.* 2001; Katz 1992). It is much more likely that the extent of muscle recruitment by the brain differs five-fold so that, for example, five times more muscle fibres are active during a few seconds of absolutely maximal exercise than are active during a maximal effort that lasts an hour or more. But this apparently obvious conclusion evaded my thinking at that time as, apparently, it has evaded the grasp of many of the world's leading exercise physiologists to this day (Bassett and Howley 1997, 2000; Bergh *et al.* 2000; Ekblom 2000; Noakes 2004; Wagner 2000).

Seven years later, I concluded the J.B. Wolffe Memorial Lecture at the 1996 Annual Conference of the American College of Sports Medicine with the proposal that whatever mechanisms limit exercise performance, there appeared to be a reason for such regulation:

[A]n alternate physiological model is proposed in which skeletal muscle contractile activity is regulated by a series of central, predominantly neural, and peripheral, predominantly chemical, regulators that act to prevent the development of organ damage or even death during exercise in both health and disease and under demanding environmental conditions. ... Regulation of skeletal muscle contractile function by central mechanisms would prevent the development of hypotension and myocardial ischemia during exercise in persons with heart failure, of hyperthermia during exercise in the heat, and of cerebral hypoxia during exercise at extreme altitude (Noakes 1997: 571).

Clearly I had still not grasped the eminently more logical proposal that the easiest way for the brain to regulate skeletal muscle power production is through the regulation of the number of muscle fibres that it recruits during exercise (Gordon *et al.* 2001, Katz 1992). This imprecise thinking was again conditioned by my continuing subconscious assumption that muscle recruitment must be maximal at exhaustion in all forms of exercise (Figure 4.5).

Predictably, since the publication of the J.B. Wolffe lecture represented a radical departure from the accepted 'foundation myth', which had not been seriously challenged for more than 70 years, it was accompanied by a detailed rebuttal (Bassett and Howley 1997). That rebuttal made the somewhat crude point that A.V. Hill was a Nobel Prize winner whose opinion was far more likely to be correct than was that of an iconoclastic Third World scientist. In preparing my response (Noakes 1998) I was forced to reread all of A.V. Hill's original papers. It was there that I uncovered his remarkable insight that had been overlooked, perhaps since he first described it in the 1920s.

For what Hill realized, and which has been ignored ever since, was that if the pumping capacity of the heart does indeed limit oxygen utilization by the exercising skeletal muscle as predicted in Figure 4.1, then the heart itself will be the first organ affected by any postulated oxygen deficiency (Hill *et al.* 1924b). This is because the blood supply to the heart is dependent on the pumping capacity of the heart; once the maximum output of the heart is reached, the heart will be unable further to increase its own oxygen supply and must therefore begin to work 'anaerobically' (Figure 4.1). The interpretation of Hill and his colleagues was unequivocal:

> Certain it is that the capacity of the body for muscular exercise depends largely, if not mainly, on the capacity and output of the heart. It would obviously be very dangerous for the organ to be able, as the skeletal muscle is able, to exhaust itself very completely and rapidly, to take exercise far in excess of its capacity for recovery . . .. When the oxygen supply becomes inadequate, it is probable that the heart rapidly begins to diminish its output, so avoiding exhaustion ... (1924b: 161–2).

The point identified by Hill and his colleagues (and since ignored) is that the heart is also a muscle, dependent for its function on an adequate blood and oxygen supply. But, unlike skeletal muscle, the heart is dependent for its blood supply on its own pumping capacity. Hence any intervention that reduces the pumping capacity of the heart, or demands the heart to exceed its own maximum pumping capacity, imperils the heart's own blood supply. Any reduction in coronary blood flow will consequently reduce the heart's pumping capacity, thereby inducing a vicious cycle of progressive and irreversible myocardial ischaemia (inadequate blood supply to the heart). It would seem reasonable that human 'design' should include controls to protect the heart from ever entering this vicious circle.

Hence if (skeletal) muscle function fails when its oxygen demand exceeds supply (Figure 4.1) then, for logical consistency, the inability of the pumping capacity of the heart to 'raise the cardiac output' at the $VO_2$ max (Rowell 1993), must also result from an inadequate (myocardial) oxygen supply caused by a plateau in blood flow to the heart. This limiting coronary blood flow would cause myocardial 'fatigue', a plateau in cardiac output and hence in the $VO_2$ max leading, finally, to skeletal muscle anaerobiosis. Thus, according to this argument, the coronary blood flow must be the first physiological function to show a 'plateau phenomenon' during progressive exercise to exhaustion. All subsequent physiological 'plateaus' must result from this limiting of coronary blood flow.

Whereas the most influential modern exercise physiologists for the past 75 years have enthusiastically embraced what increasingly appears to be a mythical basis for a 'plateau phenomenon' (Day *et al.* 2003), none seems to have grasped this logical prediction of the 'plateau phenomenon', which requires that the heart fatigue first before skeletal muscle failure develops. But this was clearly a concept with which the pioneering exercise physiologists were entirely comfortable.

In addition to the conclusion of Hill and his colleagues, already quoted, the pioneering United States exercise physiologists Arlie Bock and David Dill (Bainbridge 1931) also believed that myocardial ischaemia causes a fall in the cardiac output at the point of fatigue during high-intensity exercise:

> The blood supply to the heart, in many men, may be the weak link in the chain of circulatory adjustments during muscular exercise, and as the intensity of muscular exertion increases, a point is probably reached in most individuals at which the supply of oxygen to the heart falls short of its demands, and the continued performance of work becomes difficult or impossible (Bainbridge 1931: 15).

Hence they proposed that: 'Another factor, which may contribute to the production of this type of fatigue, is fatigue of the heart itself' (Bainbridge 1931: 229).

> Although the occurrence of fatigue of the heart in health is not very clearly established, a temporary lowering of the functional capacity of the heart, induced by fatigue of its muscular fibres, might gradually bring about during exercise an insufficient blood supply to the skeletal muscles and brain. The lassitude and disinclination for exertion, often experienced on the day after a strenuous bout of exercise, has been ascribed to fatigue of the heart as its primary cause (Bainbridge 1931: 229).

Hence they concluded: 'The heart, as a rule, reaches the limit of its powers earlier than the skeletal muscles, and determines a man's capability for exertion'.

In summary, the early physiologists who believed that skeletal muscle anaerobiosis limits maximal exercise, clearly understood that any plateau in cardiac output, necessary for there to be a limiting skeletal muscle blood flow, must result from a plateau in coronary blood flow, which would expose the heart to a progressive myocardial ischaemia that would worsen if exercise continued at that intensity.

Perhaps the reluctance of modern physiologists to acknowledge these concepts stems from the current appreciation that progressive myocardial ischaemia does not occur during maximal exercise in healthy athletes (Raskoff *et al.* 1976). Thus one postulate might be that the termination of exercise must occur before the heart actually reaches its maximum capacity and hence well before skeletal muscle anaerobiosis can develop according to Figure 4.1. Hence for over 75 years, exercise physiologists may have focused on the incorrect organ as the site of any potential anaerobiosis that may develop during maximal exercise (Noakes 1998, 2000; Noakes *et al.* 2001; Noakes and St Clair Gibson 2004).

Interestingly, Hill and his colleagues seem to have been the first to suggest a solution to this dilemma as early as 1924:

> From the point of view of a well co-ordinated mechanism, . . .. it would clearly be useless for the heart to make an excessive effort if by doing so it merely produced a far lower degree of saturation of the arterial blood; and we suggest that, in the body (either in the heart muscle itself or in the nervous system), there is some mechanism which causes a slowing of the circulation as soon as a serious degree of unsaturation occurs, and vice versa. This mechanism would tend to act as a governor maintaining a high degree of saturation of the blood (161–2).

On reading this text it immediately became clear to me why Hill was not quite correct and how such a governor would likely act to protect the heart. For Hill's model requires that the heart must first fail before the governor is activated, in keeping with his idea that a catastrophic limitation must first develop before exercise terminates. But since we now know that myocardial function is not impaired in healthy persons at maximal exercise (Raskoff *et al.* 1976), any governor must act *before* the heart becomes ischaemic. At some time during this process, the scales finally fell from my eyes and I realized that the more logical conjecture would be for such a governor to regulate the function, not of the heart, but of the skeletal muscles, specifically by regulating the number of muscle fibres that can be activated during maximal exercise. Accordingly in my rebuttal I made the first tentative proposal of what has since become known as a 'central governor', that responds to sensory information about the metabolic status of the heart. This information then leads to a reduction in skeletal muscle recruitment by the motor cortex leading to a reduction in exercise performance before there is any catastrophic failure of blood flow to either the heart or skeletal muscles. Discussion with my colleagues, especially Professor Vicki Lambert, led to the suggestion that exercise in a profoundly hypoxic (oxygen-depleted) environment, for example at high altitude, would show whether or not such a control exists and, in particular whether it is sensory feedback information from the heart or the exercising skeletal muscles that regulates maximal exercise performance, especially in an hypoxic environment. For if an oxygen deficiency really does develop in either heart or skeletal muscle, its appearance will likely be more easily identifiable during maximum exercise at altitude where the oxygen content of the inspired air is much reduced. Furthermore, such experiments should identify in which organ – heart or skeletal muscle – anaerobiosis first becomes apparent; the heart, according to the ideas of the pioneering British and North American exercise physiologists (Hill et al. 1924b; Bainbridge 1931), or the skeletal muscles, according to the influential group of modern exercise physiologists (Bassett and Howley 1997, 2000; Bergh *et al.* 2000; Ekblom 2000; Wagner 2000).

But regardless of their level of commitment to the cardiovascular/anaerobic/ catastrophic model of exercise physiology, more than 65 years of work have now established two ideas that are accepted by all exercise physiologists. First, that peak blood lactate concentrations during maximum exercise fall with increasing altitude (Edwards 1936; Green *et al.* 1989; Kayser 1996) a phenomenon since labelled the 'lactate paradox' (Hochachka *et al.* 2002). Second, that maximum heart rate and cardiac output likewise fall during exercise at increasing altitude (Sutton *et al.* 1988; Calbet *et al.* 2003a, 2003b).

Interestingly Edwards (1936) interpreted the 'lactate paradox' at altitude accordingly:

> The inability to accumulate large amounts of lactate at high altitudes suggests a protective mechanism preventing an already low arterial saturation from becoming markedly lower . . .. It may be that the protective mechanism lies in an inadequate oxygen supply to essential muscles, e.g. the diaphragm or the muscles (374–5).

Hence, in as much as high muscle lactate concentrations would have to be present if the exercising muscles were contracting 'anaerobically', these studies prove that exercise at extreme altitude terminates when the exercising muscles are contracting in the presence of an adequate oxygen supply. Hence we can conclude that skeletal muscles do not become anaerobic during maximal exercise in an oxygen-deficient environment at altitude.

The finding that the maximal cardiac output and heart rate are reduced at extreme altitude is equally paradoxical according to the model which holds that the delivery of an adequate oxygen supply to the exercising muscles is the cardinal priority during exercise (Figures 4.1 and 4.2). For according to the logic of this model, if the principal responsibility of the cardiovascular system is the achievement of an (ultimately inadequate) oxygen supply to skeletal muscle, then the cardiac output must always reach the same maximal value at exhaustion regardless of the conditions in which the exercise is undertaken (Noakes 2004).

Yet here too the evidence is definitive. The heart makes the exactly opposite adjustment – maximum cardiac output falls with increasing altitude (Sutton *et al.* 1988; Calbet *et al.* 2003a, 2003b). Nor is there any evidence that the function of the heart is impaired at altitude (Reeves *et al.* 1987; Suarez *et al.* 1987) as would occur if the heart were hypoxic. Hence the conclusion must be that some currently unrecognized mechanism must exist to ensure that the heart does not become 'anaerobic' during maximal exercise at any altitude – from sea level to the summit of Mount Everest – in healthy humans. The point is that this mechanism must exert its control before the heart fails, in contrast to the predictions of Hill's model (Figure 4.1).

Interestingly, Christensen, but not Dill, interpreted this phenomenon correctly in my view:

> Christensen and I differed in our interpretation of his measurements of respiratory and circulatory function in exercise (at altitude). In his opinion, the chief limiting factor is the ventilation of the lungs. In the hardest grade of work at any station, the pulmonary ventilation reached about as high a value as at sea level, while the maximal cardiac output became less as the altitude increased. He thinks this means that the heart has an untapped reserve; it is circulating blood fast enough to carry to the tissues all the oxygen supplied by the lungs (Dill 1938: 170–1).

These studies invite two precise conclusions. First, that the oxygen demands of the skeletal muscles are not the cardinal priority and hence are not 'protected' during maximum exercise, at least at extreme altitude. Second, neither the skeletal muscles nor the heart becomes 'anaerobic' or ischaemic during maximal exercise under conditions of hypoxia. The sole conclusion must be that some form of 'governor', as originally proposed by A.V. Hill, must terminate maximum exercise at altitude even before skeletal muscle anaerobiosis or myocardial ischaemia develops (Noakes 2004).

Furthermore, it would be difficult to explain why the same control mechanism should not also act during maximum exercise at sea level. For it would indeed be surprising if the human body evolved one specific control mechanism that acts only at extreme altitude. How could evolutionary forces have acted *in anticipation* of the possibility that one day humans would choose to climb to the roof of the world? More likely this form of control has a much wider application and is also active during exercise at sea level.

In summary, a number of famous studies have shown that under the precise conditions of maximal exercise at altitude most likely to induce anaerobiosis or ischaemia in either the heart or skeletal muscles, neither the heart nor the skeletal muscle show any evidence whatsoever for 'anaerobic' metabolism. This unexpected finding can be explained only if there is a 'governor', probably in the central nervous system, whose function it is to prevent the development of an inadequate blood supply to one or more vital organs such as the brain, heart, muscles or diaphragm. The same governor could also serve the identical function at sea level, thereby preventing the development of myocardial ischaemia during maximum exercise at sea level. Dill's conclusion is therefore incorrect: 'The capacity of the heart, as has already been suggested, is restricted at high altitude because of the deficiency in supply of oxygen to it' (Dill 1938: 15). For the important point is that the heart never actually develops an oxygen deficiency at altitude or at sea level; the 'governor' acts to terminate exercise well before any such deficiency can develop.

Confirmation of the presence of this theoretical governor comes from the studies of Kayser and his colleagues (Kayser 2003; Kayser et al. 1994). They showed that the extent of skeletal muscle recruitment, measured as skeletal muscle electromyographic (EMG) activity at peak exercise, falls with increasing altitude, but increases acutely with oxygen administration. They conclude: 'During chronic hypobaric hypoxia, the central nervous system may play a primary role in limiting exhaustive exercise and maximum accumulation of lactate in blood' (Kayser *et al.* 1994: 634). Calbet *et al.* (2003a, 2003b) have also shown that inhalation of an oxygen-rich gas mixture at the point of exhaustion during maximal exercise in simulated altitude instantly reverses the fatigue and normalizes the exercise performance. Since the partial pressure of oxygen in the arterial blood ($PaO_2$) is immediately normalized with the inhalation of oxygen-enriched air, this finding suggests that the $PaO_2$ provides the sensory feedback to the central governor during exercise in hypoxia (Noakes 2004).

Interestingly, had the human body been designed to function according to the modern physiologists' cardiovascular/anaerobic/catastrophic model, which requires that anaerobiosis should first develop in skeletal muscle before maximal exercise is terminated, no climber would ever have reached the summit of Mount Everest or other high mountains, even with the use of supplemental oxygen. Rather, all would have succumbed to a combination of myocardial ischaemia and cerebral hypoxia whilst their skeletal muscles were exercising vigorously, relentlessly and unrestrainedly, in pursuit of anaerobiosis and fatigue, according to the model depicted in Figure 4.1.

## The integrated neuromuscular recruitment model of exercise physiology

In order to offer an alternative physiological model that would explain all these divergent findings, the central governor model has been developed (Chambers *et al.* 2004; Noakes 1991, 2000, 2002; Noakes *et al.* 2001; St Clair Gibson and Noakes 2004). We originally postulated that receptors may exist in the heart, muscles, brain, blood and perhaps respiratory muscles to assess the adequacy of oxygenation of those tissues. Before any of these reach some predetermined limit, the motor cortex in the brain reduces the number of skeletal muscle fibres that are recruited. As a consequence, skeletal muscle recruitment fails to rise further, or it falls, limiting the amount of power the exercising muscles can produce. Since the body's power output is regulated in this way, so the need from blood flow and oxygen use is reduced according to Figure 4.6. Thus the regulated fall in work output by the body reduces tissue oxygen demands and, as a consequence, the threat of hypoxic damage is averted.

Accordingly I have proposed that maximal exercise is limited by a regulated process that terminates exercise before the development of an oxygen deficiency in any of the tissues at risk during such exercise.

The next advance in the development of this 'central governor' model came when we found that less than 100 per cent of the muscle fibres in the active limbs are recruited during voluntary exercise (Gandevia 2001); that this amount is less the longer the duration of exercise and may be as little as 30 per cent at exhaustion during more prolonged (1–2 hours) exercise (St Clair Gibson *et al.* 2001); but that the body has the capacity to increase the number of muscle fibres that it recruits near the end of exercise, the so-called 'end spurt phenomenon' (Kay *et al.* 2001; Tucker *et al.* 2004). All these findings are compatible only with a model of exercise in which the brain regulates the performance by altering the number of muscle fibres that it recruits at all times during exercise (Figure 4.6).

We therefore concluded that the regulation of changes in power output during self-paced exercise reflects, principally, changes in the number of motor units that are active, that is, the mass of skeletal muscle that is recruited by the central nervous system (Noakes 2003). As a result, we propose (i) that it is indeed the brain that regulates performance during exercise by determining the total number of motor units that are recruited and alternatively de-recruited during exercise and (ii) that the number of motor units that are active is influenced by afferent sensory feedback to the brain from a host of peripheral receptors, only some of which are currently recognized (Figure 4.7). The goal of

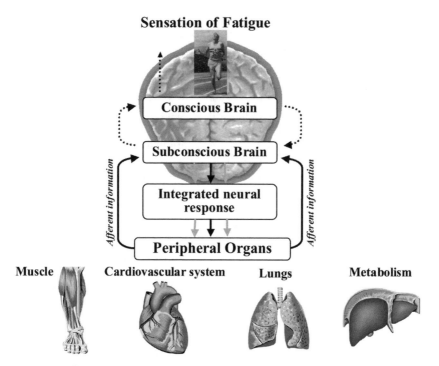

*Figure 4.7* The central governor model acknowledges the brain as the organ responsible for the regulation of exercise performance.

this sensory feedback is to ensure that the homoeostasis is regulated and that damage to vital organs is prevented (Noakes and St Clair Gibson 2004; St Clair Gibson and Noakes 2004; Lambert *et al.* 2004).

Perhaps the simplest analogy for the central governor model is that of a Formula 1 racing car which will remain stationary until the brain of its driver takes control. The decision on how fast to travel is set by the driver's subconscious and conscious brain in response to sensory feedback, including feedback from the racing team's pit crew, the nature of the racing circuit, the driver's prior experience and his perceived ability. But the control of the speed of the racing car is ultimately set by the pressure the driver's foot exerts on the accelerator pedal. This is in turn determined by the number of muscle fibres in the driver's right calf muscles that are recruited by his brain. And unless he has a death wish, the driver's ultimate consideration will always be his own self-preservation (homoeostasis) and this will set the ultimate speed that he is prepared to risk.

## Conclusion

The central conjecture that I have questioned originates from the statement by Hill and his colleagues in the 1920s, to the effect that: 'The oxygen intake (during maximal exercise) may attain its maximum and remain constant merely because it cannot go any higher owing to the limitations of the circulatory and respiratory systems'. This conjecture has exerted a profound influence on the teaching of exercise physiology for the past 70 years, for it predicts a physiological model in which exercise performance is determined solely by oxygen delivery to the exercising muscles (Figure 4.2). Thus it is believed that exercise, especially of high intensity, causes the oxygen demand of the active muscles to outstrip the available oxygen supply, requiring the muscles to contract in the face of a developing anaerobiosis. This physiological model also predicts that, since anaerobic conditions in muscle terminate maximal exercise, the principal effect of exercise training and of any other interventions that improve exercise performance must be either to increase oxygen supply to the muscles or to increase the muscles' capacity to utilize that oxygen (Figure 4.1). The model is also 'catastrophic' in that fatigue or exhaustion results only after the limitations of the system have been exceeded, causing system failure (Noakes and St Clair Gibson 2004; St Clair Gibson and Noakes 2004; Lambert *et al.* 2004).

Yet, as I have shown (Figure 4.3), Hill's own findings did not adequately support his original conclusions. Hence the original basis for this physiological model is without substance. If the basis for the model is in doubt, then it behoves us to question vigorously the further predictions of that original model. The key assumption made by A.V. Hill, and by three generations of succeeding physiologists, is that there is complete skeletal muscle recruitment during all forms of exercise, not only during progressive maximal exercise to exhaustion but also during prolonged submaximal exercise. For if skeletal muscle recruitment is not total at exhaustion, then there is no known manner by which a peripheral regulator can determine fatigue in any form of exercise. The simple reason is that a peripheral control cannot regulate the contractile function of motor units that have yet to be recruited and in which the concentration of these 'poisonous' metabolites must be low if it is the process of muscle contraction that causes the accumulation of such toxic metabolites.

To accommodate this new insight, my colleagues and I have proposed a novel model (Noakes and St Clair Gibson 2004; St Clair Gibson and Noakes 2004; Lambert *et al.* 2004) in which skeletal muscle recruitment is regulated, not limited, specifically to prevent damage to any of a number of different organs. Severe anaerobiosis is one specific endpoint that must be thwarted so that irreversible rigor and necrosis in the active muscles is prevented. But any number of other regulated processes can be imagined. Thus the function of the brain during exercise is to ensure that homoeostasis is maintained in all the organ systems so that bodily damage does not occur. This model further predicts that the sensation of fatigue that is experienced during all forms of exercise is in some way determined by the effort required to maintain that homoeostasis (St Clair Gibson and Noakes 2004; St Clair Gibson *et al.* 2003).

The challenge for the next generation of exercise scientists is to understand how the body anticipates the potential for organ damage and how skeletal muscle recruitment is regulated specifically to preclude any such calamity.

## Bibliography

Bainbridge, F.A. (1931) *The Physiology of Muscular Exercise*, A.V. Bock and D.B. Dill (eds), 3rd edn, London: Longmans, Green and Co., 1–272.

Bassett, D.R. (2002) 'Scientific contributions of A.V. Hill: exercise physiology pioneer', *J Appl Physiol*, 93, 1567–82.

Bassett, D.R. and Howley, E.T. (1997) 'Maximal oxygen uptake: "classical" versus "contemporary" viewpoints', *Med Sci Sports Exerc*, 29, 591–603.

Bassett, D.R. and Howley, E.T. (2000) 'Limiting factors for maximum oxygen uptake and determinants of endurance performance', *Med Sci Sports Exerc*, 32, 70–84.

Bergh, U., Ekblom, B. and Astrand, P.O. (2000) 'Maximal oxygen uptake 'classical' versus 'contemporary' viewpoints', *Med Sci Sports Exerc*, 32, 85–8.

Calbet, J.A.L., Boushel, R., Radegran, G., Sondergaard, H., Wagner, P.D. and Saltin, B. (2003a) 'Determinants of maximal oxygen uptake in severe acute hypoxia', *Am J Physiol*, 284, R291–R303.

Calbet, J.A.L., Boushel, R., Radegran, G., Sondergaard, H., Wagner, P.D. and Saltin, B. (2003b) 'Why is the $VO_2$max after altitude acclimatization still reduced despite normalization of arterial $O_2$ content?', *Am J Physiol*, 284, R303–R316.

Calbet, J.A.L., De Paz, J.A., Garatachea N., Cabeza De Vaca, S. and Chavarren, J. (2003c) 'Anaerobic energy provision does not limit Wingate exercise performance in endurance-trained cyclists', *J Appl Physiol*, 94, 668–76.

Costill, D.L. (1979) *A Scientific Approach to Distance Running*, Los Altos, CA: Tafnews.

Day, J.R., Rossiter, H.B., Coats, E.M., Skasick, A. and Whipp, B.J. (2003) 'The maximally-attainable $VO_2$ during exercise in humans: the peak vs. maximum issue', *J Appl Physiol*, in press.

Dill, D.B. (1938) *Life, Heat and Altitude*, Cambridge, MA: Harvard University Press.

Edwards, H.T. (1936) 'Lactic acid in rest and work at high altitude', *Am J Physiol*, 116, 367–75.

Ekblom, B. (2000) 'Editorial', *Scand J Med Sci Sports*, 10, 119–22.

Fletcher, W.M. and Hopkins, F.G. (1907) 'Lactic acid in amphibian muscle', *J Physiol*, 35, 247–309.

Friedman, N. (1994) 'Toward a new paradigm', in *Bridging Science and Spirit: Common Elements in David Bohm's Physics. The Perennial Philosophy and Seth*, St Louis: Living Lake Books, 282–3.

Gandevia, S.C. (2001) 'Spinal and Supraspinal factors in human muscle fatigue', *Physiol Rev*, 81, 1725–1789.

Gordon, A.M., Regnier, M. and Homshier, E. (2001) 'Skeletal and cardiac muscle contractile activation: Tropomyosin "Rocks and Rolls"', *News Physiol Sci*, 16, 49–55.

Graham, T.E. and Saltin, B. (1989) 'Estimation of the mitochondrial redox state in human skeletal muscle during exercise', *J Appl Physiol*, 66, 561–6.

Green, H.J., Sutton, J.R., Young, P.M., Cymerman, A. and Houston, C.S. (1989) 'Operation Everest II: muscle energetics during maximal exhaustive exercise', *J Appl Physiol*, 66, 142–50.

Hawking, S. (1989) *A Brief History of Time*, London: Bantam Press.

Hawking, S. (1993) *Black Holes and Baby Universes and Other Essays*, London: Bantam Books.

Hill, A.V. (1925) *Muscular Activity*, London: Baillière, Tindall and Cox.

Hill, A.V. (1965) *Trails and Trials in Physiology*, London: Edward Arnold.

Hill, A.V. and Lupton, H. (1923) 'Muscular exercise, lactic acid, and the supply and utilization of oxygen', *Q J Med*, 16, 135–71.

Hill, A.V., Long, C.N.H. and Lupton, H. (1924a) 'Muscular exercise, lactic acid, and the supply and utilization of oxygen – Parts IV–VI', *Proc Roy Soc B*, 97, 84–138.

Hill, A.V., Long, C.N.H. and Lupton, H. (1924b) 'Muscular exercise, lactic acid and the supply and utilization of oxygen – Parts VII–VIII', *Proc Roy Soc B*, 97, 155–76.

Hochachka, P.W., Beatty, C.L., Burelle, Y., Trump, M.E., Mckenzie, D.C. and Matheson, G.O. (2002) 'The lactate paradox in human high-altitude physiological performance', *News Physiol Sci*, 17, 122–6.

Katch, V. (1986) 'The burden of disproof . . .', *Med Sci Sports Exerc*, 18, 593–5.

Katz, A.M. (1992) *Physiology of the Heart*, 2nd edn, New York: Raven Press.

Kay, D., Marino, F.E., Cannon, J., St Clair Gibson, A., Lambert, M.I. and Noakes, T.D. (2001) 'Evidence for neuromuscular fatigue during high intensity exercise in warm humid conditions', *Eur J Appl Physiol*, 84, 115–21.

Kayser, B. (1996) 'Lactate during exercise at high altitude', *Eur J Appl Physiol*, 74, 195–205.

Kayser, B. (2003) 'Exercise begins and ends in the brain', *Eur J Appl Physiol*, 90, 411–419.

Kayser, B., Narici, M., Binzoni, T., Grassi, B. and Cerretelli, P. (1994) Fatigue and exhaustion in chronic hypobaric hypoxia: influence of exercising and muscle mass. *J Appl Physiol*, 76, 634–40.

Kuhn, T.S. (1970) '*The Structure of Scientific Revolutions*', 2nd edn, Chicago: University of Chicago Press.

Lambert E.V., St Clair Gibson, A. and Noakes, T.D. (2004) 'Complex systems model of fatigue: integral control and defence of homoeostasis during exercise in humans', *Br J Sports Med*, in press.

Le Fanu, J. (1999) *The Rise and Fall of Modern Medicine*, London: Abacus.

Miller, D.A. (1983) *A Pocket Popper*, Glasgow: Fontana Press.

Mitchell, J.H. and Blomqvist, G. (1971) 'Maximal oxygen uptake', *N Engl J Med*, 284, 1018–22.

Mole, P.A., Chung, Y., Tran, T.K., Sailasuta, N., Hurd, R. and Jue, T. (1999) 'Myoglobin desaturation with exercise intensity in human gastrocnemius muscle', *Am J Physiol*, 277, R173 – R180.

Needham, J. and Baldwin, E. (1949) *Hopkins and Biochemistry 1861–1947*, Cambridge: W. Heffer and Sons, 1–361.

Noakes, T.D. (1988) 'Implications of exercise testing for prediction of athletic performance: a contemporary perspective', *Med Sci Sports Exerc*, 20, 319–30.

Noakes, T.D. (1997) 'Challenging beliefs: *ex Africa semper aliquid novi*', *Med Sci Sports Exerc*, 29, 571–90.

Noakes, T.D. (1998) 'Maximal oxygen uptake: "classical" versus "contemporary" viewpoints: a rebuttal', *Med Sci Sports Exerc*, 30, 1381–98.

Noakes, T.D. (2000) 'Physiological models to understand exercise fatigue and the adaptations that predict or enhance athletic performance', *Scand J Med Sci Sports*, 10, 123–45.

Noakes, T.D. (2002) *Lore of Running*, 4th edn, Champaign, IL: Human Kinetics Publishers.

Noakes, T.D. (2003) Commentary to accompany: 'Training and bioenergetic characteristics in elite male and female Kenyan runners', *Med Sci Sports Exerc*, 35, 305–6.

Noakes, T.D. (2004) 'Central regulation of skeletal muscle recruitment explains the reduced maximal cardiac output during exercise in hypoxia', *Am J Physiol*, 281, in press.

Noakes, T.D. and St Clair Gibson, A. (2004). 'Logical limitations to the "catastrophe" models of fatigue in humans', *Br J Sports Med*, in press.

Noakes, T.D., Peltonen, J.E. and Rusko, H.K. (2001) 'Evidence that a central governor regulates exercise performance during acute hypoxia and hyperoxia', *J Exp Biol*, 204, 3225–34.

Nybo, L. and Secher, N.H. (2004) 'Cerebral perturbations provoked by prolonged exercise', *Prog Neurobiol*, 72, 223–261.

Pickering, G.W. (1956) 'The purpose of medical education', *Br Med J*, 2, 113–16.

Popper, K. (1969) *Conjectures and Refutations*, London: Routledge and Kegan Paul.

Popper, K.R. (1988) *Realism and the Aim of Science*, W.W. Bartley (ed.), London: Hutchinson.

Raskoff, W.J., Goldman, S. and Cohn, K. (1976) 'The "Athletic Heart." Prevalence and physiological significance of left ventricular enlargement in distance runners', *JAMA*, 236, 158–62.

Reeves, J.T., Groves, B.M., Sutton, J.R., Wagner, P.D., Cymerman, A., Malconian, M.K., Rock, P.B., Young, P.M. and Houston, C.S. (1987) 'Operation Everest II: Preservation of cardiac function at extreme altitude', *J Appl Physiol*, 63, 531–9.

Resink, T.J., Gevers, W., Noakes, T.D. and Opie, L.H. (1981a) 'Increased cardiac myosin ATPase activity as a biochemical adaptation to running training: Enhanced response to catecholamines and a role for myosin phosphorylation', *J Molec Cell Cardiol*, 13, 679–94.

Resink, T.J., Gevers, W. and Noakes, T.D. (1981b) 'Effects of extracellular calcium concentrations on Myosin P light chain phosphorylation in hearts from running trained rats', *J Molec Cell Cardiol*, 13, 753–65.

Richardson, R.S., Noyszewski, E.A., Leigh, J.S. and Wagner, P.D. (1998) 'Lactate efflux from exercising human skeletal muscle: Role of intracellular $PO_2$', *J Appl Physiol*, 85, 627–34.

Richardson, R., Leigh, J.S., Wagner, P.D. and Noyszewski, E.A. (1999) 'Cellular $pO_2$ as a measure of mitochondrial $O_2$ consumption in the trained human muscle', *J Appl Physiol*, 87, 325–31.

Rowell, L.B. (1993) *Human Cardiovascular Control*, Oxford: Oxford University Press.

St Clair Gibson, A. and Noakes, T.D. (2004) 'Evidence for complex system integration and dynamic neural regulation of skeletal muscle recruitment during exercise in humans', *Br J Sports Med*, in press.

St Clair Gibson, A., Schabort, E.J. and Noakes, T.D. (2001) 'Reduced neuromuscular activity and force generation during prolonged cycling', *Am J Physiol* 281, R187–R196.

St Clair Gibson, A., Baden, D.A., Lambert, M.I., Lambert, E.V., Harley, Y.X.R., Hamson, N D., Russell, V. and Noakes, T.D. (2003) 'The conscious perception of the sensation of fatigue', *Sports Med*, 33, 167–76.

Suarez, J., Alexander, J.K. and Houston, C.S. (1987) 'Enhanced left ventricular systolic performance at high altitude during Operation Everest II', *Am J Cardiol*, 60, 137–42.

Sutton, J.R., Reeves, J.T., Wagner, P.D., Groves, B.M., Cymerman, A., Malconian, M.K., Rock, P.B., Young, P.M., Walter, S.D. and Houston, C.S. (1988) 'Operation Everest II: Oxygen transport during exercise at extreme simulated altitude', *J Appl Physiol*, 64, 1309–21.

Swales, J.D. (1985) *Platt versus Pickering. An Episode in Recent Medical History*, The Keynes Press/British Medical Association, Cambridge University Press.

Taylor, H.L., Buskirk, E. and Henschel, A. (1955) 'Maximal oxygen intake as an objective measure of cardio-respiratory performance', *J Appl Physiol*, 8, 73–80.

Thomas, L. (1985) 'Medicine as a very old profession', In: *Cecil Textbook of Medicine*, 17th edn, 9–11.

Tucker, R., Rauch, L., Harley, Y.X.R. and Noakes, T.D. (2004) 'Impaired exercise performance in the heat is associated with an anticipatory reduction in skeletal muscle recruitment', *Pflugers Archiv*, 448, 422–430.

Van Der Werff, T.J., Noakes, T.D. and Douglas, R.J. (1985) 'The effects of changes in heart rate and atrial filling pressure on the performance characteristics of isolated perfused pumping rat hearts', *Clin Phys Physiol Meas*, 6, 205–19.

Wagner, P.D. (2000) 'New ideas on limitations to $VO_2$ max', *Exerc Sports Sci Rev*, 28, 10–14.

Waller, J. (2002) *Fabulous Science. Fact and Fiction in the History of Scientific Discovery*, Oxford: Oxford University Press.

Will, C.M. (1986) *Was Einstein Right?* New York: Basic Books.

## Note

1  I should like to acknowledge my gratitude for the dedicated financial support of the University of Cape Town, the Medical Research Council of South Africa, Discovery Health, the Founding Donors of the Sports Science Institute of South Africa, and the National Research Foundation through the THRIP initiative, to the work of this Unit.

# 5 Why doesn't sports psychology consider Freud?

*Graham McFee*

It is widely accepted that modern psychology owes a debt to Freud: he is one of its 'founding fathers'. Yet contemporary sports psychology does scant justice to that fact. This may result partly from the far from positive relationship between psychoanalytically inclined psychology and the kind of empirical psychology from which sports psychology developed. Whatever its general pedigree, I shall urge here that neglect of Freud typically leads to an impoverished view of the character and potential of sports psychology: that Freud could offer a more positive model. So my thesis is not merely that contemporary sports psychology neglects Freud's work, but that it is damaged thereby. For Freud's work offers ways of viewing the mind, the person and action more plausible than many currently espoused by sports psychology; and this is especially important when we consider methodologies, as Freud's ideas can help combat a dominant scientism.

A large number of major issues from philosophy intersect with this one – concerning the nature of science, free action and determinism, the nature of the mind – most of which cannot be treated here,[1] although some of them will necessarily be broached. For that reason, much of what follows says less about sport than might, perhaps, be expected.

Here, I first show that there is a problem, sketch some views of Freud's as background, and exemplify the problem more fully, as well explaining why such neglect might come about. Then I highlight three areas where taking Freud's work more seriously could be transformative: namely, methodologically, in terms of conceptual structure, and for the account of persons.

## Does sports psychology neglect Freud?

Is the neglect of Freud's work by contemporary sports psychology that I have urged actually *the case*? Is it *true* that sports psychologists do not consider Freud? Although the right answer to both questions is 'yes', it is complicated by the *forms* the neglect takes: for clarity, I simplify by distinguishing three such forms. And, consonant with the plan to address the body of sports psychology (rather than its 'cutting edge'), my chosen texts are drawn primarily from introductory works on sports psychology, the sorts of things one's students read (and take for 'gospel' truths).

Of course, not all sports psychology is the same in this respect: I am referring to trends only. But my primary use of textbook-type sources is designed to indicate the pervasiveness of the attitude – it is the 'taken for granted' wisdom. Moreover, not *only* appeal to Freud might be efficacious here: my claim, though, is that the neglect and the damage go together.

Now to the three forms of what I am calling 'neglect'. Sports psychology has neglected Freud:

- by misrepresenting his writings;
- by denigrating his ideas, usually in the misunderstood version; and/or
- by ignoring his account of the mind and psychological phenomena (and thereby his insights).

The first of these is marked (or perhaps obscured) by poor levels of scholarship, to a degree that might even seem like wilful misrepresentation. In one bizarre example, for instance, a essay attributing various views to Freud (Toner in Diamant 1991b: 128–30) gives as the only reference the *Standard Edition* of his works, but with no sense of which pages, nor even which volume (from a 24-volume work).[2] But without knowing (accurately) what Freud said, we cannot hope to address the consistency of his thought, or its congruence with uncontentious facts. In part, my objections reinforce a general dissatisfaction with much of what passes for scholarship here: that its claim to be based on the detail of Freud's work seems contentious (Lear 1998: 19–28; Nagel 1995: 26–44).[3]

The first two of these forms of 'failure to consider' (above) that I am calling *neglect* are manifest when authors just mention Freud, and go no further. That is enough to imply both a view of Freud and the lack of importance of Freud on that view. And this is a common practice. For example, Don Davies (1989: 71) mentions Freud in passing;[4] Diane Gill (1986: 196) claims simply that 'psychoanalytic approaches [to aggression] ... are associated with Freudian concepts', without mentioning a specific text of Freud's; and a short introductory text on memory (one regularly recommended to students of sports science) attributes a brief account of 'motivated forgetting' to Freud, but comments that this 'doesn't really tie in with any other major theoretical perspective' (Moxon 2000: 7). Of course, that might show those other perspectives to be hopelessly flawed. And Moxon does concede, 'In some ways this gives it a unique appeal'. Unfortunately, it is not an appeal explored further in that text. Instead, we are reminded that 'It is very difficult to assess the validity of Freud's ideas' (Moxon 2000: 7) since they do not lend themselves to laboratory experimentation.

This idea highlights the *scientism* of such texts, where scientism is not just the worship of science (that is, a commitment to science as either the best or the only model of knowledge) but also takes a view of what is *appropriate* to science: and that will be controlled experimentation, measurement, hypothesis-testing (with contrastive null-hypotheses), and the rejection of whatever can be dismissed as 'subjective' because it is either not directly observable or involving persons' views of their world.[5] Of course, *some* science – and even some good science – might be conducted on these assumptions. The point here is simply that those assumptions do not mark out science from non-science, that some of the best science has not had this character, and that scientific enquiry (and other valuable enquiry) can be conducted from quite different assumptions. So we must be on guard against such scientism.

The first two forms of neglect identified above are also visible in more extended discussions of Freud. As we shall see, giving more extensive exposition may amount neither to not neglecting Freud nor to considering him, unless that exposition was both accurate and fair to Freud.

The third form is least easy to identify: it involves our noticing *absences*. Typical texts used by students here, such as Weinberg and Gould (1995) or Hardy *et al.* (1996), have no mention of the 'founding father', either in the body or the bibliography.[6] Yet, as we shall see, they do discuss themes to which Freud's ideas might be thought germane.

## Some Freudian ideas

Of course, *one* explanation that might be offered for such neglect – perhaps the simplest one – would be that Freud was simply *wrong*: and then critics would go on to point out in what ways; for instance, citing his crazy views about penis envy or his misvaluing of women. There are two difficulties with interpreting the responses of sports psychologists in this way: first, this would explain a *complete* neglect of Freud, not the partial neglect noted above; second, mature discussion might find these views not that wrong after all.

To respond, we would need a clearer view of Freud's commitments, located within (at least) a thumbnail sketch of his general position:[7] that is, showing us the minimum that must be accepted in order to count as a psychoanalytically inclined psychologist. I would highlight four general features. First, psychoanalysis (at least on Freud's model) recognizes that thoughts, ideas and (especially) desires not open to consciousness can seek an *indirect* expression (in slips of the tongue, in dreams, in pathological symptoms [in the worst case]): thus such ideas or thoughts can be 'latent and operative' (Wollheim 1971: 157) – they have a bearing on the person's *behaviour*, even if/when he or she has no knowledge of them. Further, one can 'track back' from the indirect expression to the underlying thought, idea or desire, since the indirect expression is connected to them along chains of association. Second, these are features of the *mind* of a *person*, rather than structures of machines or biological systems; hence, a primary mode of access to them will be by talking to (or listening to) the person. Third, people differ in these respects, reflecting their upbringing and life as well as any biological inheritance.

The fourth point is more complex: it concerns Freud's recognition of (full) rationality as an *achievement*: that reason is not something given, but something that has to be struggled for. So we should see the mind as constantly engaged in such a struggle – this is one sense in which psychoanalytically inclined psychology is concerned with a *process*, rather than a product.

Further, there is Freud's recognition of persons as agents. Although psychoanalytic psychology offers a view of the mind *as such*, it incorporates a concern with pathologies of the mind. For example, the case of the lady with the tablecloth (PFL 1: 300–2)[8] involved a woman who repeatedly called a maid into a room where the maid was sure to notice a large stain on a tablecloth, and then sent the maid away with no task or a trivial one: Freud investigated this compulsive behaviour. The point for us, though, is that his aim was to return the poor woman to normalcy – to rid her of the compulsion. So psychoanalytic thinking is centrally concerned with a return to the human condition, for there is no assumption that we all have such pathologies.

But might Freud's work be just plain wrong? Of course, any response must stress – as below – the insights Freud's work embodies. But that cannot be the whole story. A reply must also recognize, first, that what we take for 'Freud' is itself a topic for dispute – so, at best, one will be defending a 'reading' of Freud's work (as of any theorist).[9] Second, Freud's work is not necessarily seamless – one need not necessarily be committed to it all. For instance, perhaps insight from his other theoretical interventions need not depend on, say, committing oneself to the theoretical importance of *penis envy* (or better, *widdler envy*: Lear 1990: 98ff.). Moreover, finding one's way here will certainly involve rational reconstruction of Freud's ideas, based on his own writings and perhaps from periodizing those writings. Yet, third, since Freud was (as inevitably) a 'man of his times', some of his comments on the state of the world or on the lot of women should be read as describing the world, or women's lot, *at that time*. Moreover, some commitments of Freud's will find no place in any plausible rational reconstruction we make.[10] Of course, our view of Freud's consistency will be a matter of *argument*, with reasons for preferring particular readings. These will never be absolute: still, we can appeal to the fact that

> interpretations, like ways of seeing line drawings, can be … more or less natural (as opposed to 'strained') …. To show … [that a particular 'reading'] is a very unnatural reading is not to disprove it, but it ought to make it less attractive …. (Baker and Morris 1996: 5–6)

By showing the 'strained' nature of other readings, one gives weight to one's own. However, the defence of Freud here aims to grant that, properly understood, his view of minds and persons is insightful. But to see Freud's position here we must engage in detailed reading of Freud's works, perhaps in combination with their rational reconstruction.

The explanation of why this sort of discussion is not forthcoming in sports psychology literature is, I suspect, that a neater rejection of Freud is thought to be at hand. In line with the sort of scientism identified earlier, it amounts to dismissing Freud's work as *unscientific* for the (supposed) reason that it lacks the kind of evidential base appropriate to science; in particular (as suggested above), that it does not lend itself to laboratory investigation.[11] This charge, too, will turn out to be groundless. But reaching that conclusion will require some consideration of Freud's theory and practice. We can fill in further details of some of Freud's ideas, and their evidential base (especially the section entitled 'Does Freud deserve attention? (ii) Conceptual structure' in this chapter, cf. Lear 1998: 23–7), as they arise.

## An example from sports psychology: misrepresenting Freud

Ideally, we should continue by showing how Freud's ideas are treated in contemporary sports psychological writings. Here, to make the points more concrete, it is worth exemplifying the issues from a single text. Then we can bring out how those pictures of 'Freud' in the sports-psychological literature (where they occur) differ from what Freud actually wrote. (And it should be stressed that the texts selected for discussion throughout this essay are chosen for stating *clearly* positions often only implicit in other texts.)

Thus, for example, in *Psychology in Practice: Sport*, Barbara Woods *does* mention Freud as offering a psychoanalytic theory of personality (2001: 6), a theory which can be applied to the understanding of aggression (2001: 25), and hence to sport. Now, other accounts of personality sketched in Woods (such as trait theory and social learning theory) are treated in an equally cavalier fashion – we learn neither enough about them to say what they really are, nor enough to adjudicate amongst them. In this respect, Freud's ideas fare no worse.

But Woods' discussion is worth elaborating in some detail, since doing so will also offer insight into Freud's *real* positions. And our later discussion will require an elaborated view of Freud on some (relevant) issue.

To explore the topics, then, I will highlight aspects of Woods' general discussion of Freud's ideas, the discussion of displacement, and the criticisms of Freud. To take the first of these, consider the explanation of aggression, as applied to sport. As it is short, I will quote almost all of it. We are told that, for Freud:

> [W]e have instincts which have to be satisfied. Aggression is part of what he calls our death instincts, which are destructive …. In order that these instincts can be satisfied, they create a drive, so we have to find a way of managing our aggressive drive in a way which is positive, such as … exercising or sports. These activities are *cathartic*, because they allow the release of pent-up aggression. According to Freud, participating in sports, or simply watching, would reduce aggression. (Woods 2001: 25)

In what text does Freud make these comments about *sport*? We are not told – indeed, there is no text by Freud in either the 'Further Reading' or 'References' section of this chapter. And it seems unlikely that Freud did make such comments. Towards the end of his life, when Freud came to write about aggression – most particularly in *The Ego and the Id* (1923: PFL Vol. 11) and *Civilization and Its Discontents* (1930: PFL Vol. 12) – his concerns were with war, not sport. Of course, there may be some overlapping themes here (see Gomberg 2000), but we should generally be wary about 'reading across' insights from one area to another; and be especially wary of doing so for Freud, given his attention to the detail of context.

Moreover, contrary to the suggestion above, Freud's view of aggression was not as cathartic, as we shall see. The reading offered by Woods might seem to receive support from the way Freud regularly uses *energy-based* models of psychological phenomena: that is, explains them in terms of the accumulation and discharge of what he calls 'affect' (Lear 2000: 86). Such a model might see a discharge of aggression as cathartic. But such energy-based models of the mind were common during Freud's time; so there seems no *special* inference to be drawn here. Further, it seems odd to attribute such a view of aggression to Freud, even before we come to detailed study of his work. For Freud recorded that a human inclination towards aggression 'constitutes the greatest impediment to civilisation' (*Civilisation and Its Discontents*: PFL Vol. 12: 313), and only sport's greatest fan would see it as an antidote to such a huge impediment.

Moreover, Freud does not typically treat aggression as central in this way: indeed, in much of his writing, he 'overlooked the ubiquity of non-erotic aggressivity and destructiveness and failed to give it its due place in our interpretation of life' (*Civilisation*: PFL Vol. 12: 311) That means that (later) Freud noticed a gap in psychoanalytic theory: as Lear (2000: 87) eloquently points out, the later discussion was just an attempt to paper over that gap.

Freud had resisted the idea that there was an independent aggressive instinct. He wrote: 'I cannot bring myself to assume the existence of a special aggressive instinct alongside of the familiar instincts of self-preservation and of sex, and on an equal footing with them' ('Little Hans' 1909: PFL Vol. 8: 297).

In a footnote added in 1923, Freud seemed to withdraw that judgement, in the light of the insight noted above. But, in fact, he thereafter took aggressiveness to be a characteristic of instinct, and assigned it (in the structural theory of the mind) to the id, which Woods (2001: 6) characterizes as 'the "package" of unconscious instincts (including sexual and aggressive instincts) which need immediate gratification'. But, as often, we should doubt the adequacy of her explanation.

One difficulty here, of course, is that the id is but one structure of the person's mind: perhaps it would be possible for a very small child to consider 'immediate gratification' a necessity in this way, but that is not possible for adults. Rather, adults can see that 'gratifications' may need to be delayed: that, roughly, one needs to take the time to build a trap if one is to get the food. Thus the power of the id should not be overrated. Certainly psychoanalysis 'seeks to prove to the ego that it is not even master in its own house' (Introductory Lectures: PFL Vol. 1: 326). But Freud was also careful to draw a distinction between drive (*Trieb*) and instinct (*Instinkt*) (Lear 1998: 88): drives were shaped by experience or one's environment, but were also responsive to needs, and so embody a kind of *choice* (only open to minded-creatures); while instinct (properly so called) is a rigid behavioural pattern – for example, the 'pressure' on birds to build a nest. Seen in this light, human aggression would be regarded as a *drive*. As Jonathan Lear

(1990: 170) summarizes: '[T]he world is an occasion for the satisfaction development of drives, not just a recipient of discharges' (see PFL Vol. 11: 365).

On this view, then, very little of the psychological life of a typical human being could reasonably be understood as *instinct* (rather than *drive*) since most of the behaviour turned on what was (broadly) within human power or choice. So that, for example, even human hunger does not lead to biting the first edible thing that passes before one's field of vision; and similar remarks apply for, say, human reproductive behaviour. Hence, much of the fabric of society was *chosen* in at least this sense.

Thus, even what was *instinctual* might not be unavoidable. Although interpersonal aggression was a problem which resulted from civilization (a problem that would beset even those on the top of the economic heap), dealing with it was not beyond human power. To understand how, we need a clearer picture of Freud's thought on this topic.[12] As he sees it, dealing with interpersonal aggression requires the removal of *occasions* for such aggression: this motivates Freud's enthusiasm for abolition or attrition of institutions of nationhood and property (PFL Vol. 12: 337–8; PFL Vol. 2: 218). As Richard Wollheim (1971: 233) notes, Freud thought that, in the management of aggression 'a real change in the relations of human beings to possessions would be of more help ... than any ethical commands' (PFL Vol. 12: 338).

This may be the most that can be done unless the fruits of civilization are distributed in a way that is 'not blatantly unjust' (Wollheim 1971: 234), since, 'It goes without saying that a civilisation which leaves so large a number of its participants unsatisfied and drives them into revolt neither has nor deserves the prospect of a lasting existence' (PFL Vol. 12: 191–2).

But, once these external pressures are removed, aggression *can* be internalized – the superego is invested with the 'instinct' (more technically, the drive: *Trieb*) that the individual renounces: the superego functions as a moral guardian. Finally, there can be the replacement of 'instinct' by intellect,[13] the possibility of what Freud called 'the dictatorship of reason' (PFL Vol. 12: 359) or the idea that 'reason ... [may] establish a dictatorship in the mental life of man' (PFL Vol. 2: 208): the target here is 'morality freed from anxiety' (Wollheim 1971: 222). And there is some reason for hope, since 'in the long run, nothing can withstand reason and experience' (PFL Vol. 12: 238).

So Freud's own account of aggression (and how it might be mastered) is very different from that which Woods ascribes to him. In particular, the aim is not cathartic; rather, mastery of aggression is a step humans take towards becoming rational (if they can). In that sense, Freud's own picture here – as often – gives far more weight to human powers and capacities (and to human agency) than ascribed to him. For he treats those involved as persons who can make choices, and can genuinely *learn*, as *capable* of becoming rational, of reaching 'the dictatorship of reason', even if he is not optimistic about the likelihood of such an outcome.

So the account urged here offers not so much the *content* of Freud's picture of aggression for – as Lear (2000: 87) notes – Freud does not really have a picture of aggression *as such*. Rather, it exploits the particularist and person-oriented methodology which Freud developed; and does so in ways that recognize the psychological priority of action.

If we view persons (and emotions, and so on) in a certain way, we shall never be able to see how persons – as opposed to robots, with 'pullable strings' (see 'Does Freud deserve attention? (i) Methodology' on page 97) – function in sporting contexts. And if our understandings of persons do not make sense in any research design that involves persons, we are in difficulty. For Freud, persons are (or, at least, can be) rational agents: if we do not see *that* about them, we shall view them as trapped in aggression – exactly what Freud denied.

Interestingly, the same kind of mistake clouds the influential thinking of Bredemeier and Shields (1986: 25) on this point:[14] they argue that sports typified by aggressive acts tend to attract participants with lower levels of moral reasoning, and may inhibit moral growth. Freud might well stress the opposed view: that, since *mastering* aggression is of crucial importance, the opportunity to confront it in relative safe contexts should be beneficial.

## Misunderstanding continued: more on aggression

Woods' account continues by discussing how Freudian ideas might explain our interest in sport:

> Freud ... maintained that when we want to do something that we know is not acceptable, we use techniques such as *displacement* . . .. If the boss makes you really angry you might want to hit him, but you do not. Instead you are very aggressive in your five-a-side match that evening, which is a more acceptable way of releasing aggression. This is an example of displacement – redirecting an emotional response from a dangerous target to a safe one. (Woods 2001: 25)

Freud's is here classified as an instinct theory, such that 'Taking part in sport should reduce aggression' (Woods 2001: 25). It is easy to see that this is nothing like Freud's own account (as sketched above): far from seeking the release of aggression through displacement, Freud aims at mastery of aggression.

A similar level of misunderstanding besets Woods' attempt to adjudicate among accounts of aggression:

> The key element of ... psychoanalytic theories is that sport should lead to reduced levels of aggression. However, critics argue that this is not generally supported by the evidence, as shown by Berkowitz (1972) who reviewed research . . .. (Woods 2001: 26)

It seems as though this might be evidence against Freud's views. Here, though, we are simply told that such evidence exists, and that we should take Berkowitz's word for both the soundness of the research and the interpretation of its conclusions – although in this instance we do at least have the details of the paper listed in the 'References'! Further, the connection to psychoanalytic theory here is not a direct one: that is, it is not to the theory of aggression (as Woods misdescribes it), but to the account of displacement. So, at many levels, this remains contentious. Woods (2001: 26) then urges: 'Many have argued that watching sport actually increases aggression . . .'.

This would be contrary to the characterization of the psychoanalytic account by (say) Woods as cathartic. Moreover, we are not told how one identifies such 'increases [in] aggression'. So such remarks seem problematic from the start. Woods (2001: 26) continues:

> but this may be dependent on the sport. In research by Arms, Russell and Sandilands (1979), some participants watched aggressive sports (such as ice-hockey and wrestling) and others watched a swimming meet. Those watching the aggressive sports experienced increased feelings of hostility whereas those watching swimming did not. (Woods 200: 26)

But it is far from obvious how 'increased feelings of hostility' (towards whom?) have any bearing on the matter.

Notice, too, that this account of 'Freud' on aggression exactly parallels the one that Weinberg and Gould, who do not mention Freud, ascribe to the *instinct theory of aggression* (1995: 471). As with Woods' account, this theory stresses the 'innate instinct to be aggressive' (1995: 471) as well as the idea of *catharsis*. So this text exemplifies the *third* kind of neglect identified initially, and perpetuates mistakes by now familiar. In a vein similar to Woods', they point out that 'no biologically innate aggressive instinct has ever been identified and no support has been found for the notion of catharsis' (1995: 471).

If this is right, we should be glad that this summary does not represent Freud's view of aggression. Similarly, Gill (1986: 197)[15] simply characterizes *instinct theories*: 'Instinct theories predict that all individuals and cultures have the same innate urges, similar levels of aggressive energy, and should exhibit similar levels of aggressive behaviour.' Even were this true of 'instinct theories', it is not true of Freud, especially in ascribing a transcultural dimension. For Freud explicitly provides a role to just such cultural specificity (see sections in this chapter, 'More on methodology – determinism' and 'A complexity of structure: the social character of individuals' below).

Moreover, Gill (1986: 200) makes the connection here whereby 'instinct theories support and advocate sport as a catharsis'. But, since Gill goes on to offer (what at least she takes as) a demolition of the credentials of catharsis, it may be no bad thing that the idea is not one of Freud's! So we should conclude (again) that – if these are indeed the contours of *instinct theories* – it is no bad thing that Freud's own view differs so markedly from those here characterized as *instinct theories*.

These, then, typify the sorts of neglect of Freud's meticulous exposition commented on initially. (One is sometimes left wondering whether these authors have actually *read* any Freud – at least, whether they have read him carefully.) All in all, this example of the discussion of aggression illustrates in some detail the kind of thing I am calling 'neglect', and does so, interestingly, in an area where Freud's own views are significantly more interesting than those ascribed to him.

## What is the basis for the neglect?

I speculate as to three (related) possible sources of this 'neglect'. First, Freud's work is viewed as inappropriate for sports psychology because it is, somehow, not *scientific*. We have already noted this criticism: as I shall urge, there is something right in this 'accusation' – Freud's work certainly does not fit the *scientistic* models of scientific knowledge and understanding common in sports psychology. Indeed, this accusation is one from psychology more generally: the enthusiasm for the white coat of the laboratory scientist seems to preclude the humanistic, in ways I will come to. Nevertheless, this objection is wide of the mark since research may be realistic *without* adherence to this scientistic model, as I urged earlier. Freud not only exemplifies such ideas, but – as we shall see – explains and motivates them.

Second, sports psychologists wish to distance themselves from 'the couch', and from any connection with *psychiatry*. Indeed, one motive for the demand for *science* is to put aside the less rigorous practices sometimes thought to be part of therapy. But, while this second point is sound – sports psychology is not primarily concerned with pathological conditions[16] – the same is true of psycho-analytically inclined accounts of the mind (or of persons). So that, while much of Freud's material derived from his study of cases of neurosis, psychosis, and the like, not *all* of it did (dreams and slips of the tongue, for example, are not pathological); and the origin of the ideas is irrelevant, but their impact is not. Thus, even if Freud used clinical data in formulating his accounts of the mind (given his own concerns), that is no reason to reject those accounts.

The third issue concerns intervention, where sports psychology aims not just at *understanding* what is going on in sporting situations (a theory or account of the person) but at *improving* performance! Perhaps this characterization is a little crude. Nevertheless, it highlights some problems for using techniques of psychoanalysis with sports players or athletes: in line with the point above, the sports player or athlete is not typically the subject of any pathology – or, when there is something pathological, there is no necessary connection between it and poor performance. Further, the methods of psychoanalysis require the presence of an analyst, rather than being something the sports player or athlete can operate or practice for him/herself. This seems problematic (when not impossible) in a practical sporting context. Moreover, psychoanalytic techniques often take years to reach completion: as the Woody Allen character in *Sleeper* (who has just been revived after 200 years cryogenically preserved) asks, 'What about my analyst? He was a strict Freudian. I'd almost have been cured by now'.

This last point – about the duration of 'cure' – is actually irrelevant: if a Freudian account of the mind (or person) is lacking from sports psychology, such an account need not *only* be harnessed through psychoanalysis. This turns on its head the earlier point: our sports players and athletes do not typically need psychoanalysis *because* they do not typically suffer from the pathologies for which it is arguably the appropriate therapeutic technique. More simplistically, the conditions of sports players and athletes are not typically pathological (despite both the incomprehensibility of their motivation, to some of the rest of us, and the few obvious counter-cases – I'd cite Mike Tyson, but others might prefer the footballer Roy Keane). But that says nothing about the benefits (or otherwise) that might follow from integration of Freud's view of persons.

Moreover, the emphasis on intervention highlights a positive feature of Freud's thinking: for Freud was keen to recognize individual difference – that people differ as to what would be a suitable intervention for them. So Freud's conceptions here would militate against *blanket* 'treatment' of athletes and sports players, as though they were all the same. Instead, and in line with some contemporary practice, it would suggest an emphasis on the individual.

Unclarities here derive from uncertainty as to the exact *aims* of sports psychology. Woods (2001: 1), for example, writes of 'the application of psychology to the sports environment', which later becomes the application of 'psychological theories and models ... in a systematic way'. Similarly, Weinberg and Gould (1995: 8) take sports psychology to involve identifying 'principles and guidelines that professionals can use to help adults and children participate in and benefit from sport and exercise activities'. This remains pretty unclear. For example, is sports psychology only good if (or when) it *improves* performance? Although Woods (2001: 3) speaks of sports psychology helping 'sports participants and coaches to become more effective', the accounts above suggest a 'no' answer. Certainly the value of physics is not circumscribed by its positive applications: part of the benefit lies in the knowledge itself. But the activities of the sports psychologist must be seen as *purposeful* – and that purpose, especially for (say) national teams, will be cashed-out in terms of success. Thus, when Hardy *et al.* (1996: 4) write about the 'necessary psychological skills', our first thoughts might be to ask, 'Necessary for what? Necessary to whom?'; but considered reflection will typically answer those questions in terms of sporting success.

Interestingly, Woods (2001: 2) recognizes two conflicting accounts of the ultimate nature of sports psychology. The first, already sketched, draws directly on the application of ideas and models from psychology – roughly, sports psychology does whatever general psychology does, but in relation to sport. The benefits, then, will be those of 'applied psychology'; we might still question what *exactly* these were. The second, contrasting view regards sports psychology 'as a sub-discipline of sports science' (Woods 2001: 2). In aligning itself in this second way, sports psychology will tend towards scientism – and we have noted that tendency in the emphasis on experimental situations conceived a certain way (see 'Does Freud deserve attention? (ii) Conceptual structure' on page 101).

This seems to return us to the explanation of the neglect, within sports psychology, of ideas from Freud: namely, that Freud is mistaken about this or that – that his ideas are neglected because they have been superseded. Yet such criticisms – were they sustainable – imply that there are clear ways to arbitrate between competing theories in psychology in general (and hence in sports psychology). But, in fact, psychology has regularly had difficulties with issues of theory-choice: Wittgenstein's diagnosis (for psychology in general but applicable when sports psychology appropriates its ideas) was that 'in psychology there are experimental methods and *conceptual confusion*' (Wittgenstein 1953: 232)

As an example, consider for a moment theories of imagery. Such imagery is widely used in sports psychology, so that it is 'a major component of every sports performer's preparation for performance' (Hardy *et al.* 1996: 27).[17] But the effectiveness of imagery-based techniques must be explained: they are certainly not transparent. As one might expect, there are competing accounts to be given, so how do we discriminate among such theories? Conceptual confusion will preclude our doing so. For instance, suppose it were important to distinguish *imagery* from *mental rehearsal*:

> [I]magery is a mental process . . . . Mental rehearsal, on the other hand, is defined . . . as the employment of imagery to mentally practice an act. Thus, mental rehearsal is a *technique* as opposed to merely a *mental process*. (Hardy *et al.* 1996: 28.)

One might, with justice, find this difficult to grasp. Is mental rehearsal then *not* a 'mental process'? Can one really 'mentally practice' an act, as opposed to, say, imagining that one was performing the act? Certainly, many of the usual implications of the expression 'to practise' are missing here: one cannot, for instance, ask how I did in practice, or what my practice score was. Now, my point is not that such questions cannot be addressed. But our addressing of them is not helped by *assuming* that we know what, say, mental processes are like.

A primary issue here will connect the theories of sports psychology to the practice of sports psychology: that is, to practical interventions. For instance, do theories of imagery *impact* on the use of mental imagery (or mental rehearsal) etc. by sports performers or athletes? If the answer is 'no', then the imagery etc. is just used, at best, as mumbo-jumbo; it works but we do not know how, because which (if any) theoretical account is correct makes no difference. Moreover, we do not *really* care (as we have imagined it, *knowing* would not make a difference, since theory does not impact . . .). We treat it a bit like, say, faith-healing: if it keeps working, well and good – but we don't understand how.

If, by contrast, the answer were 'yes' (that theory can impact on practice) – and this *must* be the right answer if sports psychology is to deserve an academic pedigree – then using or getting the *wrong* theory will have a negative impact. It will make us unclear what to do, or yield misguided principles for intervention. Then it becomes important to select the *true* or *correct* theory (or, at least, the best approximation). But how can we choose among candidate theories?

Conceptual confusion means that we have no reliable basis for selecting one theory as preferable to another.

As a way forward, I suggest that we put aside questions about which theory is *true* in its entirety – as though any might be! – and turn instead to the sorts of factors we might appeal to when confronting competing theories: does Freud's work suggest raising different sets of factors, or different examples?

I will mention three ways in which Freud's ideas deserve more attention, ideas to be explored. For Freud's work is important *methodologically*, *conceptually* and *substantively*: all three points can be sketched, although to do so requires detailed engagement with Freud (of a kind often lacking in sports psychology, as we have seen). Hence, it moves us some way outside the context of sport.

## Does Freud deserve attention? (i) Methodology

The first insight, then, concerns the *methodology* of psychology: Freud's work was *particularist* in dealing with individuals, and denying a kind of generality. Popular misunderstandings of his work assume the opposite view. For instance, Freud is often supposed to believe that there were wholly general symbols ('Freudian symbols') to be found in dreams, stories and the like. In fact, Freud explicitly recognized that most of the images that are used in this way are personal – deriving from the person's life, and from what is of value to that person. Occasionally, symbols were more generally applicable but, typically, that fact could be explained. For example, Freud explains some commonalities discovered in dreams, in the following ways:

- '[T]his symbolism is not peculiar to dreams' (*Interpretation of Dreams*: PFL Vol. 4: 467). There is a fund of such symbols in myths, folklore, and so on. This is where we learn symbols, which partly explains generality; so 'we' read the same myths, etc. and myths drawn on what is human (feelings, etc.).
- '[M]any of the symbols are habitually or almost habitually employed to express the same thing' (PFL Vol. 4: 469). So one could generalize, but carefully – any such generalization will not be exceptionless (as 'cheetahs can run faster than men' is true without being exceptionless).

And, even then, these commonalities were just places analysis could *start* – to be potentially rejected by further consideration of *this* person! Thus, as his discussion of the way to make sense of dreams illustrates, Freud's strategy is a particularist one, not the universalist one usually ascribed to him. So that, asked whether we should interpret *all* dreams in this fashion, Freud replies: 'No, not at all ... ' (PFL Vol. 2: 4).

As already noted, Freud was especially good – by and large – at recognizing and acknowledging individual differences. This is not readily accommodated within certain models of scientific understanding: scientists do not care about the difference between *this* hydrogen molecule and *that* one (because, insofar as we regard them just as having the properties typical of hydrogen molecules, both are equivalent) – and if a particular flower lacks the characteristic colour then, for purposes of our biology class, it may be dismissed as *wrongly* coloured. In a not dissimilar way, an idealized (biomechanical) model of, say, a golf swing is used to criticize the actual swing of real golfers: for it is *supposed* to be the general pattern to which the *lame* efforts of Tiger Woods *et al.* approximate. And, of course, the point is not applied simply to those (say, John Daly) with unorthodox golf swings, but to all swings. So that, even when individual difference is noted, it is dismissed or minimized. Freud's thinking would militate against such a tendency.

Indeed, there is just the beginning, within sports psychology, of a stress on the need for a person-to-person relation between sportsperson and sports psychologist (for example, Gilbourne 1999; Holt and Strean 2001; Knowles *et al.* 2001[18]). A related idea, already pioneered in social psychology, comes from Rom Harré's slogan that one should treat people, for research purposes, as though they were human beings (Harré 1983: 160–1; Harré and Secord 1972: 101–23). On this picture, (i) our athletes are first-and-foremost people, who can be asked about what is going on, and whose judgements should be taken seriously, if not always accepted; (ii) what sometimes seems natural (or inevitable) should be recognized as contingent. So that it is a fact about *us*, in this set of social settings, that we see such-and-such as natural or inevitable. But those values have a social dimension: in another place, they might no longer seem inevitable. Here again, Freud's work, properly understood, can remind us of this contingency – that things might easily have been different, without minimizing that they are as they are. For example, consider the correct reading of Freud's views on aggression, from *Civilization and Its Discontents* (PFL 12), in contrast to the idea of the supposed inevitability of aggression: for Freud, social inequalities were fundamental to aggressive tendencies, although (of course) these were not the ones he set out to study. But his choice of methodology – to study those whose social position obviated these needs – precisely reflects his recognition of the contingencies of human life.

## More on methodology – determinism

Equally important in Freud's impact on *methodology* is his *humanistic* commitment: as we have noted, at its heart, Freud's work recognizes that people make choices, that they can do *this* or *that*. His picture of the mind (or the person) was not therefore deterministic: it did not assume that the behaviour of persons was the inevitable outcome of the working-out of the kinds of 'laws of nature' science identifies. Throughout, the (potential) *rationality* of persons was stressed. The contrasting view argues that the notion of choice is really an illusion: that persons' behaviour is not simply the outcome of factors beyond those persons' control. In this sense, it is often called an opposition to *free will*. Yet, in fact, the central thought rejects the idea of *agency*:[19] of people being able to intervene so as to change what happens. The first premise of this argument will be that every event has a cause. But only by reaching that conclusion does one count as a *determinist* (McFee 2000: 21[20]). Now, Freud does not use the term in only that sense. Instead, in some places, he writes as though all he was discussing was the explicability of psychological events; namely that 'nothing in the mind is ever arbitrary or undetermined' (PFL Vol. 5: 303). Moreover, 'the whole *Weltanschauung* [world-view] of science' would be overthrown if one believed in 'occurrences which might just as well happen as not happen' (PFL Vol. 1: 53). For Freud, then, the contrast *here* seems to be just with randomness.

In some cases, though, Freud seems to go further and write as if free will (or free action) is an illusion. But did Freud really need (for consistency) to take that further step? There seems no reason to suppose he does. Yet Freud often writes about 'determinism' (although not in our sense): '[Y]ou nourish a deeply rooted faith in undetermined psychical events and in free will, but ... this is quite unscientific and must yield to the demands of a determinism whose rule extends over mental life' (PFL Vol. 1: 136). Such remarks should be read either as an overstatement of his case for emphasis or as reflecting typical assumptions of his time, or both.

Genuine determinism on Freud's part would align him with much contemporary theory; and imply that *all* behaviour is *always* determined (in the sense of being the inexorable working out of causal laws) – rather than implying that *some* behaviour is *sometimes* determined. The contemporary explanation would invoke the dependence of psychological events on neural ones. And *that* does not seem to be Freud's view, since he explicitly refuses to reduce psychology to neurology.[21] For example, Freud avoids the mistaken ideas that knowledge of brains has much to do with psychology. As he puts it:

> We know two kinds of things about what we call our psyche (or mental life): firstly, its bodily organ and scene of action, the brain (or nervous system), and, on the other hand, our acts of consciousness, which are immediate data and cannot be further explained by any kind of description. Everything that lies between is unknown to us and the data do not include any direct relation between these two terminal points of our knowledge. If it existed, it would at the most afford an exact localization of the processes of consciousness and would give us no help towards understanding them. (PFL Vol. 15: 375–6)

Instead, we should begin from a conception of agency, rather than viewing this human power as something to be discovered, say, empirically. That is, Freud begins from what Lear has called the fact of our 'being minded', which recognizes the restlessness of minds by acknowledging that they are 'not mere algorithm performing machines ... do not merely follow out the logical consequences of an agent's beliefs and desires ...' (Lear 1998: 84). So the activities of minds are not linear (etc.), as, say, computers are. Instead, 'it is part of the very idea of a mind that a mind must be able to make leaps, to make associations, to bring things together and divide them up ...' (Lear 1998: 84–5). Therefore it would be odd to offer a 'reconstruction' of thought processes (of a kind required if computers did 'that thinking') as though one's mind were going through those same steps.

Consider a case, from a television programme, which claimed that a water-skier was making many thousands of calculations as she kept her balance. My reaction would be that elaborate mental arithmetic is quite a feat for someone simultaneously engaged in water-skiing; and my advice would be to keep her attention on what she is doing! The television programme, of course, meant something quite different: roughly, that if we chose to *simulate* the skier's behaviour using a computer – or perhaps a computer-controlled robot – and if we understood computers in a fashionable way, then *the computer* would be doing such calculations. Now, even this is not obviously true; but, either way, it has no obvious bearing on what that *person* was doing. For that person is not a computer, nor do we have any reason to model her behaviour as computation: if we think we do, it is because we have been listening to too much 'popular science'.

But what makes the computer modelling idea so attractive? Here, we should recognize that philosophy has regularly understood the person (roughly equivalent to the mind) on the model of the most complicated thing one could imagine at the time: for Descartes (1984 Vol. 1: 101), water features in ornamental gardens; for philosophers in the 1950s, telephone exchanges; for the 1990s/2000s, computers. Much recent philosophy seems to take for granted that minds (or persons) *resemble* computers in some important respects. John Searle[22] has dubbed the key project here 'Strong AI' (roughly, the view that mind is to brain as programme is to hardware; and hence that computers can genuinely be said to know, understand etc., rather than just to 'know', 'understand' etc.). We see more clearly the oddity of the underlying assumptions of this view when we recognize this focus on the most 'sophisticated' as the *real* reason for our analogy of mind (or, worse, brain) to computer. (And, of course, this will be another way to put aside the credentials of some putative *science* here.)

Of course, being able to argue seamlessly from brain processes to mental ones would – were it possible – suggest that there could be causal laws for the mind. This assumption (much beloved of some contemporary psychology) Freud insists on giving up. If we cannot argue from brain processes to mind processes (as Freud's comment above implies), we cannot have causal laws – or any other kind – here. But how might this be *demonstrated*?

Freud's argument draws on at least two kinds of cases. The first invokes ideogenic conditions (and similar): that is, generated by ideas (Wollheim 1971: 23). For example, people who (as a result of some trauma) had lost the use of a limb could regain its use under hypnosis. So any problem was not straightforwardly physical, in the sense of involving broken bones, tendons and the like. Since his time working with the French neurologist Charcot, Freud took such conditions to provide clear evidence for mental activity where forces were somehow 'latent and operative' (Wollheim 1971: 159). And Freud also noticed that such a loss of use of a limb from traumatic injury can be based on a *conception* of how the body works: so that paralysis of the leg might not reflect the fact that the socket for the head of the femur is in the groin. As Freud[23] puts it, the condition '*behaves as though anatomy did not exist or as though it had no knowledge of it*' (original italics). And similar points could be made about post-hypnotic suggestion.[24] Ideogenic conditions (etc.) of this sort are incompatible with a determinism based on, say, brain-states alone.

Freud's second case is yet more fundamental: that patient choice is incompatible with determinism. For patients must *choose* to visit the psychoanalyst – and granting such choice is granting agency. Of course, what this grants is not choice unlimited: we do not need to choose every little thing. So there is a need quite generally, and especially in sport, for 'automatic responses': that is, for 'grooved' responses, as when the sound of the car's engine straining prompts me to change gear – but I do so without noticing, and with no break in our conversation. Here we have become trained (etc.) to make choices, but without needing to think about them. Still, first, they are my choices, and I would be responsible if they were the wrong choices; second, I have the capacity to think beyond that training, to confront new situations – although that may take more time.

In conclusion, then, we have seen how Freud's methodological intentions work against some versions of the 'scientistic' view of sports psychology – a point made eloquently by Jim Parry (1998: 210), there applied directly to aggression in sport! Further, we have noted how accepting Freud's view would lead to the rejection of determinism (and some of its associated 'computer-modelling' of persons), and how it would speak for particularism, against a drive towards abstraction.

## Does Freud deserve attention? (ii) Conceptual structure

If Freud's work incorporates a powerful methodological insight for psychology, it also generates a very different conceptual structure from that regularly assumed. So, second, Freud's work deserves attention *conceptually*. He places great importance on psychological structure – that we cannot understand the mind without paying psychological structure due attention. Or, to put it another way, that the mind is rarely transparent.

In addition, a central relevance of this topic lies in its illustrating the evidential base for Freud's work, highlighting that it *is* empirical but without becoming scientistic, by helping us to understand the nature of clinical evidence.

We can usefully begin from some misplaced criticisms of Freud. For example, Grünbaum (1984) suggests that psychoanalysis is threatened by the mere *possibility* that (as Wollheim 1993: 110 puts it), 'it is impossible to free the evidence from the taint of suggestion by the analyst.' Were this so, Grünbaum concludes, psychoanalysis would be 'clinically unconfirmable' (Wollheim 1993: 110), since *suggestibility* might provide a possible explanation of 'why the patient recalls his past as he does, why he free-associates as he does, why he recounts his dreams as he does ... and, most sobering of all, why he gets well if he does' (Wollheim 1993: 110) Freud was aware of this potential problem.[25] But Grünbaum's version of the worry simply reflects his failure to grasp the place of psychological structure, as Freud reconstructs it, combined with a failure to grasp the logic of the situation. For what is the status of Grünbaum's suggestion that there might be *suggestion*?

Grünbaum's strategy here is sceptical: that the mere possibility of *suggestion* must be ruled out, if we are to trust what our patient says. But the starting place of scepticism is simply *justified* scepticism in *this* case (Descartes 1984 Vol. 2: 12: 'with respect to objects that are very small or in the distance . . .'), for *this* reason – there is no basis for generalizing. So the fact that, in some special circumstances, we do have *reason* for scepticism gives us no general reason to be sceptical in an area (see McFee 2000: 141).

Of course, sometimes we have just such a genuine reason for scepticism, where something about this case raises the question of whether (in *this* case) we do know, or gives reason to be hesitant. And there is a *parallel* in the psychoanalytic case: if I have *reason* to doubt that this patient is genuinely remembering (or genuinely working through), I have reason to be hesitant. But, lacking such a reason, there is no basis for doubt. So the question is: *Why should you rule it in?* rather than *How do you rule it out?* As with scepticism, *in reality* doubt must always be *grounded* doubt – if we have no (specific) reason to suspect suggestion by the analyst in the case, we have no basis for raising the possibility:

- In a situation where suggestion is *likely* (compare lying), we have a reason *in that case*.
- In a situation where there is no such likelihood, we have no reason.

So, like lying, suggestion by the analyst is a serious *practical* worry – but no more than that.

Thus Grünbaum misconceives the nature of clinical evidence by treating it in too attenuated a fashion. For example, the Rat Man's pacing up and down ('A Case of Obsessional Neurosis', 1909: PFL Vol. 9: 89–90) is, for Freud, important in understanding what occurred in the particular clinical setting – what events took place. Here, what the Rat Man's pacing displays has a profound significance for his psychological state, especially his dissatisfaction with the penetrating nature of the analysis. Of course, the behaviour at issue (pacing up and down) is not obviously psychological, nor does it seem obviously to suggest the kinds of psychological states discussed by those who begin by contrasting the mental with the physical. Rather, it reflects Freud's commitment to the idea of a 'bodily ego' (PFL Vol. 11: 364: Wollheim 1993: 64–78). Moreover, we should be clear that sports psychology – in its desire for repeatability (see, for example, Woods 2001 11–13) – will find it hard to regard *this* pacing (and not [necessarily] other examples) as *data*.

Once we start to doubt it, though, it is just a small step from *justified* scepticism to something more fundamental. Thus, Wollheim (1993: 111) follows Fine and Forbes in noting how:

> [S]uggestibility starts off . . . as a mere place-holder for sceptical doubt. But gradually it escalates. Its claims upon our credence grow: its content is

inflated. Soon it appears as an alternative theory to psychoanalysis, replete with its own hypotheses. (Wollheim 1993: 111)

For Grünbaum, then, the mere possibility of suggestion can soon generate an alternative picture of the clinical setting; and one which does no justice to Freud's account of what occurs in that setting.

In part, then, the debate turns on the nature of the evidence here. Thus, as Grünbaum (1984: 253) points out, in understanding the event Freud drew on material (ostensibly) from the Rat Man's mother. Yet Freud had never met her. But this material was provided by the Rat Man, and helped Freud make sense of which among competing ways of understanding the Rat Man was preferable. That is, it functioned as one might look to something else that was said and, by giving it credibility, choose to understand other behaviour a certain way. ('She flashed her headlights; that probably wasn't a joke, wasn't without significance; and it is towards dusk; so I probably don't have my own headlights on'.) So, again, Freud's attitudes to understanding seem straightforward. There, as here, one has an 'hypothesis' one might 'test'!

This example shows that, in the clinical situation, the question 'What happened?' cannot be reduced to some 'lowest common denominator' (say, of bodily motions) if it is to be genuinely understood. For what happened may need to be seen in psychologically complex terms. And this is what Grünbaum fails to do: in particular, through his seeking accounts of the clinical sessions *detached* from central Freudian concepts. Instead: '[I]f the hypotheses that clinical testing tests are to be restored to anything like a recognisably Freudian character, they have to have a great deal more psychological structure restored to them or built back into them . . .' (Wollheim 1993: 108).

For only then will we see, in (say) the Rat Man's pacing back and forth, what is thereby visible of his psychology. And once this restoration is done, as Wollheim (1993: 109) notes, the possibilities of the clinical session in particular, its evidential possibilities – become far greater: 'Put structure in, and then clinical testing has to become ingenious enough in its procedures to tell us not only whether, given an initial condition, a further condition comes about, but how it does so or along what route'.

No doubt there is a danger here. For, if Freud's account is completely misconceived, to require its being taken seriously will hinder us – as though we could only grasp the significance of the earth's flatness by first believing it! The problem, though, is one familiar in the philosophy of science:[26] that asking questions about, say, forces and accelerations involves the application of those concepts – that Greek science (which lacked those concepts) could not even understand the question, let alone answer it. And, lest we get too complacent, recall that putting similar questions *once* we have recognized Einstein's insights into, for example, the meaning of the term 'straight line' will be similarly problematic: our accounts of all such vectors is transformed. So there is a note of warning to be struck here: care is needed. But nothing here need preclude our going forward.

What we see, then, is the improbability of success for any psychological theory that fails to recognize, or ignores, psychological structure in this way. Of course, the selected psychological structure might not be Freud's: that would be a matter for further detailed discussion. But Freud's insight here lies in recognizing the need – within our understanding of happenings (clinical or non-clinical) – for a sophisticated view of psychological structure. In contrast, sports psychology typically has assumed that describing behaviour (almost) automatically yields *data*.

## A complexity of structure: the social character of individuals

As well as stressing, in this way, the importance of *recognizing* psychological structure, Freud emphasizes a dimension to the psychological less individualistic than is often assumed: that is, he recognizes that individuals cannot be viewed atomistically. Instead Freud's account of the acquisition of rule-related understanding, and of morality, has a social dimension that is absent from much sports psychology (cf. Wollheim 1984: 198–205). For example, the 'internal agent' of morality, the super-ego, 'represents more than anything the cultural past' (*Outline of Psychoanalysis*: PFL Vol. 15: 443). And Freud is even more explicit:

> [I]t represents the influence of a person's childhood, of the care and education given to him by his parents and his dependence on them . . .. And . . . it is not only the personal qualities of these parents that is making itself felt, but everything that has a determining effect upon them ... [for example] the taste and standards of the social class in which they lived. (PFL Vol. 15: 442)

Further, the activities of the super-ego should be seen as regularly following that person's sense of him/herself: so that, for example, shame and/or guilt should be understood as arising from a person's coming to think less well of him/herself. One chief insight here is that the prohibitions and concerns (for example, of morality) are partly internal and partly external; but not as they are often theorized. For what is external is, in effect, what is learned – and, while some of that learning may be reducible to training when young, some is genuine learning (and hence the province of personal agents). Moreover, what is internal *really* is: in favoured cases, I genuinely hold the moral prohibitions I espouse (against, say, cheating, deception and so on), even though they may have been learned, and even built on training. Likewise, I am the one who espouses such-and-such as a virtue: it is certainly not reducible to what others believe or accept. In these ways, then, we see how Freud's account reinstates the *person*.

Moreover, persons are not thought of as isolated from one another: although there is something individualistic here – there are no super-individual concepts – the individuals are not treated atomistically.[27] Further, this 'social' conception of agency is explained through the development of our understanding: in particular, its dependence on sets of values which antedate us, and into which we grow.

The argument here is complex: roughly, that the kinds of regularities that are tracked by *causal laws* are inadequate for the theorization of action – that one must distinguish the case of following, or failing to follow, the rule ('yes, he was on-side') from cases where the particular rule-following action was adventitious or not ('yes, it was a legitimate move in chess; shame it was a bad one!' – where, again, the speaker could be wrong). As it might be put, such rules (and similar) import *normativity* (McFee 2000: 88–9). The behaviour of trained seals can *conform* to rules; but only agents can genuinely follow rules – and, where they do, that rule-following can be adventitious or not (McFee 2000: 88–9).

When we come to consider how sports behaviour should be understood – which is as a *process* – this conception is just what one needs: it makes us see *people*, not systems or processors, and it recognizes the *social* character built into all human interaction. Yet a huge problem here concerns how this recognition is developed in practice. Moreover, we have stressed that human behaviour must be seen as the activity of rational agents. But our Freudian picture recognizes the holistic nature of much human understanding; as such, it works against the 'boxes' mentality prevalent in sports psychology, where what is hoped for is a graphical model of *boxes* connected by *arrows* – as though we knew what the boxes or arrows meant!

This point can be difficult to illustrate: begin by looking at, say, a schematic information-processing model of perception (see Figure 5.1).

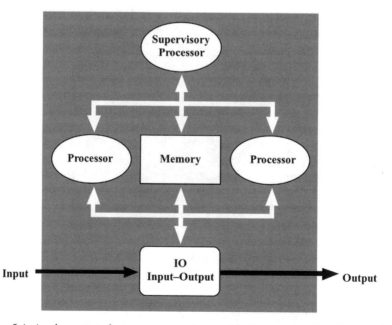

*Figure 5.1* A schematic information-processing model of perception (based on Lindsay and Norman 1977: 603).

Now, the term 'perception' here is just a catch-all for seeing, hearing, tasting, touching, smelling; activities of persons. And what is being perceived would typically at least *begin* from objects: tables, chairs, glasses of beer, watches. If the question were, 'How do humans see objects?', the diagram obviously cannot help, since it just ascribes all the hard work to one of the boxes (with its associated arrows): in this case, one of the boxes marked 'processor' or that marked 'supervisory processor'. For, if we begin from 'information in' (that is, I see stuff) and conclude either with 'information out' (I remark, 'I see a so-and-so') or with action (I grab it), the crucial issue is how the first gets 'turned into' the second: how my seeing the beer and my drinking it are related. That is to say, how do *I* mediate between the perception and the action? We can put the question more fully, by importing further assumptions (for the sake of argument): How do *I* turn the information from my perception into action? And, if we put the question in terms of the diagram, and conclude that either one of the processors or the supervisory processor does it by processing the information (perhaps storing it, drawing on other information, and so on), we have really made no progress. We still want to know how the perception is mediated to lead to the action, and that is not the sort of question such a model *could* answer.

In a humorous moment in a book on consciousness, Dan Dennett (1991: 38) includes a cartoon in which two scientists confront a blackboard covered with equations and the like (Figure 5.2): the caption reads, 'I think you should be

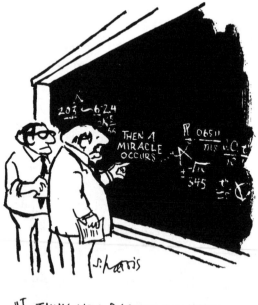

"I THINK YOU SHOULD BE MORE
EXPLICIT HERE IN STEP TWO."

*Figure 5.2* A humorous moment from 'Consciousness Explained' (Dennett, 1991).

more explicit here in step two' – step two reads, 'Then a miracle occurs'. Obviously, that remark is not an explanation within science – perhaps not an explanation at all. In one sense, the problem I am identifying is just this one: the 'processor'/'supervisory processor' boxes in Figure 5.1 simply stand in for the person doing the 'processing'. If we think of the problem in this way, it instantiates the *homunculus fallacy* (Kenny 1984: 125–36), on which we explain how people are able to do such-and-such by postulating a little person (a homunculus) 'inside' each of us, who actually does the thing. But if the little person inside can just *do* whatever, why can't the ordinary person? In this way, granting power to the homunculus *but not* the person simply repeats the problem.

In another way, our case is really the reverse of this one for, rather than having something completely unexplained at work, we have an ordinary explanation for my beer-drinking behaviour, in seeing and picking up the beer – featuring, say, my eagle-eyes and my fondness for beer – which seems to leave out very little. And, again, the comparison with the homunculus brings this out. For what *seemed* to be needed was an explanation of how person *did* such-and-such: it turns out the explanation might just be that persons can do such things!

I have been juxtaposing Freud's account, which stresses humans' rational powers and the capacity to act, with a particular example of the 'box-and-arrow' models of psychology: of course, not all models embody precisely this mistake. But there are, as it were, versions of this same set of mistakes: we need to understand what the boxes and the arrows represent – and the models themselves cannot help us with that, since they are what stands in need of explanation. This is one of the many places where a picture is worth a thousand words only if accompanied by the thousand words.

Consider a 'model' of adherence to psychological skills training, in Figure 5.3 (Shambrook and Bull 1999: 185): the *exact* meaning of its arrows may remain unclear. The stated purpose of this model is to guide sports psychology consultants providing psychological skills training to athletes; some of the arrows represent 'influences' while others show the 'structure'. The danger lies in thinking that the picture does more work than it can in making these ideas clear to their target audience.

The difficulty, though, is not simply the unclarity of some key ideas presented here. Rather, the difficulty lies in how, within sports psychology, to give weight to the social nature of human life – what Freud picks up as the social character of the individual. That means, roughly, that one's understanding of human life needs a social element which operates pervasively (and differentially) across all of the boxes in a model. For Freud's work brings out the logical dependence of our values on theirs (even when we differ), even when we seem most unconnected to our fellow humans.

Here, then, Freud's general commitment to the importance of psychological structure, and his specific commitment to the social character of such structure, should be contrasted with certain influential positions within contemporary sports psychology. In particular, of course, it should be contrasted with any behaviouristic account of psychology, on which the concern is with patterns of

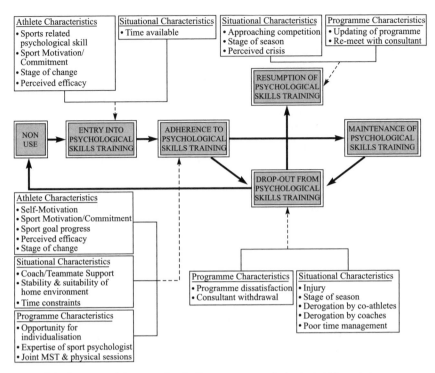

*Figure 5.3* Conceptual framework of adherence to psychological skills training.

dispositions to behave in characteristic ways under certain physical conditions. No doubt such conceptions most readily yield experimental protocols for psychology; but they precisely ignore much that Freud took to be crucial. Instead, he is considering people; and, typically, in social contexts.

### Does Freud deserve attention? (iii) A view of persons

So, third, Freud's work deserves more attention *substantively*. For central to the insights that sports psychology could have got from Freud – therefore, central to its present lack – is the view of persons possible within a psychoanalytically inclined psychology. In contrast, Ted Honderich (2001: 9) speaks for many in the philosophical community when he dismisses Freud by writing of his own view of 'minds, which is to say mainly about consciousness'. Yet the mind is not always best approached via discussion of consciousness. But this need not endorse starting from the *unconscious*: rather, we should recognize that any account of the mind must do justice to, say, *dreaming* – but dreaming has neither a bodily 'face' (of presently dreaming) nor an obvious connection to consciousness.[28] This illustrates that there are more and less illuminating ways to talk about persons' powers and capacities. Following Wollheim,[29] the suggestion is to augment one's account of the mind by drawing on ideas from Freudian psychoanalysis. These should include at least four, already mentioned: first, the idea of a 'bodily ego' (PFL Vol. 11: 364; Wollheim 1993: 64–78) will stress the essential embodiment of persons; second, the social character of a super-ego, thought of in terms of 'the growth of moral sentiments. moral beliefs, moral habits in the typical life-history of the individual' (Wollheim 1984: 198) since it 'represents more than anything the cultural past' (*Outline of Psychoanalysis*: PFL Vol. 15: 443).

The third element recognizes persons as rational agents: as our retelling of Freud's discussion of aggression (above) highlighted, this possibility is fundamental to any account of what we might achieve, and of how we might go about it.

The fourth feature is a connection to the history of one's psychological development. For example, as Wollheim's (1999: see also Young 2001) thinking here elaborates, the emotions are best understood historically, in their origination, development and interaction with other things. For emotions are complex phenomena, not easily dismissed (as in much philosophy) as mere *propositional attitudes*: that is, as attitudes (such as beliefs) towards propositions or other 'representations'. So central here will be the recognition of the importance of a history for what can truly be said of a particular person (even if that history is not Freud's). Saying this emphasizes the developmental character of our powers and capacities, plus our ability to learn: the possibility of learning is especially important for persons, and should be contrasted with, say, *socialization*, since learning is a rational process. Moreover, this stress on the powers and capacities of persons works against a predominant rationalism. For what is at issue is what persons can do: and this, one might think, is just what sports psychology requires.

One importance of *history* here is that it recognizes the *process* character of human psychology. For instance, we *come to* a particular emotion, etc., sometimes through learning, sometimes through training (that is, causally). For example, if the mastery of depressive anxiety requires 'the concept of a whole object or a whole person' (Wollheim 1984: 207), while persecutory anxiety does not, I must come to frame that distinction if I am to experience depressive anxiety. The emotion is a cognitive achievement. So, importantly, there was a time when we did not possess it, and a time when we possessed it only to some degree (or possessed some strongly similar proto-emotion etc.), as well as the case when we have it in its full-blown form. And Freud is among a handful of thinkers – I would also mention Aristotle and Wittgenstein[30] – who take seriously the fact that all adults were once children; that is, Freud integrates this thought into a view of the mind.

A fifth feature grows from these: for learning here will often involve being able to do certain things – we should not imagine that, for Freud, psychological activity was to be sharply contrasted with physical activity. Indeed, how could it be, for a *bodily ego*?

In Freud, then, we find a picture of agents whose interaction with other agents should be seen in precisely that way: agents who can learn from and rationally influence others, but also be trained by them.

In these ways, Freud recognizes persons as central to the project of psychology, as changeable (and therefore process-directed), and as having essential social connections. Each of these represents a departure from some of the rampant individualism of much sports psychology.

## Conclusion

So, in summary, why is Freud's work neglected in sports psychology (for surely I have shown that it is, at the least, under-represented)? The reasons offered, or the objections made, are revealing about assumptions entertained. To recapitulate: one set of *candidate* reasons would be that Freudian ideas make sports psychology too hard (because too tailored to individual athletes); that they conflict with an understanding of the scientificity of psychology; and that they don't allow genuine interventions – either things cannot be changed readily, or changing them is unreasonably time-consuming.

My reply began by highlighting the scientistic model of psychology from which such criticisms begin: rejecting that model will change the balance of probabilities here. Further, once we recognize the individual or particular character of many *useful* interventions from sports psychology, and the humanistic conception of sports psychological knowledge and research that these subtend (Sparkes 1992: 24–9), these objections obviously represent nothing more than adherence to a certain model of science and of knowledge. And that model seems highly suspect, given developments in the philosophy of science.[31] Rejecting that scientistic model makes logical space for Freud. And I have shown how this might be done. I have also implied that one cannot simply dismiss Freud's work as wrong-headed: that, at the least, there was something to be said for his work as a whole, even when details are rejected.

My real point, though, is that the sets of objections raised could not *justify* the neglect of Freud by sports psychology, even if they go some way towards explaining that neglect, especially once the (suspect) connection of psychoanalysis to therapy or 'the couch' is factored-in. Still, if these are the best that opponents can offer as objections, they are pretty lame.

In contrast, I have suggested that taking seriously Freud's work *methodologically*, *conceptually*, and *substantively* has the capacity to reshape one's sports psychology by making it more particularist, less deterministic, more socially inflected, and more person-centred. Precisely what these might amount to for sports psychology in practice remains a good question; and certainly not one answered conclusively here. So one big task remains to identify some of the potential impact, for a revitalized sports psychology, of (re)introducing Freudian ideas. Often, this is less a question of *doing* something different than of understanding it differently. For example:

- a focus on individuals, rather than on groups – practised at present (at least by some sports psychologists) but now explained in Freud's terms;
- the impact on methodology: for instance, use of case-evidential models –

part of a general liberalization, and a move away from the statistical (this is partly a move away from a certain view of scientific 'validity').

It might seem that this is a non-specific outcome: that I have not suggested specific changes that could be made, nor specific theories (or accounts) of sport that should be deployed. But this is a *feature* of my position, not an objection to it. The emphasis here has not fallen on specific *ideas* that sports psychology should develop, because to do so would go against Freud's particularist message – that improvements in both applied sports psychology and in the underpinning theory can only be case-by-case. For the evidential base will include the parallel to Freud's clinical evidence.

As a consequence, there will be less we can say in the abstract – hence, less we can say about *all* those who are engaged in sport. Therefore this is (explicitly) a recipe for a kind of particularism, the kind both needed (if considerations from Freud are well-taken) and currently lacking. But a detailed study of Freud's *own* writings should have done more. We must conclude that Freud's critics failed to make clear this particularism; that they offered, at best, simplified versions of his key ideas. Indeed, this is an outcome Freud (1966)[32] foresaw:

> [Q]ualifications and exact particularisation are of little use with the general public; there is very little room in the memory of the multitude; it retains only the bare gist of any thesis and fabricates an extreme version which is easy to remember.

His point is that what is *taken* from his theoretically precise accounts of human beings is, instead, something inexact; and where that inexactness follows from how Freud's works are presented to a general audience.

So the stress has fallen rather on general concerns, especially methodological ones, that sports psychology should seek to address. For these are all one can write in the abstract. Still, we can see how – if, say, one's goals related to adherence to mental skills training – one's practice, and one's theory, might become more athlete-centred, and might move away from dealing with the team *en masse*, and how this emphasis might need to be accommodated within one's bidding for contracts to provide sports psychology support to (for instance) national teams.

Would such a conclusion *really* spell a return to Freud? I would answer 'no': but it would spell a return, at the abstract level, to various themes foregrounded in Freud's work – a *process* conception of psychology, a person-centred conception of the mind (beginning from *agency*), a particularist picture of theory and application. No doubt these could have been arrived at elsewhere. The need for a view of minds or persons might well be satisfied through an account similar to Freud's. At the least, there must be promise in asking that psychology treats *as agents* (and hence as rational) the aggressive athletes in one's squad or team. But, in Freud, we have both a 'founding father' and a meticulous writer who, when properly understood (and rationally reconstructed), exemplifies just these methodological virtues.

One response here would dispute that I have *really* characterized sports psychology, in the examples discussed. These are *my* examples but, as was said initially, they were chosen to best exemplify trends I discerned. Of course, both my examples and my discernment might be challenged. The structure of this chapter involves disputing concrete claims: hence my use of real examples. Since the examples were not selected by any respectable research method, they have only the force of having been found. But to the degree that they are typical, my critique is justified.

Might a more sophisticated version of sports psychology avoid the criticisms voiced here concerning some themes from the contemporary literature of sports psychology? Well, the whole idea behind this chapter is to aid in producing a legitimate sports psychology which does just that. My thought has been to highlight some central issues by drawing on Freudian ideas, but nothing in the discussion requires that the *conclusions* be Freud's – my thought was only that, without Freud, the *issues* might go unnoticed. Also, having no clear view of the purposes, or resources, of sports psychology, one must not conclude that a sports psychology *cannot* ignore Freud. Equally, one must look (as here) at the consequences of doing so. But, just as later philosophy might be Platonist without mentioning, or even reading, Plato, any plausible sports psychology should not avoid acknowledging the points here drawn from Freud. That need not make it Freudian – nor even Freud-influenced. But the impact of ideas we have located in Freud seems fundamental. In these ways, then, ignoring, neglecting, misinterpreting or not considering Freud might still be some of the many paths towards misunderstanding in sports psychology.

## Bibliography

Appignanesi, L. and Forrester, J. (1992) *Freud's Women*, London: Virago Press.

Baker, G. and Morris, K. (1996) *Descartes' Dualism*, London: Routledge.

Bredemeier, B.J. and Shields, D.L. (1986) 'Athletic aggression: an issue of contextual morality', *Sociology of Sport Journal*, 3, 15–38.

Chalmers, A.F. (1982) *What is This Thing Called Science?* 2nd edn, Milton Keynes: Open University Press.

Davies, D. (1989) *Psychological Factors in Competitive Sport*, London: Falmer Press.

Dennett, D. (1991) *Consciousness Explained*, Harmondsworth: Allen Lane.

Descartes, R. (1984) *The Philosophical Writings of Descartes*, three vols (trans. J. Cottingham, R. Stoothoff and D. Murdoch), Cambridge: Cambridge University Press.

Diamant, L. (ed.) (1991a) *Psychology of Sports, Exercise and Fitness*, London: Hemisphere Publishing.

Diamant, L. (ed.) (1991b) *Mind-Body Maturity*, London: Hemisphere Publishing.

Evans, L., Hardy, L. and Fleming, S. (2000a) 'Intervention strategies with injured athletes: an action research study', *The Sports Psychologist*, 14, 188–206.

Evans, L. Fleming, S. and Hardy, L. (2000b) 'Situating action research: a response to Gilbourne', *The Sports Psychologist*, 14, 296–303.

Feyerabend, P. (1993) *Against Method*, 3rd edn, London: Verso.

Freud, S. (various dates) *The Penguin Freud Library*, 15 vols, Harmondsworth: Penguin.

Freud, S. (1966) *The Standard Edition of the Complete Psychological Works*, 24 vols, London: Hogarth Press.

Gilbourne, D. (1999) 'Collaboration and reflection: adopting action research themes and processes to promote adherence to changing practice', in S. Bull (ed.) *Adherence Issues in Sport and Exercise*, Chichester: Wiley, 239–61.

Gilbourne, D. (2000) 'Searching for the nature of action research: a response to Evans, Hardy and Fleming', *The Sports Psychologist*, 14, 207–14.

Gill, D.L. (1986) *Psychological Dynamics of Sport*, Champaign, IL: Human Kinetics.

Gomberg, P. (2000) 'Patriotism in sports and in war', in T. Tännsjö and C. Tamburrini (eds) *Values in Sport*. London: Routledge, 87–98.

Gough, R. (1998) 'Moral development research in sports and its quest for objectivity', in M. McNamee and S.J. Parry (eds) *Ethics and Sport*, London: Routledge, 133–47.

Grünbaum, A. (1984) *The Foundations of Psychoanalysis: A Philosophical Critique*, Berkeley: University of California Press.

Hackford, D. and Spielberger, C.D. (eds) (1989) *Anxiety in Sports*, London: Hemisphere Publishing.

Hardy, L., Jones, G. and Gould, D. (1996) *Understanding Psychological Preparation for Sport: Theory and Practice of Elite Performers*, Chichester: Wiley.

Harré, R. (1983) 'An analysis of social activity', in J. Miller (ed.) *States of Mind: Conversations with Psychological Investigators*, London: BBC, 154–72.

Harré, R. and Secord, P. (P.F.) (1972) *The Explanation of Social Behaviour*, Oxford: Blackwell.

Holt, N.L. and Strean, W.B. (2001) 'Reflecting on initiating sports psychology consultation: a self-narrative of neophyte practice', *The Sports Psychologist*, 15, 188–204.

Honderich, T. (2001) *Philosopher: A Kind of Life*, London: Routledge.

Kenny, A. (1984) *The Legacy of Wittgenstein*, Oxford: Blackwell.

Knowles, Z., Gilbourne, D., Borrie, A. and Nevill, A. (2001) 'Developing reflective sports coaches: a study exploring the processes of reflective practice within higher education coaching programmes', *Reflective Practice*, 2, 185–207.

Kremer, J. and Scully, D. (1994) *Psychology in Sport*, London: Taylor and Francis.

Kuhn, T.S. (1970) *The Structure of Scientific Revolutions*, 2nd edn, Chicago: University of Chicago Press.

Kuhn, T.S. (2000) *The Road Since Structure*, Chicago: University of Chicago Press,

Lear, J. (1990) *Love and Its Place in Nature*, London: Macmillan.

Lear, J. (1998) *Open Minded*, Cambridge, MA: Harvard University Press.

Lear, J. (2000) *Happiness, Death and the Remainder of Life*, Cambridge, MA: Harvard University Press.

Lindsay, P.H. and Norman, D.A. (1977) *Human Information Processing*, 2nd edn, New York: Academic Press.

McFee, G. (1993) 'Reflections on the nature of action research', *Cambridge Journal of Education*, 23, 173–83.

McFee, G. (1994) 'The surface grammar of dreaming', *Proceedings of the Aristotelian Society*, XCIV, 95–115.

McFee, G. (2000) *Free Will*, Teddington: Acumen.

McFee, G. (2002) 'The place of philosophy in the study of sport', in J. Sugden and A. Tomlinson (eds) *Power Games*, London: Routledge, 117–37.

Mitchell, J. (1975) *Psychoanalysis and Feminism*, Harmondsworth: Penguin.

Moxon, D. (2000) *Memory*, London: Heinemann.

Nagel, T. (1995) *Other Minds*, Oxford: Oxford University Press.

Parry, S.J. (1998) 'Violence and aggression in contemporary sport', in M. McNamee and S.J. Parry (eds) *Ethics and Sport*, London: Routledge, 205–24.

Searle, J. (1980) 'Minds, brains and programmes', *Behavioural and Brain Science*, 3, 417–57. (This article is also available in Boden, M. (ed.) (1990) *The Philosophy of Artificial Intelligence*, London: Oxford, 67–88; and in Bourne, R. (ed.) (1987) *Artificial Intelligence: The Case Against*, London; Routledge, 18–40.)

Searle, J. (1984) *Minds, Brains and Science*, London: BBC, 32–8.

Searle, J. (1992) *The Rediscovery of the Mind*, Cambridge, MA: Bradford Books.

Shambrook, C. and Bull, S. (1999) 'Adherence to psychological preparation in sport', in S. Bull (ed.), *Adherence Issues in Sport and Exercise*, Chichester: Wiley, 169–98.

Sparkes, A. (1992) 'The paradigm debate: an extended review and a celebration of difference', in A. Sparkes (ed.) *Research in Physical Education and Sport: Exploring Alternative Visions*, London: Falmer Press, 9–60.

Vealey, R.S. (1994) 'Current status and prominent issues in sports psychology interventions', *Medicine and Science in Sports and Exercise*, 26, 495–502.

Weinberg, R.S. and Gould, D. (1995) *Foundations of Sport and Exercise Psychology*, Champaign, IL: Human Kinetics.

Williams, C. and James, D. (2001) *Science for Exercise and Sport*, London: Routledge.

Wittgenstein, L. (1953) *Philosophical Investigations*, Oxford: Blackwell.

Wollheim, R. (1971) *Freud*, London: Fontana.

Wollheim, R. (1984a) *The Thread of Life*, Cambridge: Cambridge University Press.

Wollheim, R. (1984b) *The Mind and Its Depths*, Cambridge, MA: Harvard University Press.

Wollheim, R. (1999) *On the Emotions*, New Haven: Yale University Press.

Woods, B. (2001) *Psychology in Practice: Sport*, London: Hodder & Stoughton.

Young, J.O. (2001) Review of *On the Emotions*, *Journal of Aesthetics and Art Criticism*, 59, 336–7.

## Notes

1   A good example: the discussion of the place (if any) of *paradigms*, in Kuhn's sense, in sports psychology. Hardy *et al.* (1996: 257) state that 'Kuhn (1962) *defined* a scientific paradigm as a school of thought relative to the nature of knowledge and how one goes about studying the world' (my emphasis). This is quite wrong, and could scarcely have been written by someone familiar with Kuhn's work – in particular, with *The Structure of Scientific Revolutions* (1962; 2nd edn 1970) – which stresses that paradigms function sometimes within what Kuhn calls 'normal science', where there is one paradigm in place (within a particular area of science). During such a period, the scientist works to make explicit the implications of that paradigm. So Kuhn (1970: 10) explains that *normal science* is: 'firmly based upon one or more scientific achievements, achievements that some particular scientific community acknowledges for a time as supplying the foundation for its future practice'.

Indeed, that foundation just is the paradigm: thus, the practitioner of normal science 'has … assimilated a time-tested and group-licenced way of seeing' (Kuhn 1970: 189). A paradigm, then, just is 'a time-tested and group-licenced way of seeing': and, in his later writing especially, Kuhn was at pains to clarify each of these ideas.

In contrast, there might be periods of crisis (or of *revolutionary science*) where, within a particular area of science, no one paradigm held sway. And the history of any particular area of science should be seen as fluctuating between phases of 'normal science' and 'revolutionary science'. Indeed, this was a fundamental characteristic of (natural) science, on Kuhn's view (see McFee 1993: 183).

These ideas are radically misunderstood by those who do not recognize, or fail to give weight to, the place of normal science. Kuhn was very clear that the idea of *normal science* had no role outside natural science; and hence that the idea of a *paradigm* did not either. As he wrote: '[T]he practice of astronomy, physics, chemistry or biology normally fails to evoke the controversies over fundamentals that today often seem endemic among, say, psychologists or sociologists' (Kuhn 1970: viii).

That is, the idea of 'normal science' (central to Kuhn's account) makes no sense outside natural science – contrary to what many commentators write, and contrary to the widespread use of the term 'paradigm' in social scientific contexts. (For a very different view, see Sparkes 1992.)

2  And even when somewhat more detailed notations are supplied (as in Diamant 1991a: 122–3), we are still left in the dark as to the precise pages.

3  To demonstrate the point, though, may make some early sections here seem slightly pedantic.

4  We are told that: 'It was Sigmund Freud who stressed the anticipatory nature of anxiety' (Davies 1989: 71), without any sense of whether this was insight or blunder, or how we might decide.

5  See, for instance, the view of science offered in Williams and James (2001: 4–5).

6  Similar points could have been made about, for example, Kremer and Scully (1994); or the essays in Hackfort and Spielberger (1989).

7  The beginner here could usefully begin from Wollheim (1971).

8  Reference to Freud's works will usually be to the *Penguin Freud Library* (15 vols) – cited as 'PFL' followed by volume and page number.

9  An additional problem: the question of translation.

10  Partly, this might require little more than avoiding gross misperceptions or misunderstandings of what Freud actually said (and meant). For instance, the widely heard accusation of misogyny might be met by the view of Juliet Mitchell (1975: xv): '[A] rejection of psychoanalysis and of Freud's work is fatal to feminism ... if we are interested in understanding and challenging the oppression of women, we cannot afford to neglect it'. (For more down this particular road, see Appignanesi and Forrester 1992: 460–2.)

11  We should also note, in passing, a confusion inherent within this attitude: Freud's work is both seen as not amenable to *proper* evidence, and yet some of his views are clearly false. This cannot be right. If there is enough evidence to assess Freud's claims, then they do submit to evidential assessment.

12  Here I follow Wollheim (1971: 232–4), who lays out Freud's answer here in a clear fashion, under four headings.

13  However, these last two may not be so distinct: at the end of *Why War?*, Freud writes of 'strengthening of intellectual life *and* renunciation of instinct' (PFL Vol. 12: 362: my emphasis). (Note: 'renunciation' is not really 'getting rid of': PFL Vol. 12: 358.)

14  See Gough (1998) to highlight other errors in the account they favour, and in their methodological assumptions.

15  Gill is probably the source of many of these discussions, to judge by the citations.

16  Although, as Woods (2001: 2), among others, notes, there can be a clinical aspect to the sports psychologist's work, dealing with emotional or behavioural problems such as depression, addiction, etc.

17  As an aside: is this really true? *Every?*

18  One impetus for these ideas is found in Vealey (1994); see also Evans *et al.* (2000a, 2000b); Gilbourne (2000).

19  This technical notion includes omissions, and might be contrasted with the kind of movement of, say, clouds: further, the issue here concerns whether or not there is agency (or choice) in the world, not how much there is (see McFee 2000: 8–9).

20  This is a terminological point: I use the term 'determinism' to apply to the conclusion of the argument; roughly to the effect that therefore the notion of human agency makes no sense.

21  Freud was generally very clear in separating questions of biology from those of psychology: we see this most clearly when he goes on to apologize for failing to do so. 'I try in general to keep psychology clear from everything that is in general different from it, even biological lines of thought' (PFL Vol. 11: 71).

22  Searle (1984: 32–8; 1980: esp. 417–19; 1992: 42–5; 201).

23  'Some Points for a Comparative Study of Organic and Hysterical Motor Paralyses' (1893) *Standard Edition* Vol. 1: 169 – not in PFL: see also Wollheim (1971: 23).

24  As Freud puts it:

The real stimulus to the action being the order of the physician, it is hard not to concede that the idea of the physician's order became active too. Yet this last did not reveal itself to consciousness, as did its outcome, the idea of the action; it remained unconscious, and so was active and unconscious at the same time. (PFL Vol. 11: 51–2.)

25  For example, in a footnote of 1924 he writes that, at an earlier time 'I had not yet found out how to distinguish between the patients' phantasies about their childhood and real memories' ('Further Remarks on the Neuro-Psychoses of Defence' (1896) *Standard Edition* Vol. 3 – not in PFL).

26  See in particular Kuhn (2000: esp. 16–32).

27  Hence, it is not something a methodological individualist could endorse. Against methodological individualism, see McFee (2002: 124–6).

28  Thus, writers who believe that (real) dreams occur during REM sleep may then talk about 'dreamlike mentation' faced with the well-documented cases of what the rest of us would call dreams, but no REM sleep (see McFee 1994: 103–4). If we are willing to 'move the goalpost' as to our area of interest, it is hard to know if one is really investigating what seemed fascinating about humans.

For more on the idea of giving dreaming a more central place in one's philosophy of mind, see McFee (1994).

29  Especially Wollheim (1984); also Wollheim (1993).

30  See, for example, Lear (2000: 8–10).

31  See Chalmers (1982) for a general account: Kuhn (2000); Feyerabend (1993) more specifically.

32  Freud, 'On Psychotherapy' (1905) *Standard Edition* Vol. 7: 267 – not in PFL.

# 6   Do statistical methods replace reasoning in exercise science research? How to avoid statistics becoming merely a solution in search of a problem

*Stephen-Mark Cooper and Alan M. Nevill*

## Introduction

The nature of research in the exercise sciences can be described as lying along a continuum, at one end of which lies basic research and at the other applied research. Basic research is concerned with the corroboration or discounting of the theories that underpin the mechanisms pertaining to a particular phenomenon. It is this type of research that is typically involved in modelling physiological or psychological mechanisms. The kinds of theory-driven research questions developed by exercise scientists are typically analysed using classical *hypothetico-deductive* (Nevill 2000) methodologies. Here a hypothesis is formulated, an experiment is designed, data are collected and statistical methods are applied to test the hypothesis with respect to these data. Generally, this type of research asks *binary* questions, such as: if all other factors are controlled, does X explain Y? Basic research principles should allow the exercise science researcher to apply fundamental statistical theory and be fairly certain that, if all other factors other than X were controlled, then any changes in Y that are not due to a chance occurrence must therefore be due to X (Atkinson and Nevill 2001).

Conversely, applied research refers to the investigation of factors that impinge upon variables in 'real-world' settings. Atkinson and Nevill (2001) maintain that applied researchers ask more evaluative questions, such as: whatever the mechanisms of its action, in the real world, does X make a worthwhile difference to Y? Once again in applied research, the exercise scientist formulates a hypothesis and designs an experiment, data are collected and statistical methods are applied to test the hypothesis with respect to these data. It is important that exercise science researchers appreciate that basic research and applied research should not be considered as dichotomous but that, as we indicated earlier, they lie at opposite ends of a continuum. There are, however, differences in approach taken along the basic–applied research continuum, particularly with respect to the outcomes and the conclusions drawn from these outcomes. Because applied research takes place in a 'real world' setting, where variables are not easily controlled, the consequence is that in making decisions about whether X makes a worthwhile difference to Y, the exercise scientist must account for many other plausible alternative explanations for the outcomes from their research.

Research in the exercise sciences, conducted along the basic–applied continuum, is oriented predominantly towards the quantitative paradigm. The consequence of this has been an emphasis upon testing hypotheses and testing the statistical significance of the analysis outcomes. Together, these two are the fundamental data-analysis methods used by exercise science researchers today. Setting hypotheses, collecting quantitative data and testing the hypotheses with respect to these data by the application of statistical methods are not, however, without their problems.

The roles of hypothesis testing and tests of statistical significance are often misunderstood and misinterpreted (Shultz and Sands 1995; Atkinson and Nevill 2001). Commenting directly about these common misunderstandings and misinterpretations, Nevill (2000) reported that in every issue of the *Journal of Sports Sciences*, containing an average of 40 significant results ($P \leq 0.05$), there will be on average two false conclusions drawn where authors are reporting significant findings when in reality no significance actually exists. As a result of the potential confusion that can arise from misinterpretation of the term tests of statistical significance, Meehl (1978) has suggested that adoption of both the term and the procedures inherent in tests of statistical significance have actually slowed down the rate at which scientific knowledge has been acquired. Others, such as Carver (1978) and Weitzman (1984), have called for scientists to abandon tests of statistical significance completely. More moderately, Chow (1988) considered that tests of statistical significance do have a role to play in basic research studies that aim to corroborate scientific theories, but are limited when the nature of the study is applied or is purely descriptive. Shultz and Sands (1995) pragmatically concluded, however, that tests of statistical significance are, by now, so well inculcated into the processes of scientific research (including exercise science research) that their presence would be hard to reject, even if the promises of the method are never fulfilled.

Rather than reconsidering the statistical methods typically used by exercise scientists in resolution of their hypotheses, the aim of this chapter is primarily to develop a conceptual understanding of the issues surrounding the appropriate application of these methods. We hope that the interrogation of these issues will help to reduce confusion and, further, to reduce the sources of errors when conclusions are being drawn about the data collected. Second, we shall consider the manner in which these analytical results are reported by exercise science researchers in an effort to move away from what we feel is an undue focus on the hypotheses. The chapter has seven main sections, the first of which deals with approaches to research in the exercise sciences. The second section deals with issues surrounding the hypothesis and statistical significance. Section three considers the types of errors that can be made when testing the hypothesis. The fourth section investigates the importance of choosing an appropriate level of statistical significance. Section five deals with the types of errors that can be made when considering the hypothesis using statistical tests that are predicated on collected data following a Normal distribution. Section six argues for the inclusion of confidence intervals, as helpful interpretative indices, in studies where the results of hypothesis tests are being reported. The final section outlines the conclusions that we draw from the arguments developed in the chapter.

## Approaches to research in the exercise sciences

From reviewing the literature, it would seem that when conducting research, most exercise scientists adopt a *confirmation bias* approach – the confirmation of a theory or hypothesis – rather than the *falsification* approach as advised by philosophers of science such as Karl Popper (1968). The logic underpinning such an approach is the assumption that a theory or a hypothesis (the *antecedent*) is correct and then the formulation of an expected experimental outcome (the *consequent*). Shultz and Sands (1995) maintain that tests of statistical significance provide the minor premise in the logical argument (the *conditional* or *implicative syllogism*) used in testing a theory or hypothesis.

It was the celebrated statistician, Sir Ronald A. Fisher (1890–1962) who developed the idea of the *statistical hypothesis* or *null hypothesis* ($H_0$). It should be clearly differentiated from the exercise scientist's *research hypothesis*. The $H_0$ is the hypothesis that is tested by the application of statistical tests with respect to the data collected by the scientist. The research hypothesis is the scientist's research question – the idea that prompted the study to be developed initially, the nature of which is usually formulated on ideological grounds.

Based on the statistical analysis of their collected data, many exercise science researchers reject the $H_0$, believing that this provides support for an alternative hypothesis. In so doing, they are making an assumption that this supports the outcome predicted by the theory or hypothesis, thus affirming the consequent. Conceptually, the major premise of the *conditional argument* is that *if* the exercise science researcher's theory or hypothesis is true, *then* this expected outcome should be the result. However, if the minor premise – the results of the test of statistical significance – supports the expected outcome, then the conclusion is that the theory or hypothesis is supported. The unfortunate thing is that this is an illogical argument and is called *affirming the consequent* (Shultz and Sands 1995).

Philosophers of science would prefer that exercise scientists approach their research by applying a method that the philosophers call *modus tollens*, or *denying the consequent*. Here, a prediction (the *consequent*) is formulated from a theory or hypothesis (the *antecedent*). If the evidence is eventually shown to refute the prediction, then the theory or hypothesis is also refuted (Shultz and Sands 1995). This approach to scientific research is that typically employed in the physical sciences, and might, therefore, be more commonly applied in biomechanics research than in the behavioural disciplines of exercise science research – exercise physiology and exercise psychology. Indeed, Shultz and Sands (1995) believe that the method of denying the consequent results in both a rapid acquisition of knowledge as well as the elimination of inappropriate theories. They go on to suggest that the easiest way in which *modus tollens* can be achieved is by associating the exercise scientist's research hypothesis with the statistical hypothesis and predicting an outcome that cannot occur. If the study produces the outcome that cannot occur, then the researcher's hypothesis has, in effect, been falsified.

## The hypothesis and statistical significance

### The relationship between the null hypothesis and the alternative hypothesis

Broadly speaking, there are two fundamental $H_0$s commonly proposed and then tested by statistical methods in exercise science research. These are: (i) that variable $X$ and variable $Y$ are *not* related in a linear fashion,[1] and, (ii) that there is *no* difference between the means of two sets of scores.[2] The latter $H_0$ can be expanded to consider one that says that there is *no* difference between the means of three or more sets of scores.[3] In recent years, it has become quite a common practice amongst exercise science researchers to postulate a $H_0$ and, in doing so, also to offer an *alternative hypothesis* ($H_1$). If, as a result of the data analysis, the $H_0$ is rejected, then the $H_1$ is the most likely explanation. It is common to see the $H_1$ directionalized such that if there is evidence in the collected data for a linear relationship between variables $X$ and $Y$ the $H_1$ might be $r_{XY} > 0$ (the correlation is significantly greater than $0$ – it tends towards $+1$) or $H_1$: $r_{XY} < 0$ (the correlation is significantly less than $0$ – it tends towards $-1$). With respect to evidence in the collected data for a difference between means, we might see, for example, an $H_1$: $\mu_2 > \mu_1$ (the population mean for group 2 is significantly greater than that for group 1 in relation to a variable of interest).

Many exercise science researchers believe that, in writing up the results of their research, when they reject their $H_0$ they are doing just as Popper (1968) suggested and falsifying the hypothesis. In *modus tollens*, however, it is falsification of the exercise scientist's research hypothesis that is required and not falsification of the $H_0$. The former situation might well be due to the remnants of Fisher's (1971) own approach to statistical methodology. Fisher was actually trained in logic, and he theorized that a valid form of logic could come about from falsifying a hypothesis. He therefore created the idea of the $H_0$ (the only hypothesis in Fisherian statistics) for that reason. Further, as far as the Neyman–Pearson[4] approach to statistical inference is concerned, the research-er's hypothesis is related to the $H_1$, and the $H_0$ is falsified (Shultz and Sands 1995). It is little wonder, therefore, with all these different approaches towards the application of statistical methods in research that exercise scientists are apt to be confused and to make errors of judgement as to the exact nature of the outcomes from their research.

### Testing the hypothesis and testing the statistical significance

Even though Fisher (1971) clearly distinguished between these two ideas (*testing the hypothesis and testing the statistical significance*), it would be fair to say that contemporary exercise science researchers tend to treat the two synonymously. It is worthwhile here, then, considering the underpinning nature of each.

The term *hypothesis test* emphasizes the *deductive* elements of exercise science research, as it requires the exercise scientist to deduce a hypothesis and then to examine the degree of agreement between their own expectations and the observed outcomes from their study. On the other hand, the term *significance test* emphasizes the *inductive* elements of exercise science research – the inductive reasoning behind the hypothesis test is provided by the test of statistical significance. The latter test also provides the exercise science researcher with the rules that are used to reject (or fail to reject) the $H_0$ (Shultz and Sands 1995).

The word *significance* in the term *tests of statistical significance* is derived from the concept of *level of statistical significance*. From reviewing the literature, there seems to be some confusion over what this actually means. With reference to this issue, Shultz and Sands (1995) identify two groups of exercise science researchers: (i) those that associate the level of statistical significance with alpha ($\alpha$), or the probability of making a *type 1* error (i.e., rejecting the $H_0$ when it is true), and (ii) those that associate it with the P-value – the *associated probability*.

This associated probability is the probability (normally expressed as a percentage[5]) that the statistical outcome[5] (or a more extreme value) of applying the chosen test to the data collected has come about by chance under the assumption that the $H_0$ is true. As a result of using statistical software run on a modern personal computer, the exact P-value is normally generated and reported as part of the analysis output. It is a *conditional probability*, and Shultz and Sands (1995) have summarized it as the probability of the collected data (D) or an outcome of a particular value (or more extreme) assuming the $H_0$ is true as: $P = D/H_0$. The statistical outcome of the analysis is then compared with a *critical value* for the distribution of that outcome.[6] This critical value has become known as the *alpha level* ($\alpha$-level) or *level of statistical significance*, and is reflective of the maximum risk that the exercise scientist is willing to tolerate for falsely rejecting the $H_0$. Shultz and Sands (1995) summarized this scenario as the decision (D*) to reject the $H_0$ based on a particular outcome, assuming the $H_0$ to be true as: $P = D*/H_0$. In making such a decision, the exercise science researcher is concluding that some effect exists in the data that they have collected (i.e. there *is* evidence for a linear relationship or there *is* evidence for a difference between two or more means).

## Types of error

Whenever the $H_0$ is tested, there are two kinds of errors that can be made in rejecting the stated hypothesis, or not. A *type 1* error is committed when the $H_0$ is true but is erroneously rejected. The second type of error is known as a *type 2* error and it occurs when the $H_0$ is false but the researcher incorrectly interprets it as being true. Table 6.1 details the conditions under which *type 1* and *type 2* errors can be made, and is often called the *truth table* (Thomas and Nelson 2001).

Hopkins (1998) has offered a differentiation between the two types of error by suggesting that a *type 2* error is only an error in the sense that an opportunity to

*Table 6.1* Conditions under which *type 1* and *type 2* errors can be made

|  | *The $H_0$ is true* | *The $H_0$ is false* |
| --- | --- | --- |
| Do not reject the $H_0$ | No error is made – the conclusion is correct | A *type 2* error is made – the conclusion is incorrect |
| Reject the $H_0$ | A *type 1* error is made – the conclusion is incorrect | No error is made – the conclusion is correct |

Adapted from Thomas and Nelson (2001).

reject the $H_0$ correctly was lost. He goes on to say that it is not an error in the sense that an incorrect conclusion was drawn, since no contextualized conclusion is drawn (i.e. a generalization (inference) of the results from the sample to the population studied) when the $H_0$ is not rejected. It is simply that the exercise science researcher reports that there was insufficient evidence in their data for a linear relationship or a difference between means. Conversely, a *type 1* error is an error in every sense of the term, and the drawing of contextualized conclusions when a *type 1* error has been made is certainly far more serious.

The critical issue for exercise science researchers to appreciate is that errors can never be totally eliminated. It is up to the individual researcher to do their utmost to protect against making an error. The research design, in terms of the sample's size ($n$), the representation of the sample to the population, the reliability (consistency and accuracy) of the measurements made and appropriate data analysis and interpretation provides the means by which the probability of making an error can be reduced. If, having collected and analysed their data, the researcher concludes that there is evidence for a significant linear relationship, or evidence for a significant difference between means, when there is not (a *type 1* error), the worst-case scenario is that this conclusion could prove likely to risk human life. At the very least, the researcher might commit large amounts of resources to what is a false conclusion. On the other hand, if evidence for a *real* linear relationship (i.e. it was not a chance occurrence) does exist, or there is evidence for a *real* difference between means (i.e. it was not a chance occurrence), and the study fails to identify them as significant (a *type 2* error), consumers of the research might never have the opportunity to take advantage of this new knowledge – knowledge that might actually serve a positive function. Consequently, exercise science researchers should more frequently ask themselves the question: 'If I have to make an error, which type of error am I willing to make?', or put another way: 'If I'm going to make an error, would I rather reject an $H_0$ that is true (make a *type 1* error) or not?'

## Choosing a level of statistical significance

The appropriate setting of the level of statistical significance, or the alpha level, is another way in which the exercise science researcher can help protect against possible errors (Hopkins 1998; Vincent 1999). In contemporary exercise science research, it seems to have become common practice to set $\alpha$ at the 0.05 or 5 per cent level (i.e. odds of 5-in-100 that the result came about by chance). Indeed, Munro (1997) concludes that this value has, by repeated practice, become enshrined as a 'threshold value' for the declaration of statistical significance. Hopkins (1998), however, suggests that there is nothing particularly special about the choice of the 0.05 $\alpha$-level at all. Even so, exercise science researchers should appreciate the importance of the $\alpha$-level that they set in their research design, and to set $\alpha$ at a particular level without offering any justification for doing so in their studies, in our view, is wholly inappropriate.

If the $\alpha$-level is set at 0.10 or 10 per cent[7] rather than at 0.05 (5 per cent), then the researcher is setting $\alpha$ at a level that will provide statistical significance when a lower relationship exists between variables $X$ and $Y$, or a smaller difference exists between the means of two or more groups of scores. By increasing the $\alpha$-level, however, the researcher also runs the risk of rejecting the $H_0$ when it is true – making a *type 1* error. Conversely, if the researcher reduces the $\alpha$-level from 0.05 to say 0.01 (1 per cent)[8] or even 0.001 (0.1 per cent),[9] it becomes less likely that a false $H_0$ will not be rejected. The negative effect of following this latter course of action is that by requiring stronger evidence for rejection of the $H_0$, the researcher runs the risk of failing to reject the $H_0$ when it is in fact false; there is a *real* linear relationship or a *real* difference between means and they end up making a *type 2* error. In using the term 'real' we mean that the results were not chance occurrences – they were not due to variations in sampling or measurement error.

The level of statistical significance that the researcher chooses actually reflects the type of error that they are willing to make. Few exercise scientists seem to acknowledge this by justifying their choice in the methodology of their studies. Thomas and Nelson (1990: 101–2) give an example of a researcher studying the effects of a drug that might cure cancer. Here the researcher would not want to accept the $H_0$ of no effect if there was the remotest chance that the drug might work. Consequently, the researcher might set their level of alpha at 0.30 (30 per cent) even though (s)he knows that the chances of making a *type 1* error will be increased. By doing this, the researcher is ensuring that there is every chance that the drug will be seen to exhibit its effectiveness. Conversely, if the researcher was to set alpha at 0.001 (0.1 per cent) (s)he is reducing the odds of misleading other researchers as it lowers the chances of making a *type 1* error.

With regard to this issue, Franks and Huck (1986) describe two 'camps' of exercise science researchers as clearly existing. Firstly, they describe the 'camp 1' researcher (the *hypothesis tester*) who sets the $\alpha$-level at 0.05 before data collection (*a priori*). Once the 'camp 1' researcher's data have been collected and analysed, a statement is made regarding the $H_0$ based upon whether the calculated test statistic falls into the established range of critical values for that test. From this evidence alone the researcher simply makes a decision on whether to reject, or fail to reject, the $H_0$. The 'camp 1' researcher makes their decision regardless of how far into the critical value range the test statistic is positioned.

'Camp 2' researchers (the *significance testers*) approach decisions about the $H_0$ from a different perspective. In 'camp 2' the $\alpha$-level is set tentatively *a priori* (usually at 0.05) but when the data are collected and analysed, it becomes clear that $\alpha$ was viewed merely as a reference point on a continuum. If the $H_0$ can be rejected at a more stringent $\alpha$-level (0.01 or even 0.001), the 'camp 2' researcher reports the level of statistical significance at 'the most impressive "beatable" value' (Franks and Huck 1986: 245).

We might add a third 'camp' of exercise science researchers (the *technocrats*) to those described by Franks and Huck (1986). The 'camp 3' researcher is one that ignores the setting of an $\alpha$-level *a priori*, collects their data, analyses them, and then simply reports in their study the exact level of statistical significance generated in the output from their analysis package. In such cases, it is not uncommon to see significance quoted as high as $P = 0.0000$ (actually $P = 0.00005$).[10] None of the approaches to choosing the level of statistical significance outlined above is any more appropriate than any of the others. It should be noted, however, that the setting of alpha, *a priori*, is the approach taken in classical statistical methods. What is important for the exercise science researcher to be aware of, is that the $\alpha$-level chosen should be justified in terms of the type of error that the researcher is willing to make. It is our opinion that the level of statistical significance should be set *a priori*, then, when the computer software being used generates the outcomes from the analysis on the collected data, the $P$-value can be compared with the chosen $\alpha$-level and reported (together with other important illustrative results such as effect size, statistical power and confidence intervals) at the value computed by the software. We see nothing wrong with this approach as it merely demonstrates how far the computed $P$-value exceeds the stated $\alpha$-level. Finally, if borderline results are to be reported, then the exercise science researcher needs to clearly label them as such in their report (Thomas and Nelson 1990).

Shultz and Sands (1995: 260) have identified that to some exercise science researchers, the concept of statistical significance has been misinterpreted to the extent that to these researchers it implies that their results are 'meaningful, important or large'. Indeed, it would seem from the literature that this is quite a common occurrence with numerous examples of exercise scientists reporting in their research articles that their results were 'highly' significant. Such situations can often lead to the equating of statistical significance with *scientific significance* and the assumption that the results support the *research hypothesis*. We must, however, never lose sight of the fact that *statistical significance* is indicative of whether a linear relationship, or a difference between means, is large enough that it *needs* explaining. On the other hand, *scientific significance* is indicative of whether a linear relationship, or a difference between means, is *worth* explaining (Shultz and Sands 1995).

# Type 1 and type 2 errors and Normally distributed data

## Normal distribution

As we have seen, the statistical analysis of data collected in exercise science research is based upon the general idea that the researcher develops a research question that they then summarize as a statistically testable hypothesis ($H_0$). The researcher then makes some measurements or observations on a sample of subjects, and then they apply a statistical analysis to test the $H_0$ postulated for the data collected in their research. From the results of this test, the exercise science researcher makes some contextualized inferences (generalizations) about the population of subjects from which the measured sample was drawn on the variable (or variables) of interest. The most commonly applied statistical methods in exercise science research are known as *parametric*, or *category one tests*. The term 'parametric' refers to the fact that in order for these tests to be correctly applied, there are a number of key factors concerning the nature of the data collected (often known as *assumptions*) that need to be confirmed about the data collected before data analysis can begin. In other words, researchers need to know something about the *parameters* of the distribution of the scores in the population from which the sample of subjects were drawn on the variable (or variables) of interest.

Winter *et al.* (2001) believe that exercise science researchers have a major responsibility to confirm the assumptions made about the parameters of their data, in order to reduce the chances of making an error in interpreting the outcomes of their data analyses, and thereby drawing false conclusions from them. Consideration of many of these assumptions about the nature of the distribution of the data collected should form part of the exercise science researchers' planning and experimental design.

The appropriate application of the great majority of parametric statistical tests is predicated primarily upon the assumption that the variable (or variables) of interest are drawn from one of the family of distributions that are known as *Normal distributions* in the population from which the sample data were drawn (Bland 2002). With the statistical software that is available to the exercise science researcher today, a confirmatory test that collected data follows Gauss's curve of Normal distribution, such as the *Anderson–Darling test*, the *Kolmogorov–Smirnov test* or the *Shapiro–Wilks test*, is a relatively straightforward procedure. Despite this, however, from reviewing the literature in the exercise sciences, it seems that very few exercise science researchers actually bother to confirm the likelihood that the data generated by their research samples are Normally distributed in the populations from which those samples were drawn, let alone report it in their studies. Instead, *Normality* tends to be assumed. This assumption might well jeopardize the accuracy of using parametric statistical tests in resolution of the $H_0$, in the first instance, and the research hypothesis in the long-term, because the misappropriation of the test might well lead to a spurious outcome being produced.

If the exercise science researcher finds that the major assumption (i.e. data Normality) for the appropriate application of parametric statistical tests, outlined on p. 125, cannot be confirmed in the data that they have collected, they might consider testing the $H_0$ by using a *non-parametric* statistical test[11] instead. There are non-parametric equivalents available for all of the parametric tests identified in this chapter (see Table 6.2), as well as many others. *Statistical power* is the probability of rejecting the $H_0$ when the $H_0$ is false (a correct outcome), and it is an often-neglected concept in exercise science research (Bland 2002). We fully acknowledge that most authorities believe that, if at all possible, parametric statistical tests should be the first choice tests in resolution of the $H_0$, primarily because they are more *powerful*, and therefore their use will reduce the chances of making either a *type 1* or a *type 2* error. In addition, exercise science researchers should be aware that whilst the non-parametric tests

*Table 6.2* Parametric statistical tests and their non-parametric equivalents, used to test the three most common hypotheses set in exercise science research

| | Statistical hypotheses ($H_0$) | | |
|---|---|---|---|
| Type of data | Relationships (bivariate) | Differences between two variables | Differences between three or more variables |
| Ratio | $H_0$: $r_{XY} = 0$ Pearson's correlation coefficient ($r_{XY}$) | $H_0$: $\mu_1 = \mu_2$ Dependent analysis = paired *t*-test Independent analysis = independent *t*-test | $H_0$: $\mu_1 = \mu_2 = \mu_3 = \ldots = \mu_k$ Dependent analysis = one-way ANOVA RM Independent analysis = one-way ANOVA |
| Interval | $H_0$: $r_{XY} = 0$ Pearson's correlation coefficient ($r_{XY}$) | $H_0$: $\mu_1 = \mu_2$ Dependent analysis = paired *t*-test Independent analysis = independent *t*-test | $H_0$: $\mu_1 = \mu_2 = \mu_3 = \ldots = \mu_k$ Dependent analysis = one-way ANOVA RM Independent analysis = one-way ANOVA |
| Ordinal | $H_0$: $\rho_{XY} = 0$ Spearman's rank-order correlation ($\rho$) | $H_0$: $\eta_1 = \eta_2$ Dependent analysis = Wilcoxon (W) test Independent analysis = Mann–Whitney (U) test | $H_0$: $\eta_1 = \eta_2 = \eta_3 = \ldots = \eta_k$ Dependent analysis = Friedman's two-way ANOVA Independent analysis = Kruskal–Wallis (H) test |
| Nominal | Chi-squared ($\chi^2$) as a test of association | Chi-squared ($\chi^2$) as a test of independence | Chi-squared ($\chi^2$) as a test of a $k \times n$ contingency table |

ANOVA = analysis of variance.
ANOVA RM = analysis of variance for repeated measurements.

used to test $H_0$s of no difference do consider the *central tendency* of the data, they do not test differences between means. Often, these non-parametric methods test the differences between *medians* ($\eta$), or *average ranks* ($\bar{R}$), or sometimes *sums of ranks* ($\sum R$).

### Why are the outcomes of confirmatory tests of Normality omitted from studies?

Ultimately, the responsibility for justifying the use of parametric statistical tests in resolution of the $H_0$ postulated for their collected data rests squarely with the exercise scientists that submit their theses for assessment or their manuscripts to learned journals in the hope of getting their studies published. Moreover, it is highly likely that part of the problem is due to the fact that too few thesis supervisors, and too few exercise science journal reviewers and editors, ask for such confirmations to be made in manuscripts presented for assessment or publication. If supervisors, reviewers and editors do not insist that authors make the confirmation of important assumptions about their collected data, such as Normality, in manuscripts, authors are unlikely to include them. This situation is often confounded by journals restricting the length of articles, which can often prohibit expansion of the theoretical explanation of the statistical methods utilized, as well as a confirmation of the underpinning assumptions (Mullineaux *et al.* 2001).

## The case for the inclusion of confidence intervals in exercise science research reports

One of the unfortunate consequences of reporting statistical results in exercise science journals has been the shift in emphasis away from the basic results towards an undue concentration upon hypothesis testing. This, as we have seen, is due to the common procedure in exercise science where researchers examine their data in relation to a $H_0$, which, in turn, has led to the mistaken belief that studies should aim at obtaining statistical significance. There is a natural tendency for exercise science researchers to only submit for scrutiny studies that can show significant findings (Nevill 2000). This situation might well have arisen because journal editors have a bias, albeit subconsciously, towards publishing significant results, thereby treating statistical significance as a condition for publication. Whatever the reasons for this bias, we believe that it has four important ramifications:

1   It has resulted in exercise scientists taking fewer risks in refuting research hypotheses.
2   It supports the perpetuation of the confirmation bias approach to research.
3   It has led to the too often cited 'fall-back' conclusion that non-significance emanates from studies where *n* is too small and that are underpowered (Schultz and Sands 1995).

4   It leads to lazy thinking, particularly in young or inexperienced exercise science researchers, because it suggests that they believe that their results should have produced a significant outcome, but did not. Such researchers are therefore guilty of ignoring the fact that even though the results were *statistically insignificant* they might well have proved to be significant from at least a *practical* perspective.

The unfortunate consequence of this excessive use of hypothesis testing has led to levels of significance often being quoted alone in dissertations and journal articles, no mention being made of the actual study results (Altman *et al.* 2000). The implication of testing the $H_0$ – that there can always be a 'yes' (reject) *vs* 'no' (not to reject) answer – is clearly false. Used only in this way, hypothesis testing is of limited value. Statements such as: $P \leq 0.05$, $P \geq 0.05$, $P = 0.006$ or $P = NS$ (i.e. not significant), convey little information about a study's findings, and, as we have seen, the former two statements rely upon the arbitrary use of a conventional level of statistical significance (usually 5 per cent). These statements only define two alternative outcomes: (i) that the result was significant, or, (ii) that the result was non-significant. We believe that this is not helpful because it encourages lazy thinking, not only on the part of the researcher, but also on the part of the consumer of the research. For the exercise science researcher to report that $P = 0.006$ tells the reader of the study nothing about (say) the size of the differences between the study groups. In this way, reporting of the *P*-value is often given more merit than it deserves, and consumers of the researcher (and even the researchers themselves) end up equating statistical significance with importance or even relevance.

When a test statistic is computed from sample data and used as an estimate of that characteristic in the population, it is called a *point estimate* (PE). Point estimates are imprecise estimates of the chosen characteristic in the overall population – the $\bar{x}^{12}$ is therefore a *PE* for $\mu$. Fortunately, this imprecision can also be estimated, and we believe that this estimate should be incorporated into the presentation of the exercise science researcher's findings. We also agree with Altman *et al.* (2000) in that presenting findings on the original scale of measurement, with estimates of the imprecision due to sampling errors, is a sounder course of action than just providing *P*-values alone to indicate statistical significance or non-significance.

Another useful adjunct to the *P*-value therefore is the *confidence interval* (CI) for a given statistic. A *CI* is a range of values that the population parameter might take for that statistic, and it indicates the precision (or imprecision) of the sample study estimate as population values. Point estimates and *CI*s are statistics that will allow the exercise science researcher to infer the true value of an unmeasured population parameter from data gathered from a randomly drawn sample of that population. These estimates will relate to summary characteristics and *not* individual characteristics. The calculated interval gives a range of values within which the exercise science researcher can have a chosen confidence (normally 95 per cent or 99 per cent) of it containing the population value.

Imprecision is indicated by the width of the interval – the wider the interval, the less the precision. These estimates therefore become relevant whenever the exercise science researcher wants to report the results of a test of the $H_0$. They can also be calculated for some non-parametric hypotheses.

The width of the CI (the index of the statistic's precision) is dependent upon three things:

1 the *sample size* (n) – larger n give more precise results with narrower CIs – they represent the population better, whereas wide CIs emphasize the unreliability of results based on small n;
2 *variability* in the characteristic of interest – less variance (between subjects, within subjects, from measurement error etc.) results in a more precise PE of the statistic and a narrower CI;
3 the *degree of confidence* required – the more confidence required (e.g. 99 per cent ($CI_{0.01}$) *vs* 95 per cent ($CI_{0.05}$)) the wider the confidence interval.

Consider, for example, a situation where an exercise physiologist has developed a new training intervention aimed at reducing per cent body fat in a group of middle-aged women. To assess the worth of this intervention, the exercise physiologist randomly selects a cohort of 40 volunteers from the target population of middle-aged women ($n = 40$), whom they pre-test for percent body fat prior to the application of 10 weeks of the training intervention. After the intervention, the 40 middle-aged women are post-tested for percent body fat. The exercise physiologist proposes to test the $H_0$: $\bar{x}_{PRE} = \bar{x}_{POST}$, at $\alpha = 0.05$ using a paired *t*-test. The *mean difference* ($\bar{x}_{diff}$) for percent fat obtained between $\bar{x}_{PRE}$ and $\bar{x}_{POST}$ is 6.0 per cent (*standard error* of this difference ($SE_{diff}$) = 2.5 per cent). This $\bar{x}_{diff}$ in percent fat is only an estimate (a point estimate) of what the exercise physiologist really needs to know – the result obtained had all the eligible subjects (the total population of middle-aged women) been treated with the training intervention (i.e. $H_0$: $\mu_{PRE} = \mu_{POST}$). Additionally, what any interested user of this research wants to know is by how much the treatment modified the mean percent fat, not only that $P \leq \alpha$. Indeed, the purpose of most research in the exercise sciences is to determine the magnitude of some factor(s) or another.

If the exercise physiologist also calculated the $CI_{0.05}$ for the population difference between means, they could report that whilst they found (from their study) that the $\bar{x}_{diff} = 6.0$ per cent ($SE_{diff} = 2.5$ per cent), there was also a 95 per cent chance that the range bounded by the $CI_{0.05}$ (from 1.1 per cent to 10.9 per cent) includes the population difference in mean percent fat – the value that would have been obtained by including the total population of middle-aged women at which the study was aimed. The exercise physiologist could summarize the results of this experiment as: $\bar{x}_{diff} = 6.0\%$ ($SE_{diff} = 2.5\%$); $t_{39} = 2.4$; $P = 0.008$; $CI_{0.05} = 1.1\%$ to $10.9\%$; *effect size* = 0.38; $power_{0.05} = 38.8\%$.

It becomes perfectly clear from this summary of the results of the study that the immediate impact of the initial *t*-test outcome indicating that the $\bar{x}_{diff}$ for percent fat recorded for this research study was statistically significant needs to be tempered somewhat by considering an interpretation of the additional information provided. First, the $CI_{0.05}$ is wide, and it suggests a 95 per cent confidence that the population $\bar{x}_{diff}$ for percent fat would lie somewhere between 1.1 per cent and 10.9 per cent. Second, even if we applied the subjective interpretation of the size of the effect provided by Cohen (1988: 40), this difference would be classified as being somewhere between small and moderate. Finally, we could use Table 6.3 to help us interpret the power of this test of the $H_0$ in the studied population. If there was an effect of the treatment it would only be detected about 39 times out of 100 cases. In conclusion, whilst the initial test of the size of the $\bar{x}_{diff}$ for percent fat was statistically significant ($P = 0.008 = a$ difference of this size would occur erroneously only eight times in 1000 cases) the latter interpretative results, which expand the evaluation from the sample data to that of the wider population, really do question whether it was actually worth the exercise physiologist, and the 40 subjects, spending the 10 weeks on this training intervention in order to gain this limited effect in reducing percent fat.

The exercise science researcher should be aware however, that whilst CIs indicate the precision of the sample statistic as an estimate of the overall population statistic, and therefore, the effects of sampling variation, CIs cannot control for non-sampling errors in study design or application. Confidence intervals are not relevant to report in all cases, as sometimes data are purely descriptive, and sometimes, techniques for obtaining the CI for a particular statistic are complex or even unavailable (Altman *et al.* 2000).

## Conclusions

In this chapter we have attempted to show that when conducting objective, quantitative exercise science research that is based upon data collected from samples drawn from populations of subjects, there will always be a risk of making an error of judgement. By attempting to protect against one type of error,

*Table 6.3* The relationship between *type 2* error rate and statistical power

| Power | Rate of type 2 error | Conclusions |
|-------|----------------------|-------------|
| 1.00 | 0.00 | If there is a linear relationship (an effect), or difference between means (an effect), it will be detected every time |
| 0.80 | 0.20 | If there is an effect it will be detected 80 times out of 100 |
| 0.50 | 0.50 | If there is an effect it will be detected 50 times out of 100 |
| 0.20 | 0.80 | If there is an effect it will be detected 20 times out of 100 |
| 0.00 | 1.00 | If there is an effect it will never be detected |

exercise science researchers often leave themselves open to committing the alternative. However, exercise scientists are not always eager to consider the 'peripheral' issues that relate to their collected data; issues that might help in reducing the risks of making an error of judgement about the research outcomes. Even if the exercise science researcher does consider these issues, they often seem reluctant to report the outcomes in their studies.

It is the responsibility of the exercise science researcher to ascertain, before any data are collected, which type of error is of most concern to them, and, for some contingency to be implemented in the research design in an attempt to reduce the probability of its occurrence. The research design, the methods employed to collect the data, and the statistical tests chosen to analyse the collected data, should provide the researcher with ample opportunity to produce significant results without compromising the validity of the research. It is evident that some exercise science researchers can leave themselves open to making *type 1* errors in their quest to establish statistical significance. These exercise science researchers should be, however, aware that a failure to find a real linear relationship, or a real difference between means, does not necessarily render their research worthless.

Finally, we have also attempted to show the relative importance of reporting confidence intervals, in addition to the ubiquitous level of statistical significance (P-value) for a given test statistic in exercise science research. We feel that without these important additional indices, users of the research will be unable to judge appropriately the merits and demerits of the research outcomes as well as the practical usefulness of the work.

## Bibliography

Altman, D.G., Machin, D., Bryant, T.N. and Gardner, M.J. (eds) (2000) *Statistics with confidence*, 2nd edn, London: BMJ Books.

Atkinson, G. and Nevill, A.M. (2001) 'Selected issues in the design and analysis of exercise performance research', *Journal of Sports Sciences*, 19(10), 811–27.

Bland, J.M. (2002) *An Introduction to Medical Statistics*, 3rd edn, Oxford: Oxford University Press.

Carver, R.P. (1978) 'The case against statistical significance testing', *Harvard Educational Review*, 48, 378–99.

Chow, S.L. (1988) 'Significance test or effect size?', *Psychological Bulletin*, 103, 105–10.

Cohen, J (1988). *Statistical Power Analysis*, 2nd edn, New Jersey: Lawrence Erlbaum Associates.

Fisher, R.A. (1971) *The Design of Experiments*, 8th edn, New York: Hafner Press.

Franks, B.D. and Huck, S.W. (1986) 'Why does everybody use the 0.5 significance level?', *Research Quarterly for Exercise and Sport*, 57(3), 245–9.

Hopkins, W. (1998) 'A scale of magnitude for effect statistics,' Internet Society for Sports Science. http://www.exercisesci.org/resources/stats/effectmag.html.

Meehl, P.E. (1978) 'Theoretical risks and tubular asterisks: Sir Karl, Sir Ronald, and the slow progress of soft psychology', *Journal of Consulting and Clinical Psychology*, 46, 806–34.

Mullineaux, D.R., Bartlett, R.M. and Bennett, S. (2001) 'Research design and statistics in biomechanics and motor control', *Journal of Sports Sciences*, 19, 739–60.

Munro, B.H. (1997) *Statistical Methods for Health Care Research*, 3rd edn, Philadelphia, PA: Lippincott, Williams and Wilkins.

Nevill, A.M. (2000) 'Just how confident are you when publishing the results of your research?' (editorial), *Journal of Sports Sciences*, 18(8), 569–70.

Popper, K.R. (1968) *The Logic of Scientific Discovery*, rev. edn, London: Hutchinson.

Shultz, B.B. and Sands, W.A. (1995) 'Understanding measurement concepts and statistical procedures', in P.J. Maud and C. Foster (eds) *Physiological Assessment of Human Fitness*, Champaign IL: Human Kinetics, 257–87.

Thomas, J.R. and Nelson, J.K. (1990) *Research Methods in Physical Activity*, Champaign, IL: Human Kinetics.

Thomas, J.R. and Nelson, J.K. (2001) *Research Methods in Physical Activity*, 3rd edn, Champaign, IL: Human Kinetics.

Vincent, W.J. (1999) *Statistics in Kinesiology*, 2nd edn, Champaign, IL: Human Kinetics.

Weitzman, R.A. (1984) 'Seven treacherous pitfalls of statistics, illustrated', *Psychological Reports*, 54, 355–63.

Winter, E.M., Eston, R.G. and Lamb, K.L. (2001) 'Statistical analyses in the physiology of exercise and kinanthropometry', *Journal of Sports Sciences*, 19(10), 761–75.

## Notes

1　This is summarized as $H_0$: $r_{XY} = 0$ (the data are orthogonal).
2　This is summarized as $H_0$: $\mu_1 = \mu_2$ (the means are equivalent). The symbol $\mu$ is used by statisticians to indicate the mean for a population of scores.
3　This is summarized as $H_0$: $\mu_1 = \mu_2 = \mu_3 = \ldots = \mu_k$.
4　This refers to the 1933 work on hypothesis testing and statistical inference reported in: *The testing of statistical hypotheses in relation to probabilities a priori*, by the statisticians Jerzy Neyman (1894–1981) and Egon Sharpe Pearson (1895–1980), who was the son of the celebrated Sir Karl Pearson (1857–1936).
5　For the $H_0$: $r_{XY} = 0$ the outcome is $r$, for the $H_0$: $\mu_1 = \mu_2$ the outcome is $t$, and for the $H_0$: $\mu_1 = \mu_2 = \mu_3 = \ldots = \mu_k$ the outcome is $F$.
6　When collected data follow a Normal distribution the critical values for the hypotheses in the previous footnote are $r_{CR}$, $t_{CR}$ and $F_{CR}$.
7　The probability that the $H_0$ will be erroneously rejected 10 times in repeating the same study on 100 similar samples drawn from the same population, assuming the $H_0$ to be true.
8　Ditto, once in 100 cases, assuming the $H_0$ to be true.
9　Ditto, once in 1000 cases, assuming the $H_0$ to be true.
10　The result would have come about by chance or error alone five times in repeating the same study on 10,000 similar samples drawn from the same population, assuming that the $H_0$ was correct.
11　A statistic applied to test a $H_0$ where the researcher makes no assumptions about their data being Normally distributed. These techniques are often called 'distribution free' statistics.
12　The symbol is used by statisticians to signify a mean computed from sample data. It signifies the sample mean.

# 7 What are the limitations of experimental and theoretical approaches in sports biomechanics?

*M.R. Yeadon*

## Introduction

In these days of the soundbite and the buzzword we often hear the phrase 'World Class Sports Science Support'. This seems to conjure up the notion of 'World Class Sports Science' but actually refers to the 'Sports Science Support' provided to world class sports competitors. The phrase 'Sports Science Support' suggests support that is based on the results of sports science research. There is much to be said for this intention, but there are a number of factors that limit the theoretical underpinning of such support in sports biomechanics and other branches of sports science. First, it should be noted that, while there are some findings that are applicable to the majority of sports, the most useful results are often sport-specific. For example, the requirements for success in gymnastics from the perspectives of biomechanics, physiology, psychology and sociology of gymnastics are all quite different from the corresponding requirements for success in field hockey. This means that in order to provide well-informed advice on a particular sport from the perspective of a particular discipline it is necessary to have a body of research for that discipline–sport combination. Second, while the amount of sports science research is steadily increasing, the disciplinary study of individual sports is limited both by the large number of sports and by the relatively small number of sports scientists undertaking such research. As a consequence 'World Class Sports Science Support' will continue to be support that has a relatively weak foundation of relevant research. This will remain the situation until such time as some agency takes responsibility for the funding of sports science research.

So what is sports science research? What can it achieve? What are its limitations? This chapter will attempt to address such issues in the context of sports biomechanics research.

## Scientific method

Scientific method is often thought to be the basis of all scientific research investigations. While this idea might be somewhat distant from many current approaches to research it is worth reviewing its structure here. After some preliminary investigation of an area, a research hypothesis or theory is proposed.

Predictions are made on the basis of this theory, giving potentially new knowledge that is then tested against the results of an appropriate experiment. The hypothesis is then accepted or rejected on the basis of the likelihood of the results occurring by chance. The basic structure is outlined in Figure 7.1. It should be noted that the above description is that of 'experimental method' rather than 'scientific method'. In Exercise Physiology, for example, so much of the research is experimentally based that a student might assume that 'science' is 'experimental science' but this neglects an important aspect of scientific investigation, namely 'theoretical science'.

The idea of 'theoretical method' may be thought to have the same basic structure as 'experimental method' (Figure 7.1). Instead of employing a concise hypothesis with readily obtainable implications, an underlying theory is proposed that may lead to conclusions only after much development and analysis. An example of a hypothesis is that 'more training will result in better performance', whereas Einstein's Theory of General Relativity is an example of a theory that cannot be defined completely using a single phrase. The first example might lead us to expect that if running 100 miles each week enhances performance then running 200 miles per week will result in even better performance, while the second example makes possible the accurate location of an athlete using the Global Positioning System. The way in which the comparison is made between experimental and theoretical results is also different in the theoretical approach. While experimental science makes a judgement using the likelihood of the experimental results arising by chance, theoretical science makes a judgement on the basis of how accurate the prediction is and how much hitherto unexplained phenomena can be accounted for. For example, an experiment on the relationship between the amount of training and subsequent performance may involve an experimental group and a control group and will assess the difference in performance of the two groups using statistical tests. On the other hand, Einstein's General Theory of Relativity

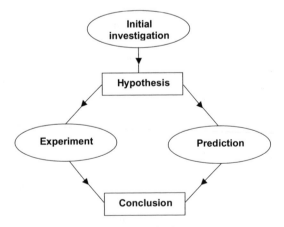

*Figure 7.1* The structure of the Scientific Method.

predicted that the sun would bend light from a distant star through 1.74 seconds of arc (0.0005°) rather than half this amount as predicted by Newtonian mechanics. Measurements taken during an eclipse of the sun gave estimated deviations of 1.61 and 1.98 seconds and supported the adoption of the model of Einstein rather than that of Newton. The general acceptance of this theory is based on its ability to explain many other results that cannot be accounted for by Newtonian mechanics.

The types of question that can be addressed by experimental and theoretical approaches also differ, as do the challenges posed by each method. These issues will be considered with reference to experimental and theoretical studies in biomechanics.

## Experimental studies

Typically an experiment attempts to test causal relationships between variables – for example, the relationship between approach speed and distance jumped. In an ideal experiment the effect of changing just one variable (approach speed), the independent variable, on the outcome (distance jumped), the dependent variable, is determined. If it were possible to change only one variable then changes in the outcome would have to be a consequence of changes in this independent variable. Although it may be possible to design such ideal experiments in certain branches of the natural sciences, the complexity of the human system prevents such tight control within the sports sciences. In sports biomechanics, attempts to change just one aspect of technique in the sports performance of an individual will inevitably result in other changes and this will require a large number of trials in order to isolate the effects of each variable.

Another feature of a well-designed experiment is that the conclusions will be applicable to the real world. The tighter the control of an experiment to remove unwanted variance, the more likely that the experiment will differ from a natural setting. In other words, the stronger the internal validity, the weaker the external validity. Obtaining data from performances in a natural setting such as competition may yield only a small number of attempts on a single day. Using intervention to manipulate technique in other settings may itself render the performance untypical due to the 'Hawthorne effect' whereby the mere knowledge of participation in an experiment may affect the outcome (Rothstein 1985). Such intervention may not be possible due to concerns of the athlete and coach or allied ethical concerns. For example, there may be issues of potential injury or disruption of learned technique arising from experimental interventions. Despite such problems, it may be still possible to obtain clear results from an experiment with an athlete. For example, Greig and Yeadon (2000) used data on 16 high jumping trials from a training session of one athlete to establish quadratic relationships between approach speed and height jumped and between leg plant angle and height jumped.

Because of the difficulties in obtaining sufficient data on a single athlete, some researchers use combined data from several athletes. Hay (1987) cautions against statistical analyses in which several jumps by each of a number of athletes are treated as if they were single trials performed by different athletes, since trials by the same athlete cannot be regarded as independent trials. A more appropriate approach would be to use a repeated measures design. Additionally, it should be recognized that the relationships between variables may be very different when the best performances of a number of athletes are taken rather than a number of performances from a single athlete. The relationship between height reached and approach speed in high jumping is quadratic for an individual (Alexander 1990), so that there is an optimum approach speed for which the height jumped is greatest. On the other hand, the relationship is linear for a group of athletes (Dapena *et al.* 1990) so that the height jumped increases with the approach speed. In other words, while there is an optimum approach speed for an individual, the better jumpers are stronger, faster and jump higher. Confusion in this area can lead to relationships that are unrelated to individual performance.

Even when data are collected on an individual athlete in a natural setting, such as competition, the search for relationships between variables is likely to be frustrated, since performances have been optimized. In long jumping it is accepted that approach speed is strongly related to distance jumped. In competition, however, all performances are likely to be close to optimum. This results not only in a small range of variable values but also in a flat response. Near an optimum a performance variable such as distance jumped will be quadratically related to a variable such as approach speed, so that the theoretical graph will resemble an inverted U (Figure 7.2). Around the optimum, therefore, data will exhibit a flat linear trend rather than an inclined linear response. As a consequence, linear regression analysis will yield no relationship. On the other hand, quadratic regression analysis will also yield little due to the small amount and range of data. Failure to recognize such effects will result in abortive attempts to reveal underlying relationships.

Linear regression is sometimes used in a fishing expedition to find relationships between variables by investigating every pair of variables. This 'shotgun'

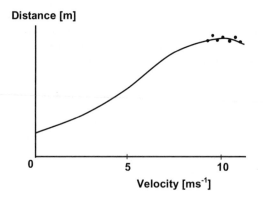

*Figure 7.2* A hypothetical data set showing approach speed and distance jumped for long jumping.

approach has the drawback that it may identify 'significant' relationships when, in reality, no such relationships exist. For example, if the level of significance is set at 5 per cent and all 45 pairs from 10 variables are regressed in turn, it may be expected that two 'significant' regressions will occur by chance. If there are three significant regressions in such a study then it may be that there is a real relationship between a pair of variables but which pair of the three will not be known. Extreme examples of this type report the expected number of random correlations as significant (Williams *et al.* 1988).

Hay and Reid (1982) proposed a hierarchical deterministic structure for identifying potential causal relationships prior to performing regressions of one variable against another. While this procedure is certainly an improvement upon regressing each variable against all others, implementations include a number of the weaknesses described above. First, the deterministic model is implicitly based on the performance of a single athlete, whereas implementations of the method typically use data from several athletes. Second, linear regression is typically used without thought, even in cases where the theoretical relationship between variables is known to be non-linear. The reason for this is over-reliance on computer packages without an understanding of what they provide and the consequence is failure to find a relationship when one exists. Finally, the search for relationships around an optimum will usually be unrewarding since the response is flat and the range of data usually too small to reveal curvature as described earlier.

The aim of research is to bring understanding to an area of study by way of providing explanations. Such explanations should do more than establish relationships between variables – they should explain how and why these relationships arise. The benefit of using an arm swing when jumping for height may be explained by showing that the arm swing puts the leg extensors in slower concentric conditions and so greater force can be exerted (Hill 1938). To demonstrate that this is so is not possible using a kinetic analysis of jumps with and without arm swing. It may be possible to demonstrate experimentally that jumps with arm swing allow greater leg extensor force to occur and that greater jump height occurs. To demonstrate that the leg extensors are in slower concentric conditions as a consequence of the arm swing requires the use of a theoretical model (Dapena 1999). As a consequence, studies aiming to reveal mechanisms using experimental studies of whole body movement either speculate on the mechanisms (Lees *et al.* 1994) or conclude that the mechanisms are unclear (Feltner *et al.* 1999).

The interpretation of experimental results is often a function of how the world is viewed. The leap from an experimental result that more training results in better performance to a general conclusion to this effect arises from an (unstated) belief that response is linear, when in general it is not. Komi and Mero (1985) express surprise that the increase in javelin range is disproportionately larger than the increase in release velocity. This error arises from an implicitly linear view of the world. As Hubbard (1989) wryly observes, a basic theoretical understanding that range is a quadratic function of velocity would lead to the opposite conclusion.

In a final observation on experimental studies, it should be noted that human response to a changed situation may be individual and somewhat unpredictable. For example, the responses to changes in surface cushioning when running can be highly individual (Dixon *et al.* 2000) and the effects of shoe inserts on gait can be unpredictable (Nigg *et al.* 1998). Additionally, the assessment of cushioning materials for running can give quite different results when subject tests are used rather than material tests (Kaelin *et al.* 1985). In an experiment in which weights were attached to a runner, the maximum vertical force recorded by a force plate, rather than increasing with increased weight, did not change (Bahlsen and Nigg 1987). This was a consequence of the runners modifying their technique, presumably to achieve a similar pressure sensation on the foot. Adaptations of technique such as these can complicate what may appear to be a simple intervention.

## Theoretical studies

As noted in the above section, experimental studies have inherent problems arising from real-world effects such as the limitations of humans in making ideal changes to technique. In this section, the advantages of using a theoretical model will be discussed along with the inherent difficulties of such an approach.

A model is a representation of a real-world system such as a human body. Such a representation is necessarily a simplification, since a model that is accurate in all respects in representing a human body will be indistinguishable from a human body. Since a model cannot reproduce all aspects of the real system it is first necessary to identify which elements of the real system should be included and how they should be represented. This is not a straightforward task as there is no guarantee that a carefully constructed model will perform in the required manner. A typical model in sports biomechanics might comprise a number of body segments connected by simple pin joints together with some mechanism for exerting torque about each joint (e.g. Hatze 1981). Often a process of iteration is necessary in which modifications are made until the model is able to match an actual performance. For example, wobbling masses may be included within the model to represent soft tissue movement within the segments (Gruber *et al.* 1998). Without such wobbling masses the forces calculated by a model may overestimate the actual forces in a movement. In order to assess when modifications result in an adequate model, a quantitative method of model evaluation is required. Typically data obtained from a real performance will be used as input to the model and the model output will be compared with the corresponding values from the actual performance. The cycle of model improvement is shown in Figure 7.3.

This step of model evaluation is essential before attempting to use the model to address research questions. Failure to do so will render any results uncertain and may lead to insights peculiar to the model rather than the real world and this will lead to misunderstanding rather than to understanding. Panjabi (1979) cautioned against evaluating a model in one situation and then using the model

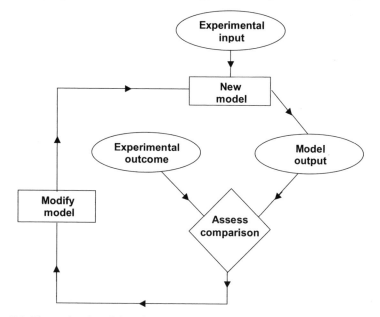

*Figure 7.3* The cycle of model evaluation and model modification.

in a quite different situation. He also observed that most models in biomechanics are not evaluated and, sadly, this still remains the case today (Gerritsen *et al.* 1995; Pandy *et al.* 1990; van Soest *et al.* 1993; Spagele *et al.* 1999; Sprigings 1998). While a number of models demonstrate some general agreement with experimental results (Alexander 1990), very few determine subject-specific model parameters (King and Yeadon 2002) and then assess the output of the model in a quantitative manner by comparison with individual performances (Yeadon and King 2002).

The term 'validation' rather than 'evaluation' of models is often used. While evaluation may be relatively well defined in terms of measuring the difference between experimental and simulated results, validation is often used to mean that the model reflects the way the world 'really is'. As Oreskes *et al.* (1994: 642) comment, 'the establishment that a model represents the "actual processes occurring in a real system" is not even a theoretical possibility.' They also observe that 'models are most useful when they are used to challenge existing formulations, rather to validate or verify them' (Oreskes *et al.* 1994: 644). Bearing in mind these inherent limitations, the ways in which models may be used will now be considered.

### Applications of models

In an ideal experiment to establish causality, just one element of the system is changed to determine its effect. As noted earlier, in practical experiments with athletes this is far from possible. With a theoretical model, on the other hand, it is achievable. It is important, however, that changes to a variable are realistic and are based on experimental data. Such an approach makes it possible to answer 'What if?' questions and is able to address why things occur, without much recourse to the speculation that is inherent in experimental studies. Additionally, a theoretical approach comes much closer to establishing causality than experimental studies that are limited to the demonstration of high correlations.

Perhaps the most powerful way of using a simulation model is in optimization studies. Since a simulation model can generate a performance in one second or less it is possible to test the outcome of thousands of scenarios and come to some conclusion regarding the technique that will produce a performance that is optimal in some sense. For example, in high jumping the optimization criterion might be the peak height of the mass centre in flight. Because of the automatic nature of the search for optimal technique there are potential problems. Even with sophisticated optimization programs such as Simulated Annealing (Goffe *et al.* 1994) there is no guarantee that the global optimum will be found. The search for an optimum can be likened to the search for the highest mountain peak in a given terrain: an optimization routine may find a local rather than a global optimum – the top of a foothill rather than the summit of the highest mountain. On the other hand, the routine may be successful in finding the top of a singular pinnacle that stands on a narrow base high above the surrounding terrain. Even if this is the global optimum it is a summit that should not be attempted, since any small location error will land on low terrain. In other words, if there is an optimum technique in javelin that is surrounded by poor performances, it is a poor strategy that strives for this in the distant hope that everything will come right on one of the attempts. The likelihood is that all performances will be poor. A better strategy may be to find a high hilltop with a large plateau so that points even some distance away are high. There is much to be said for consistency when competing.

Attempts to identify an optimization criterion that is responsible for the adoption of a particular strategy can suffer from a failure to consider the context holistically. If the research focus is led by information from descriptive studies then little insight may be gained. For example, in trying to explain why a smooth movement strategy is adopted for tasks such as drawing a line between two points, demonstrating that minimizing the rate of change of acceleration results in similar strategies (Hogan 1984) does little to bring understanding to the subject. In contrast, a strategy minimizing the error in targeting leads to an explanation of Fitt's Law on the trade-off between accuracy and speed in targeted movements (Harris and Wolpert 1998) giving real insight into movement strategy. In a similar vein, van Soest (1994) showed that optimum strategy in vertical jumping is dependent upon initial position but there exists a strategy that is close to optimal for a wide range of starting positions, suggesting that an element of robustness to change may be included in optimization strategies adopted by humans. In other words, it is likely that human movement strategies are best in the sense that small perturbations do not cause a large degradation in performance. Following this idea, Hiley and Yeadon (2003) identified the margin for error for timing release as an important determinant of high bar circling technique in Men's Artistic Gymnastics. Attempts to assess sensitivity of human performance using a theoretical model are likely to overestimate the sensitivity, since if this is a critical element in the performance, the athlete (as opposed to the model) will adopt strategies to reduce the sensitivity. While a theoretical model can attempt to replicate such strategies, it will do so in a way that is a simplified representation of the real system and will have less flexibility in the search for robustness of performance in response to perturbations in the timing of muscle contractions, for example.

## Postscript

While the case for a particular conclusion may appear clear, it should be remembered that research is conducted by humans and that humans are fallible. This is true for the natural sciences no less than for the social sciences. For example, in astronomy, telescopic observations of Mercury taken at different times showed the same face of Mercury facing the sun, and it was concluded that the planet rotated once about its own axis for one revolution about the sun. Since this result was consistent with the theoretical expectation of gravitational lock it was generally accepted as conclusive. The observations, however, were taken at intervals of 6 months during which Mercury had completed two orbits of the sun (Dyce *et al.* 1967). Subsequently it was discovered from radar measurements that Mercury rotates three times about its own axis for every two orbits of the sun. As a consequence, after an interval of 6 months Mercury was again in the same orientation. From a theoretical perspective a 3:2 ratio is understandable as well as a 1:1 ratio as in the case of the moon orbiting the earth. Thus a myopic interpretation of both experimental and theoretical data led to a false conclusion that was generally accepted from 1882 until 1965.

Our conceptual frameworks constrain the kind of questions that can be formulated and the kind of answers that are considered. The search for a single mathematical optimization criterion to explain the strategy adopted by the central nervous system to achieve a specific task will give way to somewhat different considerations when it is appreciated that robustness of response to perturbations is necessary. The idea that offspring must exhibit an intermediate blend of parental characteristics persisted in the nineteenth century due to the idea that the world was smooth and continuous rather than discrete and digital. Against this mainstream, Darwin noted that offspring were distinctly male or female rather than of intermediate sex (Dawkins 2003). The problems arising from the duality of mind and body disappear once it is accepted that there is no duality. The problem of consciousness is likely to recede once the remnants of the dichotomy between man and beast are finally laid to rest. The idea that we have no free will, since ideas originate in the subconscious before reaching the conscious mind will also dissipate when it is discovered that the conscious also affects the subconscious and that a personality properly includes both. Finally the idea that 'all truth must be one' may disappear once it is accepted that the 'true' answer depends upon our conceptual framework in posing the question.

While humanity will continue to try to make sense out of what appears to be the universe, there will always be the inherent limitation that science is constrained to sit in Plato's cave and attempt to interpret the flickering shadows on the cave wall.

## Bibliography

Alexander, R.M. (1990) 'Optimum take-off techniques for high and long jumps', *Philosophical Transactions of the Royal Society*, B239, 3–10.

Bahlsen, H.A. and Nigg, B.M. (1987) 'Estimation of impact forces using the idea of an effective mass', in B. Jonsson (ed.) *Biomechanics X-B*, Champaign, IL: Human Kinetics, 837–41.

Dapena, J. (1999) 'A biomechanical explanation of the effect of arm actions on the vertical velocity of a standing vertical jump', in W. Herzog and A. Jinha (eds) *Abstracts of the XVIIth International Society of Biomechanics Congress*, Calgary, 100.

Dapena, J., McDonald, C. and Cappaert, J. (1990) 'A regression analysis of high jumping technique', *International Journal of Sport Biomechanics*, 6, 246–61.

Dawkins, R. (2003) *A Devil's Chaplain: Selected Essays*, London: Weidenfeld & Nicholson.

Dixon, S.J., Collop, A.C. and Batt, M.E. (2000) 'The influence of surface shock absorption on ground reaction forces and kinematics in running', *Medicine and Science in Sports and Exercise*, 32, 1919–26.

Dyce, R.B., Pettengill, G.H. and Shapiro, I.I. (1967) 'Radar determinations of the rotations of Venus and Mercury', *Astronomical Journal*, 72, 351–9.

Feltner, M.E., Fraschetti, D.J. and Crisp, R.J. (1999) 'Upper extremity augmentation of lower extremity kinetics during countermovement vertical jumps', *Journal of Sports Sciences*, 17, 449–66.

Gerritsen, K.G.M., van den Bogert, A.J. and Nigg, B.M. (1995) 'Direct dynamics simulation of the impact phase in heel-toe running', *Journal of Biomechanics*, 28, 661–8.

Goffe, W.L., Ferrier, G.D. and Rogers, J. (1994) 'Global optimization of statistical functions with simulated annealing', *Journal of Econometrics*, 60, 65–99.

Greig, M.P. and Yeadon, M.R. (2000) 'The influence of touchdown parameters on the performance of a high jumper', *Journal of Applied Biomechanics*, 16, 367–78.

Gruber, K., Ruder, H., Denoth, J. and Schneider, K. (1998) 'A comparative study of impact dynamics: wobbling mass model versus rigid body model', *Journal of Biomechanics*, 31, 439–44.

Harris, C.M. and Wolpert, D.M. (1998) 'Signal-dependent noise determines motor planning', *Nature*, 394, 780–4.

Hatze, H. (1981) 'A comprehensive model for human motion simulation and its application to the take-off phase of the long jump', *Journal of Biomechanics*, 14, 135–42.

Hay, J.G. (1987) 'Biomechanics of the long jump – and some wider implications', In B. Jonsson (ed.) *Biomechanics X-B*, Champaign, IL: Human Kinetics.

Hay, J.G. and Reid, J.G. (1982) *The Anatomical and Mechanical Bases of Human Movement*, Englewood Cliffs, NJ: Prentice-Hall.

Hiley, M.J. and Yeadon, M.R. (2003) 'The margin for error when releasing the high bar for dismounts', *Journal of Biomechanics*, 36, 313–19.

Hill, A.V. (1938) 'The heat of shortening and the dynamic constraints of muscle', *Proceedings of the Royal Society of London*, Series B, 126, 136–95.

Hogan, N. (1984) 'An organizing principle for a class of voluntary movements', *Journal of Neuroscience*, 4, 2745–54.

Hubbard, M. (1989) 'The throwing events in track and field', in K. Vaughan (ed.) *Biomechanics of Sport*, Boca Rotan, FL: CRC Press.

Kaelin, X., Denoth, J., Stacoff, A. and Stuessi, E. (1985) 'Cushioning during running – material tests versus subject tests', in S. Perren (ed.) *Biomechanics: Principles and Applications*, London: Martinus Nijhoff Publishers, 651–6.

King, M.A. and Yeadon, M.R. (2002) Determining subject specific torque parameters for use in a torque driven simulation model of dynamic jumping, *Journal of Applied Biomechanics*, 18, 207–17.

Komi, P.V. and Mero, A. (1985) 'Biomechanical analysis of Olympic javelin throwers', *International Journal of Sport Biomechanics*, 1, 139–50.

Lees, A., Graham-Smith, P. and Fowler, N. (1994) 'A biomechanical analysis of the last stride, touchdown, and takeoff characteristics of the Men's long jump', *Journal of Applied Biomechanics*, 10, 61–78.

Nigg, B.M., Khan, A., Fisher, V. and Stefanyshyn, D. (1998) 'Effects of shoe insert construction on foot and leg movement', *Medicine and Science in Sports and Exercise*, 30, 550–5.

Oreskes, N., Shrader-Frechette, K. and Belitz, K. (1994) 'Verification, validation and confirmation of numerical models in the earth sciences', *Science*, 263, 641–6.

Pandy, M.G., Zajac, F.E., Sim, E. and Levine, W.S. (1990) 'An optimal control model for maximum-height human jumping', *Journal of Biomechanics*, 23, 1185–98.

Panjabi, M. (1979) 'Validation of mathematical models', *Journal of Biomechanics*, 12, 238.

Rothstein, A.L. (1985) *Research Design and Statistics for Physical Education*, Englewood Cliffs, NJ: Prentice-Hall.

Soest, A.J. van (1994) 'Control strategies in vertical jumping and implications for training', in *Proceedings: Second World Congress on Biomechanics*, Amsterdam: Stichting World Biomechanics, 132.

Soest, A.J. van, Schwab, A.L., Bobbert, M.F. and Ingen Schenau, G.J. van (1993) 'The influence of the biarticularity of the gastrocnemius muscle on vertical-jumping achievement', *Journal of Biomechanics*, 26, 1–8.

Spagele, T., Kistner, A. and Gollhofer, A. (1999) 'Modelling, simulation and optimization of a human vertical jump', *Journal of Biomechanics*, 32, 521–30.

Sprigings, E.J., Lanovaz, J.L., Watson, L.G. and Russell, K.W. (1998) 'Removing swing from a handstand on rings using a properly timed backward giant circle: a simulation solution', *Journal of Biomechanics*, 31, 27–35.

Williams, K.R., Snow, R. and Agruss, C. (1988) 'Changes in distance running kinematics with fatigue', *Medicine and Science in Sports and Exercise*, 20, S49.

Yeadon, M.R. and King, M.A. (2002) 'Evaluation of a torque driven simulation model of tumbling', *Journal of Applied Biomechanics*, 18, 195–206.

# 8  Can we trust rehydration research?

*Timothy David Noakes*

## Introduction

From antiquity until the early 1970s, athletes were advised *not* to drink during exercise. But between 1975 and 1996, novel guidelines for fluid ingestion during exercise were promulgated by a number of influential organizations including the American College of Sports Medicine (ACSM) (1975, 1987, 1996a, 1996b), the National Association of Athletic Trainers (Casa *et al.* 2000; Binkley *et al.* 2002) and the United States (US) Army (Burr 1991; Montain *et al.* 1999; Gardner 2002), amongst others. These guidelines are based on five core doctrines: First, that all the weight lost during exercise must be replaced if health is to be protected and performance is to be optimized. Second, that fluid ingestion alone can prevent serious heat illness during exercise regardless of the circumstances in which the exercise is undertaken. Third, that uniquely in humans, although apparently not in any other mammal, the sensations of thirst underestimate the human's real fluid requirements before, during and after exercise. As a result, unless properly informed, athletes will always drink too little, before, during and after exercise. Fourth, that the fluid requirements of all athletes, big and small, fast and slow, are sufficiently similar during all forms of exercise that a universal guideline is possible. And fifth, athletes can safely ingest any volume of fluid at any rate both at rest and during exercise without harmful consequences. Combined, these doctrines produce the guidelines that athletes should 'replace all the water lost through sweating (i.e., body weight loss) (ACSM 1996a, p i), or consume the maximal amount that can be tolerated' (ACSM 1996b, p i) or drink between 600–1200 ml per hour (ACSM 1996a, p i). Indeed the original US Army guidelines promoted even higher rates of fluid ingestion of up to 1800 ml per hour (Burr 1991).

But none of these ideas is evidence-based; that is, they are not based on properly conducted, peer-reviewed, scientific evidence that unequivocally proves these conclusions and excludes all other possible interpretations. In particular, it has never been shown that athletes who drink only according to thirst (*ad libitum*) and who therefore develop mild levels of dehydration during competitive sport, are at increased risk of avoidable health consequences. Indeed there is no evidence that, unlike any other living being on this planet, humans have the unique inability to determine exactly how much they should drink either before, during, or after exercise. Nor is it certain that all the weight lost during exercise must be replaced immediately. Nor is there any evidence that athletes perform better during exercise if they drink at the very high rates proposed by the ACSM or the 1991 US Army guidelines. Nor does it seem likely that fluid ingestion alone will prevent serious heat illness in those environmental conditions in which heatstroke is most likely to occur, namely competitive exercise of short duration but high intensity in hot, humid, wind-still conditions and in which severe levels of dehydration do not occur. Furthermore, sustained high rates of fluid ingestion either at rest (Speedy *et al.* 2001a; Noakes *et al.* 2001) or during exercise (Irving *et al.* 1991) are not safe, since they produce a progressive fluid overload, leading ultimately to hyponatraemic encephalopathy (brain swelling and dysfunction due to voluntary overdrinking either before, during or after exercise), and even death (Noakes 2003a).

The question arises: How could such manifestly incorrect and potentially dangerous scientific information become the accepted dogma? I propose that a number of potential factors can influence the independence of scientific findings and that some or all of these could have been at work in this particular example. Here I review, in general terms, how this could possibly happen, if not in this particular example, then perhaps in other similar cases. It is likely that similar circumstances occur more frequently than we perhaps appreciate.

First is the role of what Waller (2002) has called a 'foundation myth'. This is a mythical 'scientific belief', unsubstantiated by any definitive findings, but which becomes immune to subsequent scientific scrutiny simply because it is the earliest study in a particular field and perhaps because it seems to be so logical and easy to understand. Discoverers of a 'foundation myth' inevitably become the scientific icons in their specific discipline. The 'foundation myth' in this example is that any level of dehydration during exercise has dire consequences for both health and performance (Gisolfi 1996; Sawka and Mountain 2000; Coyle 2004). Such is the status of a 'foundation myth' that, out of deference to the iconic status of its scientific originators who are usually their tutors and mentors, subsequent generations of loyal scientists fail to review the original studies with appropriate scepticism. As a consequence, they fail to notice that those early studies did not, nor could they ever, establish the veracity of the 'foundation myth'. Indeed, as teachers, supervisors, examiners, reviewers and journal editors, the original icons and their scientific progeny are perfectly placed to ensure that the 'foundation myth' is perpetuated and never challenged.

Second is the role of industrial funding of research and the conflict of interest that such funding can create. Indeed the studies that established this particular 'foundation myth' and the iconic status of its 'discoverers' were funded by the fledgling sports drink industry in the early 1970s. It is not in the interests of either that industry or its scientific icons that the 'foundation myth' should ever be re-evaluated, much less falsified. Furthermore, it is highly improbable that future industrial funding would ever be made available to scientists wishing to challenge the veracity of the original myth. Rather, one must assume that industry will favour scientists more inclined to the propagation of the established dogma.

Third is the role of industrial funding of influential scientific organizations, particularly if the actions or pronouncements of those organizations can influence the future commercial success of the products of that industry. As a consequence, any scientific organization that is heavily dependent on funding from a particular industrial 'donor' may not wish to pursue a particular scientific idea that would cause embarrassment to, and hence the potential loss of, essential income from, that particular 'donor'. In this way any scientific organization that accepts any form of funding from industry loses its full freedom of expression in those areas of science that may impact on the commercial returns of the industrial 'donor'. Even for honorable scientific organizations, there is never a 'free lunch'. When one or more of the founding icons or their scientific progeny also serve on the leadership of those scientific organizations, the absolute independence of that organization is further threatened.

Fourth is the role of the internet, which has allowed the growth of virtual organizations that pose as 'scientific' institutions but which may be completely dependent on commercial funding and which can serve as one of the marketing/advertising arms of those industries. The use of the internet by such virtual scientific organizations for the widespread dissemination of apparently credible scientific information to both the lay public and to scientists, medical doctors and sports coaches, bypasses and hence undermines the usual scientific peer review process. Since peer-reviewed scientific journals reach only thousands to tens of thousands of subscribers, whereas the internet is open to hundreds of millions, it is understandable why such virtual scientific organizations have an unmatched power to influence public perceptions and practices and why they are so attractive to industry.

Fifth, in this particular case, I would suggest there were a series of substantive methodological and other errors made by the scientists involved in this research area, and that these errors included the following:

1   Scientists failed to observe the accepted scientific process which is to attempt the falsification of the accepted wisdom, in this case, the falsification of the 'foundation myth'. Indeed some might argue that so powerful is the 'myth' and the devotion and influence of its adherents, that any studies which attempted to falsify this particular 'myth' would likely be censored by the scientific review process, overseen as it is by an apparently honourable and scrupulously independent system of peer review. But the danger of peer review is that it will tend naturally to protect the prevailing, that is 'peer', dogma.

2   Many scientists failed to explain or to study some very simple observations. For example, it must be clear even to the most biased observer, that the fastest athletes in competition drink much less than the ACSM guidelines prescribe; indeed probably little more than did élite athletes before the 1970s, who were advised *not* to drink during exercise. Yet these winning athletes do not appear to suffer from either an impaired performance or a high rate of illness, despite their frugal drinking practices. Nor was sufficient

attention paid to the finding that those athletes who do collapse usually do so only after they complete these events and with body temperatures that are not particularly elevated. These simple observations suggest that it is the act of stopping exercise and not the exercise itself that causes most cases of exercise-associated collapse. There is also evidence that athletes with exercise-associated collapse recover without the need to be cooled, indicating that they are not suffering from a heat illness. In contrast, the 'foundation myth' predicts that such collapses are due solely to 'dehydration and hyperthermia'.

3   Furthermore, scientists ignored the published evidence that humans who did not drink during 8-hour walks covering about 30 km in desert heat tolerate dehydration well and recover rapidly when allowed free access to fluid (Brown 1947). Conversely, scientists have failed to produce evidence that the mild to moderate levels of dehydration experienced by modern athletes contribute to ill-health (Noakes 1995).

4   Scientists failed to perform controlled prospective trials to ensure the safety of the new and radically different drinking guidelines introduced in the 1980s and 1990s and which encouraged athletes to drink 'as much as tolerable' during exercise. Rather in support of what, in retrospect, are industrially favourable guidelines, they emphasized the findings from three poorly designed 'foundation studies' that had not been designed to provide the unambiguous evidence necessary to support their radically novel conclusions. In short, I would suggest that the guidelines developed were not supported by evidence-based information from rigorously designed and appropriately controlled, prospective intervention trials.

5   Scientists failed to undertake studies in environmental conditions that mimic those present in out-of-doors competition. In particular they failed to recreate the facing wind speeds experienced by athletes in out-of-doors competition. As a consequence they studied the physiological consequences of 'dehydration' in experimental conditions in the laboratory that are not found in out-of-doors competition. Thus at least some of the supposedly detrimental physiological effects of 'dehydration' are an artifact of the unnatural environmental conditions in which the laboratory testing was performed (Saunders *et al.* 2004).

6   When the first case reports of significant illness were reported in a specific group of endurance athletes who religiously followed these novel and supposedly more healthy drinking guidelines, no attempts were made by scientists or the industry to place a moratorium on these new guidelines. Rather, athletes were informed that sports drinks were superior to water, since only sports drinks contain sodium chloride. The unstated inference was that drinking 'as much as tolerable' was indeed safe but only if a sports drink, but not water, was ingested. Thus the subtle message was that the presence of sodium chloride in sports drinks but not in water would protect against the development of fluid overload in those who overdrank during exercise.

7   Only after the widely publicized deaths from hyponatraemic encephalopathy
in a 43-year-old paediatric dentist and mother of three in the 1998 Chicago
42 km Marathon (Zorn 1999), of a 28-year-old cancer survivor in the 2002
Boston Marathon (Smith 2002), of another female runner in the 2002
Marine Corps Marathon in Washington DC, and of a number of military
personnel in the United States Army (Garigan and Ristedt 1999; O'Brien *et
al.* 2001; Gardner 2002) and of a rising incidence of this condition uniquely
in United States marathon runners/walkers (Davis *et al.* 2001; Hew *et al.*
2003; Almond *et al.* 2003) was the obvious reluctantly admitted; that these
deaths were avoidable and were the result of the adoption of an incorrect
dogma based on a flawed scientific process.

On 19 April 2003, United States of America Track and Field (USATF)
announced that all future running races in the United States would be run
according to new guidelines (Noakes 2003a; Noakes and Martin 2002; Noakes
2003b) which advocate that (i) athletes should drink according to the dictates of
their thirst during exercise and not to the limits of their individual tolerance and
(ii) that collapsed athletes may not receive intravenous fluids – the treatment
predicted by the 'foundation myth' – unless there is a scientifically established
reason for such treatment.

The manner in which a misguided dogma grew to become *the* accepted truth,
how the opposing view (Noakes 2003a) was, and continues to be trivialized as
the opinion of one man (Gatorade Sports Science Institute 2003), and possibly
even actively censored by the devotees of the 'foundation myth', should serve as
a warning for those who act on the basis of a poor science that is popularized for
reasons that extend beyond science.

## The evolution of contemporary drinking guidelines for athletes

Prior to 1969, athletes were advised to avoid drinking during competitive foot
races as it was believed that fluid ingestion produced specific symptoms and
impaired performance (Noakes 1993). But in that year, a South African study
reported a linear relationship between race-induced weight losses greater than 3
per cent and the post-race rectal temperatures of runners in a 32 km race
(Wyndham and Strydom 1969).

The incorrectly titled article that described those findings – 'The danger of an
inadequate water intake during marathon running' – provided the initial
incentive for the revolutionary change in drinking behaviors during exercise,
culminating in the new drinking guidelines of the 1980s and 1990s (American
College of Sports Medicine 1975, 1987, 1996a, 1996b; Casa *et al.* 2000; Binkley
*et al.* 2002; Burr 1991; Montain *et al.* 1999; Gardner 2002).

But in describing such 'danger' the scientists made three cardinal errors. First
they assumed that a mathematical relationship between two variables means
that the two are causally related; in this case that any 'dehydration' that develops
during exercise causes a dangerous elevation in body temperature. But a cross-

sectional, observational study in which the same measurements are made in the same subjects after they perform an uncontrolled experiment, in this case running 32 km without any attempt to regulate the experimental variables, cannot prove causation.

Rather causation can only be identified by a prospective intervention trial in which the chosen variable under study is controlled. In this example, the chosen variable identified for control should have been the rates of fluid ingestion during exercise, since, only by varying the rates of fluid ingestion during exercise, is it possible to produce different grades of dehydration in the same athletes who perform exactly the same exercise in identical conditions on two or more occasions. Only by comparing the effects of *different* levels of dehydration in the *same* athletes running at the their *same* speeds in the *same* environmental conditions on two or more different occasions, could the authors have determined the independent effects of dehydration when all other variables that could potentially influence that relationship were controlled and hence identical. Instead, the study controlled for none of these variables and attempted to draw conclusions by combining data from two uncontrolled studies in which athletes drank as they wished when they ran 32 km foot races at their own chosen, and hence potentially different, paces in environmental conditions that were not the same in both trials.

Second, in reaching this conclusion, the scientists had to ignore the findings from their own (Wyndham *et al.* 1970) and other studies (Saltin and Hermansen 1966; Greenhaff 1989) showing that the most accurate predictor of the body temperature during exercise is the rate of energy expenditure (metabolic rate). By ignoring this factor they failed to exclude the possibility that any relationship between dehydration and rectal temperature was likely spurious and might have been explained by at least one other, a third factor, that they failed to recognize.

This error is so common, especially amongst neophyte scientists, that it deserves special attention. Figure 8.1 shows the familiar assumption that the two variables measured in a specific study must be causally related; in this case that factor A (dehydration) determines factor B (rectal temperature).

However, the challenge of science is to *prove* and not to *assume* causality. In this case, the goal is to exclude the presence of a confounding variable (C in Figure 8.2) that explains the assumed causal relationship between A and B, perhaps by acting through a fourth factor, D.

Thus Figure 8.2 shows that, since it determines both the body temperature (factor B) during exercise (Wyndham *et al.* 1970; Saltin and Hermansen 1966; Greenhaff 1989) and the sweat rate (factor D) (Kondo *et al.* 1998; Yanagimoto *et*

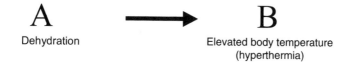

**A** ⟶ **B**

Dehydration      Elevated body temperature
(hyperthermia)

*Figure 8.1* Many believe that dehydration is the single most important cause of an elevated body temperature during exercise.

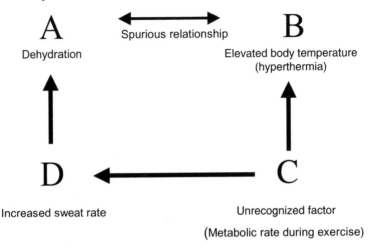

*Figure 8.2* Their co-dependence on the metabolic rate during exercise could explain a spurious relationship between dehydration and hyperthermia during exercise.

*al.* 2003), the factor C (metabolic rate) that was unrecognized and hence uncontrolled in the study of Wyndham and Strydom, could explain an apparent (spurious) relationship between dehydration and the elevated body temperature.

Thus an alternative possibility to explain this apparently causal relationship between dehydration and hyperthermia is that the faster the runners ran in that study, the higher were their metabolic rates and as a consequence their body temperatures and sweat rates. Since all the runners drank sparingly during those races, as was the custom at that time, the fastest runners with the highest metabolic rates, the highest body temperatures and the highest sweat rates would also develop the highest levels of dehydration. By failing to design an appropriately controlled experiment that could exclude this alternative explanation, Wyndham and Strydom fell head-first into the common logical trap and may erroneously have concluded the spurious relationship depicted in Figure 8.1.

The third error made by Wyndham and Strydom was that neither did the study examine a marathon race, as suggested in the title, nor did it establish any 'danger' of fluid restriction during exercise. Rather, the hottest and most dehydrated athletes won those races, as is usually the case. Indeed the post-race body temperatures of the athletes in their trial were no higher than values from other studies of marathon runners in which no reference is made to a supposed 'danger' posed by this range of body temperatures. Indeed body temperatures in their study were not elevated into the range associated with heat stroke (>41.5°C), nor does their report contain any mention of signs and symptoms of heatstroke in individual athletes with high body temperatures.

Nevertheless, one predictable consequence of Wyndham and Strydom's study was that it legitimized the value of sports drinks for ingestion during exercise. Indeed, the article's incorrect title, proposing as it did that dehydration causes 'danger' during exercise, provided the intellectual incentive for a host of studies, many funded by a fledgling sports drink industry (Gisolfi 1996), culminating in the revolutionary guidelines for fluid ingestion during exercise. Specifically, the study provided the intellectual basis for the erroneous 'foundation myth' that dehydration is the single most important factor determining the rise in rectal temperature during exercise and, hence, the risk that heatstroke or other medical dangers will develop during prolonged exercise, especially in the heat.

Influenced by this novel interpretation, the scientists advising the ACSM have, in the past 20 years, produced the four different Position Statements/ Stands pertaining to fluid ingestion and the prevention of heat injury during exercise (American College of Sports Medicine 1975, 1987, 1996a, 1996b). Each is somewhat different, particularly concerning the nature of the claims made for the benefits of such fluid replacement and the volumes of fluid that should be ingested during exercise.

In 1975, the simple advice was that athletes should 'be encouraged to frequently ingest fluids during competition' (American College of Sports Medicine 1975). 'Frequently' was considered to be every 3–4 km in races of 16 km or longer, suggesting that fluid ingestion was considered to be of lesser importance in races less than 16 km. This advice was entirely appropriate in 1975, since, for the previous 100 years, athletes had been advised to avoid fluid ingestion during exercise (Noakes 2003a; 1993). The rationale for fluid ingestion was to 'reduce rectal temperature and prevent dehydration'. No specific reference was made to the possibility that fluid ingestion alone would influence the risk of, much less prevent, heat illness during exercise. In retrospect, these guidelines contain little if anything that can be criticized.

The subsequent Position Stand of 1987 (American College of Sports Medicine 1987) introduced two additional statements of relevance to this appraisal. The first was: 'Fluid consumption before and during the race will reduce the risk of heat injury, *particularly in longer runs such as the marathon*' (current author's emphasis) (Wyndham and Strydom 1969; Costill *et al.* 1970; Gisolfi and Copping 1974). But the evidence-base for this conclusion is not sufficient for proof, since the three cited 'foundation references' do not include studies that were sufficiently well designed to support that specific conclusion. This is because all studied only the effects of different (subject chosen) rates of fluid ingestion solely on the rectal temperature either in a 32 km race (Wyndham and Strydom 1969) or during laboratory exercise (Costill *et al.* 1970; Gisolfi and Copping 1974), and none studied the influence of different (experimenter chosen) rates of fluid ingestion on the incidence of heat injury in marathon runners competing in appropriate environmental conditions out-of-doors. Therefore, none could conclude that fluid ingestion reduces the risk of heat injury, however defined, in marathoners running 42 km in appropriate environmental conditions.

Hence this Stand, which introduced a fundamentally novel concept not present in the 1975 Position Statement, was not based on new evidence that had become available after 1975. To have produced novel, evidence-based information to support these guidelines, scientists would first have had to develop unambiguous criteria for diagnosing 'heat injury', specifically to ensure that only this condition was being studied. Certain that they were diagnosing exactly and exclusively the condition they had defined as 'heat injury', the scientists would need to study the incidence of this condition in the same group of marathon runners on two or more occasions when they ran the same marathon at exactly the same pace, after exactly the same training and recovery period, under identical environmental conditions, but when they drank fluid at different rates. Instead the authors quoted a study in which runners ran for 2 hours on a laboratory treadmill drinking at different rates whilst their body temperatures were measured. This is an altogether different experiment that can only ever answer a much simpler question, specifically, what is the effect of different rates of fluid ingestion on the body temperature in laboratory exercise performed under the specific environmental conditions that were tested?

The second statement was that: 'Such dehydration will subsequently reduce sweating and predispose the runner to hyperthermia, heat stroke, heat exhaustion, and muscle cramps' (Wyndham and Strydom 1969). Nor is this statement evidence-based, since the cited reference, the original South African study of Wyndham and Strydom, studied neither the incidence of hyperthermia, heatstroke, heat exhaustion or muscle cramps in marathon runners nor, in a controlled prospective trial, the effects of different rates of fluid ingestion on the incidence of those conditions. Rather, as already described, the study simply reported a relationship between the post-exercise rectal temperature and the extent of weight loss in competitors in two 32 km running races, in which no experimental variables were controlled. In addition that study falls foul of the obvious criticism that *association does not prove causation* (Figures 8.1 and 8.2). Again, to provide evidence that the rate of fluid ingestion prevents 'hyperthermia, heat stroke, heat exhaustion, and muscle cramps', the experimental marathon studies described in the previous paragraph would need to be undertaken.

Nor interestingly is there any evidence that the dehydration that develops during exercise reduces the sweat rate (Saunders *et al.* 2004; Costill *et al.* 1970; Armstrong and Maresh 1998; Cheuvront and Haymes 2001a). Indeed one of the 'foundation studies' (Costill *et al.* 1970: 524) showed that sweat rates were the same regardless of the rate of fluid ingestion during exercise so that 'the runners' skin was sufficiently wetted by sweating to permit maximal evaporation'. Furthermore, the authors of that paper concluded that fluid ingestion reduced the rectal temperature during exercise, not as a result of superior thermoregulation but as a consequence of the cooling effect of the cold fluid that was ingested. Indeed if the sweat rate is not reduced by dehydration, it becomes increasingly difficult to believe that dehydration can have a significant effect on thermoregulation during exercise so that another explanation must be provided for the higher body temperatures in dehydrated athletes exercising in the laboratory (Saunders *et al.* 2004). This is addressed later in this chapter.

The next Position Stand of 1996 (American College of Sports Medicine 1996a) proposed that dehydration can 'predispose the runner to heat exhaustion or the more dangerous hyperthermia and exertional heat stroke (Hubbard and Armstrong 1988; Pearlmutter 1986)'. However, this statement is again not evidence-based, since the two referenced articles are literature reviews which do not provide any new findings, available since the 1987 Position Stand, that would justify this new dogma that dehydrated runners are at increased risk of 'dangerous hyperthermia' or heatstroke. Again it is necessary to emphasize that there are no reports in the scientific literature of prospective studies that have been designed specifically to determine whether the incidence of 'dangerous hyperthermia' or heatstroke is increased in runners only when they drink the least during a 42 km marathon race and that the incidence is reduced when the same runners drink more whilst performing the identical races under otherwise identical experimental conditions. Rather these new guidelines project an increasingly strident opinion, not supported by new evidence from appropriately controlled, prospective, interventional trials. Indeed one might question what extraneous factors might possibly have injected such certainty into the minds of the authors of these new guidelines.

However, the 1996 Position Stand appears to be contradictory, since it later states that 'excessive hyperthermia may occur in the absence of significant dehydration' (American College of Sports Medicine 1996a: iv), especially in short-distance races when the rate of heat production is high. That statement is indeed evidence-based. There is clear evidence that heatstroke occurs most commonly in short-distance running events in which high rates of heat production occur in environmental conditions that limit the rate at which heat can be lost to the environment and which are completed without the development of significant dehydration (Noakes 1981; Armstrong *et al.* 1996).

The 1996 Position Stand also includes the statement that: 'Adequate fluid consumption before and during the race can reduce the risk of heat illness, including disorientation and irrational behaviour, *particularly in longer events such as a marathon* (current author's italics) (Wyndham and Strydom 1969; Costill *et al.* 1970; Gisolfi and Copping 1974)'. But the statement is not evidence-based, since the same three 'foundation' references from the 1987 Position Stand are again cited and none measured, in controlled prospective intervention trials, the effects of different rates of fluid ingestion on the incidence of heat illness, disorientation or irrational behaviour in any running races, including marathon races, conducted under the appropriately controlled experimental conditions described here. The statement also proposes that athletes should be encouraged to 'replace their sweat losses or consume 150–300ml every 15 minutes (600–1200ml per hour)' (American College of Sports Medicine 1996a: i–ii). But no novel scientific rationale for that proposal is referenced.

The Position Stand also includes the statement that: 'Intravenous (IV) fluid therapy facilitates rapid recovery [in runners with heat exhaustion] (Hubbard and Armstrong 1989; Nash 1985)' (American College of Sports Medicine 1996b: iv). But that statement is also not evidence-based since it references two review articles that do not contain evidence from randomized, controlled, prospective intervention clinical trials that compared the effects of the administration of IV fluids and another form of treatment on the rates of recovery in athletes with 'heat exhaustion'. Nor is it exactly certain what constitutes 'heat exhaustion' and how this specific condition can be diagnosed correctly (Noakes 2003b). Thus no evidence-based information is provided to justify this novel dogma, which is, however, frequently promoted and practised, sometimes with unintended consequences (Eichner 1991; Noakes 1999a, 1999b, 2000).

The related 1996 Position Stand on Exercise and Fluid Replacement extends these new claims by stating that the 'most serious effect of dehydration resulting from the failure to replace fluids during exercise is impaired heat dissipation, which can elevate core temperature to dangerously high levels (i.e. > 40°C)'. Later the statement is made that dehydration during exercise 'presents the potential for the development of heat-related disorders ... including the potentially life-threatening heat stroke (Sutton 1990; Wyndham 1977). It is therefore reasonable to surmise that fluid replacement that offsets dehydration and excessive elevation in body heat during exercise may be instrumental in reducing the risk of thermal injury (Hubbard and Armstrong 1988)' (American College of Sports Medicine 1996b: ii).

But these conclusions are once again not evidence-based, as all the material quoted to support these new interpretations are review articles that represent the individual beliefs of the authors. Importantly, none of the articles provides specific data from controlled, prospective, interventional trials showing either that athletes who are dehydrated are at greater risk of heatstroke during exercise or that fluid ingestion during exercise can reduce the number of athletes who develop heatstroke under controlled experimental conditions. Given that cases of heatstroke occur so infrequently (Wyndham 1977), such research would be extremely difficult to conduct.

Influenced perhaps by the dissemination of the ACSM guidelines, two other influential organizations, the United States Army (Burr 1991; Montain *et al.* 1999; Gardner 2002) and the National Athletic Trainers Association (Casa *et al.* 2000; Binkley *et al.* 2002) published their own guidelines during the same period. Since many of the same scientists advised all three organizations, it is natural that there should be a degree of intellectual overlap in the pronouncements of all three groups.

To summarize, over the course of four revisions, the ACSM Position Statement/Stands have become progressively more strident in promoting the 'foundation myth' that high rates of fluid ingestion during exercise are necessary to prevent heatstroke and other heat illnesses and to optimize performance. But this advice is not evidence-based, since none of the Position Statement/Stands refers to specific, prospective, controlled, interventional studies from which such definite conclusions can be drawn. Furthermore, there is no evidence in the published literature to suggest that this advice is correct.

For example, there is not a single cross-sectional study – the experimental method used, for example, in the classical study by Wyndham and Strydom

(1969), and which *may identify* (Figure 8.1) *but cannot prove* (Figure 8.2) potential causal relationships – showing that runners with heat illnesses are more dehydrated than are those without such illnesses during exercise. That the majority of athletes with 'heat illness' are likely to be 'dehydrated' is a statistical certainty, since the vast majority of athletes lose weight during exercise. But the scientific question is whether athletes with 'heat illness' are more dehydrated than are healthy runners completing the same races and that this extra dehydration explains their illness. Thus the fundamental scientific requirement of a cross-sectional study is the inclusion of an appropriate control group, comprising unaffected athletes completing the same race without the development of the specific condition identified in the affected athletes under study and in whom all the same variables are measured. Therefore, the absence of an appropriate control group negates any possible scientific conclusions from any study, most especially those with a cross-sectional design.

In contrast, there is a body of published evidence from appropriately designed, cross-sectional studies showing the exact opposite, namely that there is no relationship between levels of dehydration during competitive sport and the post-race rectal temperature (Noakes *et al.* 1988, 1991b; Sharwood *et al.* 2002, 2004); nor between the level of dehydration and either performance or the development of specific medical diagnoses either during or after that race (Sharwood *et al.* 2002, 2004). In contrast, quite mild degrees of overhydration in athletes who follow the ACSM guidelines can produce significant morbidity (Noakes 2003a; Noakes *et al.* 2004).

The contrary findings of these studies are essentially never referenced by the devotees of the 'foundation myth' (Coyle 2004). In addition, there is the impression that research studies which contradict the 'foundation myth' are more likely to be rejected, perhaps censored, by a peer-review system which favours the 'peer' dogma. Yet the ultimate function of science should be to challenge the prevailing dogmas (Noakes 1997).

In summary, the conclusions of the four ACSM Position Statement/Stands are based on a 'reasonable to surmise' doctrine. Furthermore, they promote high rates of fluid replacement during exercise, sufficient to replace all the weight lost during exercise but without providing a scientific validation for that conclusion. Rather the doctrine of 'potential for prevention' is invoked. Perhaps these errors would have been understandable if they had not produced a predictable outcome (Noakes 2003a).

For the sternest criticism of these guidelines is that they elevated fluid ingestion before, during and after exercise to the status of a medicine for the prevention and treatment of a specific, albeit ill-defined, group of medical condition including 'heat illness', 'heat exhaustion', 'heat syncope' and 'heat cramps'. Yet before any medicine intervention is released for public consumption, it must be tested to ensure that it is without harmful effects in the prescribed dosage range. The organizations that developed these guidelines did not undertake controlled, prospective clinical trials to determine the safety of this medical advice.

## Commercial involvement in the public promotion and widespread adoption of guidelines that are not evidence-based

Despite the absence of an adequate evidence base, these novel ideas began to be widely promoted and liberally embellished by the manufacturers of those sports drinks that became increasingly available after the late 1970s. These drinks are actively marketed for their capacity (i) to enhance athletic performance and (ii) to prevent fatigue and heat illnesses during exercise (Gisolfi 1996; Sawka and Montain 2000). At the same time, sponsored symposia and workshops and their published proceedings have further popularized the teaching that athletes needed to drink copiously during exercise in order to aid performance and to prevent the reportedly dangerous effects of 'dehydration' (Laird and Wheeler 1988; Gisolfi and Lamb 1990; Gisolfi *et al.* 1993; Lamb *et al.* 1994; Maughan and Murray 2001).

Hence the website of the world's leading such company has carried articles claiming that: 'Dehydration can imperil health by increasing the risk of heat illnesses such as heat exhaustion and heatstroke'; that 'The goal of fluid replacement during exercise should be to fully replace sweat losses. The physiological and performance benefits of doing so are well documented'; and that: 'Although athletes and others continue to fall prey to exertional heatstroke, the frequency of deaths has been drastically reduced over the years (Murray 1996), in large part because the necessity of adequate fluid replacement has become well recognized' (Baumann 1995).

This latter statement in particular can have no factual basis, since neither the historical nor the current incidence of heatstroke in 'athletes' is known and is perhaps unknowable. Nor is this conclusion supported by any specific data in the quoted reference (Baumann 1995). In particular there is no published evidence from the appropriately controlled, prospective interventional trials showing that fluid ingestion can prevent the development of heatstroke. Furthermore, even case series find that the great majority of military heatstroke cases occur within the first 2 hours of exercise, precluding dehydration as a significant factor (Epstein *et al.* 1999).

It is of interest that many of these statements and related articles, published as they are on a commercial website of a virtual scientific organization (Gatorade Sports Science Institute 2003, 2000b; Murray 1996; Eichner 2002; Coyle 1994; Murray *et al.* 2003), are projected as if they carry the same scientific credibility as do publications in real scientific publications, whereas they may reflect a quite different bias. For example, nowhere on these websites is equal time given to the opposing belief that dehydration may not be quite as lethal as the 'foundation myth' proposes. Yet unlike the publications of those who attempt to challenge the veracity of these statements (Noakes 2000, 2003a), the opinions of a virtual scientific organization can be published instantaneously on the internet (Gatorade Sports Science Institute 2003) without passage through the established peer-review system, even when they contest material published in the accepted scientific manner and which may have required many years and multiple submissions to many journals before achieving publication.

## The practical consequences of the public promotion of novel drinking guidelines that are not evidence-based

By the late 1970s and early 1980s, a marathon-running craze had engulfed the major big cities of the world including New York, Chicago, Boston, Los Angeles, London and Berlin, amongst others. To protect against liability arising from their negligence of the, by then, accepted wisdom that dehydration is a uniquely defined and potentially very hazardous medical condition in marathon runners, the race organizers ensured that ample fluid was available at multiple aid stations along the routes of these races (Laird and Wheeler 1988). In addition, pre-race publicity, supplemented by the web-based material detailed in the previous section, emphasized the athletes' need to drink fluid at high rates to ensure that they did not suffer any of the supposedly dangerous complications of this novel sporting pandemic of the big cities.

As a result, within less than a decade, advice on drinking during exercise had changed from the idea that drinking during exercise was considered, at best, to impair performance and, at worst, to be a marker of unfitness and cowardice (Noakes 1993), to one in which athletes had been subtly conditioned to believe that they risked their lives if they failed to drink 'the maximal amount that can be tolerated' during exercise.

Simultaneously, there was also a large increase in the number of marathon runners seeking medical attention (Adner *et al.* 1988) at the finish of those, by then, populous big city marathon races. According to the 'foundation myth' it was assumed that these collapsed runners were still not drinking enough to prevent this dehydration-induced collapse. As a result, efforts to encourage athletes to drink even more during marathon races were intensified. Finally, it was also assumed that athletes who had collapsed because of 'dehydration' required resuscitation with the rapid intravenous infusion of often large volumes of fluid (Eichner 1991; Noakes 1999a, 1999b, 2000; Noakes *et al.* 1991a).

Also, in the early 1980s, the first cases of a novel, previously unreported condition – exercise-induced hyponatremia – were described (Noakes *et al.* 1985; Frizzel *et al.* 1986) shortly after the adoption of this new 'drink the maximal amount that can be tolerated' dictum. Patients with this condition develop blood sodium concentrations that are below the normal values of between 135–145 mmol.L$^{-1}$. Once the blood sodium concentration falls below about 129 mmol.L$^{-1}$, affected athletes present with varying degrees of altered levels of consciousness from mild confusion to frank coma (complete loss of consciousness), frequently associated with epileptic seizures. Other complications include fluid overload of the lungs (pulmonary oedema) with respiratory failure. The primary abnormality is excessive fluid accumulation in the brain causing an increase in the pressure within the brain. This occurs because the brain is encased in a rigid skull that does not allow any increase in volume without a steep increase in pressure. The progressive increase in pressure causes the abnormal brain function, leading ultimately to death with the cessation of certain vital functions.

By mid-2003, seven fatalities and more than 250 cases of hospitalization for this condition had been reported in the scientific literature (Hiller 1989; Noakes 2002, 2003a). It is probable that many more cases have gone unreported. During the same period, it was not possible to find a single case report of death or ill-health in an athlete in whom dehydration was established as the sole causative mechanism (Noakes *et al.* 2002; Noakes 2003b).

The earliest reports of the hyponatraemia of exercise speculated that it occurred in athletes who sustained inappropriately high rates of fluid ingestion for many (>7) hours during prolonged exercise (Noakes *et al.* 1985; Frizzel *et al.* 1986). But a more recent and unfortunately titled article suggested the reverse – that the hyponatraemia of exercise was caused by dehydration (Hiller 1989) and hence occurred in those who drank too little during exercise (Hiller 1987, 1989; Eichner *et al.* 1993). This speculation (Hiller 1989) was published in a peer-reviewed journal even though the article did not include measurements of changes in whole body fluid balance during exercise in athletes who developed the hyponatraemia of exercise. More than a decade later, review articles continue to quote that article as evidence that the symptomatic hyponatraemia of exercise can occur in those who drink too little and who lose too much salt during prolonged exercise (Maughan and Shirreffs 1998).

But this particular controversy should have been laid to rest years ago, when another South African study (Irving *et al.* 1991) established that eight comatose and desperately ill 90 km Comrades Marathon ultra-marathon runners with symptomatic hyponatraemia were all suffering from profound fluid overload. In addition, there was no evidence that abnormal losses of sodium in their sweat and urine had contributed significantly to their hyponatraemia (Irving *et al.* 1991). Since then, a series of additional studies have confirmed that this is the correct interpretation (Noakes 2002; Speedy *et al.* 2000, 2001b).

But the perplexing question remains: Why was this incontrovertible conclusion not enthusiastically embraced, especially in the United States? Was this perhaps because it conflicted with a commercial interest that benefited from the perpetuation of the 'foundation myth' that the unrestricted consumption of sports drinks under all circumstances is uniquely beneficial and scientifically proven?

The question that is yet to be answered is: How was this possible and what does it teach us about the conduct of science in the twenty-first century? One aim of this chapter is to suggest some answers to this perplexing question.

### Perpetuation of the error that hyponatraemia results from salt deficiency and can be prevented by the ingestion of sodium-containing sports drinks

Our study in 1991 showed that runners who developed hyponatraemic encephalopathy in the 90 km Comrades Marathon recovered when they excreted a fluid excess to which any sodium deficit played only a minor part

(Irving *et al.* 1991). Accordingly, it has essentially been known, at least since 1991, that hyponatraemic encephalopathy will occur only if there is a fluid overload, regardless of whether or not there is also a significant sodium deficit (Irving *et al.* 1991; Noakes 2002). Indeed the extent of the sodium deficit determines solely the extent of the fluid overload necessary to lower the blood sodium concentration (Noakes 2002). Thus even a large sodium deficit only reduces the amount of fluid overload necessary to lower the blood sodium concentration and to produce the symptoms of this condition. Yet without the fluid overload, the symptomatic brain complications – hyponatraemic encephalopathy – of this condition will not develop.

Thus the correct interpretation in 1991 should have been that hyponatraemic encephalopathy is always either a self-inflicted or, less commonly, an iatrogenic (doctor-induced) condition that occurs when affected athletes and the physicians who treat them, follow the guidelines based on the 'foundation myth' to their literal conclusion. Thus affected athletes must have drunk too much fluid either before, during or after exercise. Then when they collapse, they may also have received inappropriate IV fluid therapy that further compounds the fluid overload and drives the blood sodium concentration even lower (Eichner 1991; Noakes 1999a, 1999b, 2000; Noakes *et al.* 1991a).

Yet the 1996 ACSM guidelines for fluid replacement during exercise (1996a, 1996b) failed to acknowledge this reality. Rather than including the warning that drinking too much is dangerous, the guidelines encouraged the development of hyponatraemia by advocating that athletes should drink the maximum amount tolerable during exercise without appropriate warnings about the potential dangers of this practice.

The most recent Position Stand (ACSM 1996a: iii) does include the statement that: 'Excessive consumption of pure water or dilute fluid during exercise may lead to a harmful dilutional hyponatremia' but the message is distorted in the Position Stand on Exercise and Fluid Replacement (ACSM 1996b: iv) which concludes only that: 'One major rationale for inclusion of sodium in rehydration drinks is to avoid hyponatremia.' Yet this statement is not only *not* evidence-based but it is incorrect, since it was disproved by the study of Irving *et al.* (1991) which showed that sodium deficiency is not a factor in the development of this condition, so that the condition cannot be prevented by salt ingestion during exercise. The sole method for preventing this condition is not to overdrink during exercise as now proven in the appropriate clinical trials (Noakes *et al.* 2004, Speedy *et al.* 2000).

Indeed in my view, this historical and continuing (Murray *et al.* 2003) error that hyponatraemia is due to abnormally high sodium losses that can be prevented by the ingestion of sports drinks during exercise, has significantly delayed the acceptance that fluid overload alone causes this problem. Indeed, the only beneficiaries of this error appear to have been the manufacturers of sports drinks, who, in part, market their products on the basis that it is their sodium (and carbohydrate) content that makes sports drinks 'better' than water (Gatorade Sports Science Institute 2000c, 2000d).

In contrast, had these Position Stands properly reviewed the full range of published scientific evidence and warned already in 1996 that it is the gross overconsumption of any fluid, even those containing sodium in the low concentrations found in popular sports drinks, that causes hyponatraemic encephalopathy, it is unlikely that the epidemic of this condition that engulfed the United States Army and North American marathon runners in the mid- to late-1990s, with some fatal consequences, could have occurred (Noakes 2002; Speedy et al. 2001b).

## The contribution of laboratory studies that failed to reproduce the environmental conditions present in out-of-doors exercise

A final question that requires an answer is: Why do the ACSM guidelines specify a single ideal rate (1200 ml per hour) of fluid ingestion during exercise? Why was not some other rate chosen? The clear answer is that these guidelines are based on laboratory studies, the conclusions of which may have been influenced by a crucial difference in the environmental conditions present in laboratory versus out-of-doors exercise (Saunders et al. 2004).

Thus the original study of Wyndham and Strydom (1969) purportedly showed a linear relationship between the post-exercise rectal temperature and the level of dehydration that developed during exercise. This relationship has consistently been shown in carefully conducted laboratory studies by expert scientists (Cheuvront and Haymes 2001a; Coyle 1994; Montain and Coyle 1992). Yet we have equally consistently been unable to reproduce this relationship in field studies of real competition (Noakes et al. 1988; Noakes et al. 1991b; Sharwood et al. 2002; 2004). I have wondered why this should be so. One key difference is that rates of body cooling by convection, caused by cool air moving over the surface of the body, may be different in laboratory studies and field trials performed out-of-doors (Adams et al. 1992).

For example, the facing wind speed, the main determinant of convective heat loss, in four laboratory studies showing a relationship between the degree of dehydration and the elevation in body temperature during exercise, was either 2.1 km.h$^{-1}$ (Gisolfi and Copping 1974), 5.7 km.h$^{-1}$ (Costill et al. 1970) or 8.6 km.h$^{-1}$ (Montain and Coyle 1992) and it is not clear whether such cooling affected the whole body. All of these are well below the wind speeds generated by athletes, especially cyclists, exercising at the higher intensities necessary to cause heat injury. Since it is known that convective heat loss increases with increasing windspeed (Adams et al. 1992), the convective cooling provided in those laboratory studies was less than that found in usual exercise conditions and would have impacted on the athlete's ability to lose heat normally.

In addition, many of these laboratory studies were performed in environmental conditions that would be rated 'high risk' by the ACSM guidelines for safe exercise in the heat. Thus the two studies that most clearly establish a proportional effect of dehydration on the elevation of rectal temperature during exercise, were performed in environmental conditions (33°C; relative humidity

50 per cent (Montain and Coyle 1992); 33°C and 38 per cent humidity (Gisolfi and Copping 1974)) that constitute borderline 'very high' and 'high' risk respectively of heat injury according to the ACSM guidelines (1987). Exercise physiologists are welcome to study physiological phenomena under environmental conditions in the laboratory that have little practical application to competitive sport. But they should exhibit sufficient critical judgement not to extrapolate their data to the quite different environmental conditions under which competitive sport can be safely conducted.

Hence it makes no sense to quote these studies as proof of the 'dangers' of dehydration when they were performed under the very environmental conditions that the ACSM guidelines describe as unsafe for competitive sport. Surely there should be a consistency of logic in the pronouncements of influential scientific organizations?

Perhaps these criticisms explain why, when exercise is performed under more usual, competitively safe, environmental conditions in the laboratory (25°C; relative humidity 55 per cent and facing wind speed 13–15 km.h$^{-1}$) in a properly constructed wind tunnel so that the athlete's entire body is subjected to rapidly moving air, drinking fluid according to the ACSM guidelines did not offer any performance advantages over *ad libitum* ingestion (Daries *et al.* 2000). Indeed a number of other studies have failed to show that high rates of fluid ingestion during exercise are better than *ad libitum* intakes or those that will either replace sweat rates or 'as much as can be tolerated' (Cheuvront and Haymes 2001b; McConnell *et al.* 1997; Kay and Marino 2003). Indeed an overlooked finding in the study of Montain and Coyle (1992; Coyle 1994) that established the 1.2 L.hr$^{-1}$ ACSM drinking guidelines, was that the sole physiological advantage of increasing the rate of fluid ingestion from 712 to 1190 ml.hr$^{-1}$, which is approximately the difference between *ad libitum* and 'drinking as much as tolerable', was a reduction in the final rectal temperature after 2 hours of exercise from 38.6° to 38.4°C. It seems improbable that this small difference is of any biological significance. However, athletes who drank 'as much as tolerable' during this experiment completed the race about 800 g heavier than did those who drank only 712 ml.hr$^{-1}$. The possibility remains that athletes who 'drink as much as tolerable' incur a weight penalty that exceeds any apparent potential benefit of the small additional biological effects of such high rates of fluid ingestion. This effect would be more marked in weight-bearing activities like running and might explain why markedly dehydrated athletes can be amongst the top finishers in those races in which this relationship has been sought (Sharwood *et al.* 2002, 2004; Pugh *et al.* 1967; Muir *et al.* 1970).

Perhaps the first study to evaluate the relative importance of fluid ingestion and the facing wind speed on the rectal temperature response during prolonged cycling exercise in the hot, humid conditions tested by Montain and Coyle (1992), is that of Saunders *et al.* (2004). They showed that at low wind speeds, subjects terminated exercise prematurely even though they were not more 'dehydrated' than when they completed the full exercise bout in conditions of higher facing wind speeds. Rather, the environment limited the rate at which heat could be transferred from the exercising body to the environment; as a consequence, they accumulate body heat during the exercise leading to the premature termination of exercise.

But at wind speeds appropriate for the speed ($\sim$33 km.hr$^{-1}$) at which the cyclists would have been travelling if they were exercising out-of-doors, excessive heat accumulation did not occur. Furthermore, there was no difference in the physiological response when subjects replaced either 60 ($\sim$850 ml.hr$^{-1}$) or 80 per cent ($\sim$1100 ml.hr$^{-1}$) of their weight losses during exercise.

Thus this study proves that, because they studied unnaturally low wind speeds, most of the classic 'foundation' studies on which the ACSM guidelines are based underestimated the body's ability to adapt to mild levels of dehydration. Consequently, they overestimated the beneficial physiological effects of high rates of fluid ingestion under these unnatural environmental conditions.

## Conclusions

It is perhaps seldom that well-intentioned advice, apparently founded on impeccable science, can have produced as much avoidable damage as happened with the adoption of the ACSM and the related US Army Guidelines for fluid ingestion during exercise.

The origin of the problem begins with the failure of Wyndham and Strydom to realize that a cross-sectional study cannot prove causation (Figures 8.1 and 8.2) and their emotive and incorrect use of the word 'danger' in their classic 'foundation' paper. Historically, their study occurred at the same time that the first commercial sports drink was being developed in the United States. Interestingly, the 'foundation myth' of that product is that the US College football team for whom it had been developed subsequently became one of the best 'third-quarter' teams in US College football, implying that the prevention of dehydration in American gridiron football substantially improves performance. To my knowledge, this belief is not yet evidence-based.

The product was also developed at the precise moment that the exercise sciences were developing as a serious academic discipline, separate from the 'athletic jock' image of physical education, the branch of learning from which it arose. Under these conditions, neophyte scientists may have been particularly susceptible to industrial support that allowed them to undertake research and to acquire funding and equipment that would otherwise have been beyond their access.

Perhaps the lesson should be that industrial support for research and scientists is entirely appropriate provided that there is full transparency in all aspects of the scientific process. Those who receive such funding must declare their connection whenever there is a potential conflict of interest. Such conflicts of interest can occur whenever the recipient is involved in the academic process either as a lecturer or examiner, as a writer of influential guidelines, review articles or scientific papers, or as a reviewer of grants or journal submissions. Indeed it is essential that the approach of the *British Medical Journal* should become the world standard. That journal requires that any involvement in the academic processes, be it as an author or a journal reviewer, requires a full disclosure of all potential conflicts of interest.

Indeed in this regard, it may be of interest that, despite substantial industrial funding of this line of research (Gisolfi 1996; Gatorade Sports Science Institute 2000a), the ACSM drinking guidelines are fundamentally based on only four core studies, three of which were completed before 1974 and, as shown here, none of which is of the appropriate design to support the conclusions presented in the guidelines. Nor in the United States does there appear to have been a serious appetite to undertake the real scientific challenge, which is to attempt to disprove the prevailing 'foundation myth' (Noakes 1997). Rather the contrary studies have originated largely from laboratories outside the United States (Irving *et al.* 1991; Noakes 1995, 2000, 2002, 2003b; Noakes *et al.* 1985, 1988, 1991a, 1991b, 2004; Sharwood *et al.* 2002, 2004; Speedy *et al.* 2000, 2001b) and which therefore fall outside the influence of the North American commercial interests. For reasons that are also unclear, these studies are infrequently referenced by some influential North American exercise scientists.

The next problem was that laboratory-based exercise scientists, who may have had little exposure to clinical medicine, were responsible for the drafting of many of these guidelines and for developing treatment protocols specifically for medical conditions, in which these exercise scientists were not expert. An important error was in the definition of what constitutes a 'heat illness' and the absolute devotion to the 'foundation myth', which mandates that the sole reason why athletes require treatment after exercise is because they are 'dehydrated'. Thus when the first rash of overhydrated athletes were encountered, their identifying symptoms were missed, since the expansive range of obtuse symptoms considered to be diagnostic of 'dehydration' did not allow the distinction of those specific to overhydration.

Nor does it appear that many of these scientists could have been exposed to either the history of modern athletics or to modern-day world-class athletes. For from the history they would have learned that prior to the 1970s, athletes were advised not to drink during exercise. If dehydration is so detrimental to health and performance, one would have expected both a much higher incidence of medical problems, especially in runners in races run before the 1970s, as well as a substantial improvement in long-distance running and cycling performance after the introduction of these new guidelines. But neither seems to have occurred. Rather the proportion of athletes seeking medical attention especially after marathon races appears to have increased dramatically during this period even though these athletes run much slower than was previously the case (Noakes *et al.* 2002; Noakes 2000b). Nor do they seem to have observed that the most successful athletes in marathon and shorter running races are frequently those who drink frugally during exercise, the opposite of the predictions of the 'foundation myth'.

Finally, is the issue of simply trying to be too clever and too 'scientific'. For one obvious question might be: Why is it that, of all living beings on this planet, only humans need to be told how much they should drink during exercise? I am, for example, unaware that any American veterinary association (or similar body) has developed guidelines for fluid replacement during exercise in horses, dogs, camels, wolves and African hunting dogs, all of which frequently exercise for prolonged periods without immediate access to fluids. Perhaps their continued survival without any knowledge of such veterinary guidelines indicates that mammals have evolved with all the necessary biological signals, most particularly thirst, to ensure that, provided they have a reasonable access to fluid, they usually drink appropriately before, during and after exercise.

If this is correct, then perhaps the drinking guidelines for the most intellectual of mammals should be kept as simple as possible:

- Listen to the wisdom of the body.
- Drink if you are thirsty.
- Do not drink if you are not thirsty.
- Avoid competitive sport or intensive exercise when it is too hot.

All the rest is detail.

## Bibliography

Adams, W.C., Mack, G.W., Langhans, G.W. and Nadel, E.R. (1992) 'Effects of varied air velocity on sweating and evaporative rates during exercise', *J Appl Physiol*, 73, 2668–74.

Adner, M.M., Scarlett, J.J., Casey, J., Robinson, W. and Jones, B.H. (1988) 'The Boston Marathon Medical Care Team: ten years of experience', *Physcn Sportsmed*, 16(7), 99–106.

Almond, C.S., Fortescue, E.B., Shin, A.Y., Mannix, R and Greenes, D.S. (2003) 'Risk factors for hyponatremia among runners in the Boston Marathon', *Acad Emerg Med*, 10, 534–5.

American College of Sports Medicine (1975) 'Position Statement: Prevention of heat injuries during distance running', *Med Sci Sports Exerc*, 7, vii–ix.

American College of Sports Medicine (1987) 'Position Stand: The prevention of thermal injuries during distance running', *Med Sci Sports Exerc*, 19, 529–33.

American College of Sports Medicine (1996a) 'Position Stand: Heat and cold illnesses during distance running', *Med Sci Sports Exerc*, 28(12), i–x.

American College of Sports Medicine (1996b) 'Position Stand: Exercise and fluid replacement', *Med Sci Sports Exerc*, 28(1), i–vii.

Armstrong, L.E. and Maresh, C.M. (1998) 'Effects of training, environment and host factors on the sweating response to exercise', *Int J Sports Med*, 19, S103–S105.

Armstrong, L.E., Crago, A.E., Adams, R., Roberts, W.O. and Maresh, C.M. (1996) 'Whole-body cooling of hyperthermic runners: comparison of two field therapies', *Am J Emerg Med*, 14, 355–8.

Baumann, A. (1995) 'The epidemiology of heat stroke and associated thermoregulatory disorders', In: J.R. Sutton, M.W. Thompson and M.E. Torode (eds), *Exercise and Thermoregulation*, Sydney, Australia: The University of Sydney, 203–8.

Binkley, H.M., Beckett J., Casa D.J., Kleiner D.M. and Plummer P.E. (2002) 'National Athletic Trainers' Association Position Statement: Exertional heat illnesses', *J Athlet Train*, 37, 329–43.

Brown, A.H. (1947) 'Dehydration exhaustion', in E.E. Adolph (ed.) *Physiology of Man in the Desert*, New York: Interscience Publishers, 208–25.

Burr, R.E. (1991) *Heat Illness: A Handbook for Medical Officers*, Natick, MA: US Army Research Institute of Environmental Medicine.

Casa, D.J., Armstrong, L.E., Hillman, S.K. *et al.* (2000) 'National Athletic Trainers Association Position Statement: Fluid replacement for athletes', *J Athlet Train*, 35, 212–24.

Cheuvront, S.N. and Haymes, E.M. (2001a) 'Thermoregulation and marathon running. Biological and environmental influences', *Sports Med*, 31, 743–62.

Cheuvront, S.N. and Haymes, E.M. (2001b) '*Ad libitum* fluid intakes and thermoregulatory responses of female distance runners in three environments', *J Sports Sci*, 19, 845–4.

Costill, D.L., Cote, R., Miller, E., Miller, T. and Wynder, S. (1970) 'Water and electrolyte replacement during days of work in the heat', *Aviat Space Environ Med*, 46, 795–800. (This reference was incorrect in the original document. The correct study that the authors wished to reference is the following: Costill, D.L., Kammer, W.F. and Fisher, A. (1970) 'Fluid ingestion during distance running', *Arch Environ Health*, 21, 520–5.

Coyle, E.E. (1994) 'Fluid and carbohydrate replacement during exercise: How much and why?' *Sports Sci Exch*, 7, 1–5. Available online at http://www.gssi.com.

Coyle, E.E. (2004) 'Fluid and fuel intake during exercise', *J Sports Sci*, 22, 39–55.

Daries, H.N., Noakes, T.D. and Dennis, S.C. (2000) 'Effect of fluid intake volume on 2-h running performances in a 25°C environment', *Med Sci Sports Exerc*, 32, 1783–9.

Davis, D.P., Videen, J.S., Marino, A., Vilke, G.M., Dunford, J.V., Van Camp, S.P. and Maharam, L.G. (2001) 'Exercise-associated hyponatremia in marathon runners: A two-year experience', *J Emerg Med*, 21, 47–57.

Eichner, E.R. (1991) 'Sacred cows and straw men', *Physcn Sportsmed*, 19, 24.

Eichner, E.R. (2002) 'Heat stroke in sports: Causes, prevention, and treatment', *Sports Sci Exch* 2002; 12, 1–4. Available online at http://www.gssi.com.

Eichner, E.R., Laird, R., Hiller, D., Nadel, E. and Noakes, T.D. (1993) 'Hyponatremia in sport: symptoms and prevention', *Sports Sci Exch*, 4(2), 1–4. Available online at http://www.gssiweb.com.

Epstein, Y., Moran, D.S., Shapiro, Y., Sohar, E. and Shermer, J. (1999) 'Exertional heat stroke: a case series', *Med Sci Sports Exerc*, 31, 224–8.

Frizzell, R.T., Lang, G.H., Lowance, D.C. and Lathan, S.R. (1986) 'Hyponatremia and ultramarathons', *JAMA*, 255, 772–4.

Gardner, J.W. (2002) 'Death by water intoxication', *Milit Med*, 167, 432–4.

Garigan, T.P. and Ristedt, D.E. (1999) 'Death from hyponatremia as a result of acute water intoxication in an Army basic trainee', *Milit Med*, 164, 234–8.

Gatorade Sports Science Institute (2003) 'Gatorade Sports Science Institute refutes hydration guidelines in British Journal of Medicine' [sic], report. Press release 18 July 2003. Accessed at http://www.pepsico.com/news/gatorade/2003/20030718g.shtml on 10 August 2003.

Gatorade Sports Science Institute (2000a) Fluids 2000. Research summaries. Sports Science Center. Sports Science Topics. Available online at http://www.gssiweb.com.

Gatorade Sports Science Institute (2000b) Fluids 2000. Dehydration and heat illness. Sports Science Centre. Available online at http://www.gssi.com.

Gatorade Sports Science Institute (2000c) Fluids 2000. Sports drinks vs water. Three studies confirm sports drinks superior to water. Sports Science Center. Sports Science Topics. Available online at http://www.gssiweb.com.

Gatorade Sports Science Institute (2000d) Fluids 2000. Sports drinks: How they work. Why water leaves you empty. Sports Science Center. Sports Science Topics. Available online at http://www.gssiweb.com.

Gisolfi, C.V. (1996) 'Fluid balance for optimal performance', *Nutr Rev*, 54(suppl 4 pt 2), S564–72.

Gisolfi, C.V. and Copping, J.R. (1974) 'Thermal effects of prolonged treadmill exercise in the heat', *Med Sci Sports*, 6, 108–13.

Gisolfi, C.V. and Lamb, D.R. (1990) 'Fluid homeostasis during exercise', in *Perspectives in Exercise Science and Sports Medicine*, Vol. 3, Carmel, IN: Benchmark Press.

Gisolfi, C.V., Lamb, D.R. and Nadel, E.R. (1993) 'Exercise, heat and thermoregulation', in *Perspectives in Exercise Science and Sports Medicine*, Vol. 6, Carmel, IN: Cooper Publishing Group.

Greenhaff, P.L. (1989) 'Cardiovascular fitness and thermoregulation during prolonged exercise in the heat', *Br J Sports Med*, 23, 109–14.

Hew, T.D., Chorley, J.N., Cianca, J.C. and Divine, J.G. (2003) 'The incidence, risk factors and clinical manifestations of hyponatremia in marathon runners', *Clin J Sports Med*, 13, 41–7.

Hiller, W.D.B. (1987) 'Medical and physiological considerations in triathlons', *Am J Sports Med*, 15, 164–7.

Hiller, W.D.B. (1989) 'Dehydration and hyponatremia during triathlons', *Med Sci Sports Exerc* 21, S219–S221.

Hubbard, R.W. and Armstrong, L.E. (1987) 'The heat illnesses: biochemical, ultra-structural, and fluid-electrolyte considerations', in K.B. Pandolf, M.N. Swaka, and R.R. Gonzalez (1988) (eds) *Human Performance Physiology and Environmental Medicine at Terrestrial Extremes*, Indianapolis: Benchmark Press, 305–59.

Hubbard, R.W. and Armstrong, L.E. (1989) 'Hyperthermia: new thoughts on an old problem', *Physcn Sportsmed*, 17, 97–113.

Irving, R.A., Noakes, T.D., Buck, R., van Zyl Smit, R., Raine, E., Godlonton, J. and Norman, R.J. (1991) 'Evaluation of renal function and fluid homeostasis during recovery from exercise induced hyponatremia', *J Appl Physiol*, 70, 342–8.

Kay, D. and Marino, F.E. (2003) 'Failure of fluid ingestion to improve self-paced exercise performance in moderate-to-warm humid environments', *J Therm Biol*, 28, 29–34.

Kondo, N., Takano, S., Aiko, K., Shibasaki, M., Tominaga, H. and Inoue, Y. (1998) 'Regional differences in the effect of exercise intensity on thermoregulatory sweating and cutaneous vasodilation', *Acta Physiol Scand*, 164, 71–8.

Laird, R.H. and Wheeler, K.B. (1988) *Report of the Ross Symposium on Medical Coverage of Endurance Athletic Events*, Columbus, OH: Ross Laboratories.

Lamb, D.R., Knuttgen, H.G. and Murray, R. (1994) 'Physiology and nutrition for competitive sport', *Perspectives in Exercise Science and Sports Medicine*. Vol. 7, Carmel, IN: Cooper Publishing Group.

McConell, G.K., Burge, C.M., Skinner, S.L. and Hargreaves, M. (1997) 'Influence of fluid volume on physiological responses during prolonged exercise', *Acta Physiol Scand*, 160, 149–56.

Maughan, R.J. and Murray, R. (2001) *Sports Drinks. Basic Science and Practical Aspects*, CRC Press, Boca Raton.

Maughan, R.J. and Shirreffs, S.M. (1998) 'Fluid and electrolyte loss and replacement in exercise', in M. Harris, C. Williams, W.D. Stanish and L.J. Micheli (eds) *Oxford Textbook of Sports Medicine*, 2nd edn, Oxford: Oxford University Press, 97–112.

Montain, S.F. and Coyle, E. (1992) 'The influence of graded dehydration on hyperthermia and cardiovascular drift during exercise', *J Appl Physiol*, 73, 1340–50.

Montain, S.J., Latzka, W.A. and Sawka, M.N. (1999) 'Fluid replacement recommendations for training in hot weather', *Milit Med*, 164, 502–8.

Muir, A.L., Percy-Robb, I.W., Davidson, I.A., Walsh, E.G. and Passmore, R. (1970) 'Physiological aspects of the Edinburgh commonwealth games', *Lancet*, 2(7683), 1125–8.

Murray, B. (1996) 'Fluid replacement: The American College of Sports Medicine Position Stand', *Sports Sci Exch*, 9(4), 1–5. Available online at http://www.gssiweb.com.

Murray, B., Stofan, J. and Eichner, E.R. (2003) 'Hyponatremia in athletes', *Sports Sci Exch*, 16, 1–5. Available online at http://www.gssi.com.

Nash, H.L. (1985) 'Treating thermal injury: disagreement heats up', *Physcn Sportsmed*, 13, 134–44.

Noakes, T.D. (1981) 'Heatstroke in the 1981 SA National Cross Country Championships', *S Afr Med J*, 61, 145.

Noakes, T.D. (1993) 'Fluid replacement during exercise', *Exerc Sports Sci Rev*, 21, 297–330.

Noakes, T.D. (1995) 'Dehydration during exercise: What are the real dangers?', *Clin J Sports Med*, 5, 123–8.

Noakes, T.D. (1997) 'Challenging beliefs: *ex Africa semper aliquid novi*', *Med Sci Sports Exerc*, 29, 571–90.

Noakes, T.D. (1999a) 'Perpetuating ignorance: intravenous fluid therapy in sport', *Br J Sports Med*, 33, 296–7.

Noakes, T.D. (1999b) 'Letter to the Editor', *Am J Sports Med*, 27, 688–9.

Noakes, T.D. (2000) 'Hyponatremia in distance athletes. Pulling the IV on the "Dehydration Myth"', *Phys Sportsmed*, 28, 71–6.

Noakes, T.D. (2002) 'Hyponatremia in distance runners: Fluid and sodium balance during exercise', *Curr Sports Med Rep*, 4, 197–207.

Noakes, T.D. (2003a) 'Overconsumption of fluids by athletes. Advice to overdrink may cause fatal hyponatraemic encephalopathy', *Br Med J*, 327(7407), 113–14.

Noakes, T.D. (2003b) 'Position statement. Fluid replacement during marathon running', *Clin J Sports Med*, 13, 309–18.

Noakes, T.D. and Martin, D. (2002) 'IMMDA-AIMS Advisory statement on guidelines for fluid replacement during marathon running', *New Stud Athlet*, 17, 15–24.

Noakes, T.D., Goodwin, N., Rayner, B.L., Brankin, T. and Taylor, R.K.N. (1985) 'Water intoxication: A possible complication of endurance exercise', *Med Sci Sports Exerc*, 17, 370–5.

Noakes, T.D., Adams, B.A., Greef, C., Lotz, T. and Nathan, M. (1988) 'The danger of an inadequate water intake during prolonged exercise', *Europ J Appl Physiol*, 57, 210–19.

Noakes, T.D., Berlinski, N., Solomon, E. and Wright, L.M. (1991a) 'Collapsed runners: blood biochemical changes after IV fluid therapy', *Physcn Sportsmed*, 19(7), 70–81.

Noakes, T.D., Myburgh, K.H., du Plessis, J., Lang, L., Lambert, M., van der Riet, C. and Schall, R. (1991b) 'Metabolic rate, not percent dehydration predicts rectal temperature in marathon runners', *Med Sci Sports Exerc*, 23, 443–9.

Noakes, T.D., Wilson, G., Gray, D.A., Lambert, M.I. and Dennis, S.C. (2001) 'Peak rates of diuresis in healthy humans during oral fluid overload', *S Afr Med J*, 91, 852–7.

Noakes, T.D., Sharwood, K., Collins, K. and Perkins, D.R. (2004) 'The dipsomania of great distance. Water intoxication in an Ironman Triathlete', *Br J Sports Med*, 38 (August), E16.

O'Brien, K.K., Montain, S.J., Corr, W.P., Sawka, M.N., Knapik, J.J. and Craig, S.C. (2001) 'Hyponatremia associated with overhydration in U.S. Army trainees', *Milit Med*, 166, 405–10.

Pearlmutter, E.M. (1986) 'The Pittsburgh marathon: playing weather roulette', *Physcn Sportsmed*, 14, 132–8.

Pugh, L.G., Corbett, J.L. and Johnson, R.H. (1967) 'Rectal temperatures, weight losses, and sweat rates in marathon running', *J Appl Physiol*, 23, 347–52.

Saltin, B. and Hermansen, L. (1966) 'Esophageal, rectal, and muscle temperature during exercise', *J Appl Physiol*, 21, 379–84.

Saunders, A.G., Dugas, J., Tucker, R., Lambert, M.I. and Noakes, T.D. (2004) 'Air velocity influences heat storage and core temperature independently of fluid ingestion in humans running in hot, humid conditions', *Acta Physiol Scand*, in press.

Sawka, M.N. and Montain, S.J. (2000) 'Fluid and electrolyte supplementation for exercise heat stress', *Am J Clin Nutr*, 72, 564S–72S.

Sharwood, K., Collins, M. Goedecke, J., Wilson, G. and Noakes, T. (2002) 'Weight changes, sodium levels, and performance in the South African Ironman triathlon', *Clin J Sports Med*, 12, 391–9.

Sharwood, K., Collins, M., Goedecke, J., Wilson, G. and Noakes, T.D. (2004) 'Weight changes, medical complications and performance during an Ironman Triathlon', *Br J Sports Med*, October 2004.

Smith, S. (2002) 'Marathon runner's death linked to excessive fluid intake', *New York Times*, 13 August.

Speedy, D.B., Rogers, I.R., Noakes, T.D., Thompson, J.M.D., Guirey, J., Safih, S. and Boswell, D.R. (2000) 'Diagnosis and prevention of hyponatremia in an ultradistance triathlon', *Clin J Sports Med*, 10, 52–8.

Speedy, D.B., Noakes, T.D., Boswell, T., Thompson, J.M., Rehrer, N. and Boswell, D.R. (2001a) 'Response to a fluid load in athletes with a history of exercise induced hyponatremia', *Med Sci Sports Exerc*, 33, 1434–42.

Speedy, D.B., Noakes, T.D. and Schneider, C. (2001b) 'Exercise associated hyponatremia: A review', *Emerg Med*, 13, 13–23.

Sutton, J.R. (1990) 'Clinical implications of fluid imbalance', in C.V. Gisolfi and D.R. Lamb (eds) *Perspectives in Exercise Science and Sports Medicine*, Vol. 3. *Fluid Homeostasis During Exercise*, Carmel, IN: Benchmark Press, 425–55.

Waller, J. (2002) *Fabulous Science*, Oxford: Oxford University Press.

Wyndham, C.H. (1977) 'Heatstroke and hyperthermia in marathon runners', *Ann N Y Acad Sci*, 301, 128–38.

Wyndham, C.H. and Strydom, N.B. (1969) 'The danger of an inadequate water intake during marathon running', *S Afr Med J*, 43, 893–6.

Wyndham, C.H., Strydom, N.B., van Rensburg, A.J., Benade, A.J.S. and Heyns, A.J. (1970) 'Relation between $VO_2$ max and body temperature in hot humid conditions', *J Appl Physiol* 29, 45–50.

Yanagimoto, S., Kuwahara, T., Zhang, Y., Koga, S., Inoue, Y. and Kondo, N. (2003) 'Intensity-dependant thermoregulatory responses at the onset of dynamic exercise in mildly heated humans', *Am J Physiol*, 285, R200–R207.

Zorn, E. (1999) 'Runner's demise sheds light on deadly myth', *Chicago Tribune*, 11 October.

# 9 Is sport and exercise science a man's game?

*Celia Brackenridge, Nanette Mutrie and Precilla Y.L. Choi*

## Introduction

It would be easy to both open and close this chapter in a single word – 'yes'. That this chapter exists is, in itself, an indictment of sport and exercise science (SES). If SES were a gender-inclusive activity then (i) there would be a better gender balance among the contributors to the book and (ii) there would be no need for this chapter. One glance through the list of contributing authors reveals exactly the gender bias (whether that be intentional or not) that we have been asked to explore here. More than 10 years ago the need for sports science to evaluate gender issues was identified, but our worry is that this evaluation has not yet occurred.

> There is clearly a need for the sports science community to eliminate the bias inherent in its work by conducting more studies with women athletes, by reappraising its methods and approaches, and by including gender in its analyses. The genuine inclusion of women as subjects and as researchers should bring a more balanced and rounded perspective, and further the pursuit of knowledge in the sports sciences. (Anita White, English Sports Council, 'Women in Top Level Sport' 2nd IOC Congress on Sport Science 1991.)

Gender representation is not a new topic, however, even in the somewhat conservative ranks of sport scholars. In 1986, Miracle and Rees edited a book called *Sport and Social Theory*, described on the jacket as offering 'a fresh approach to the study of the sociology of sport'. All 21 contributing authors were male, so obviously the 15 years or so of second-wave feminist theorizing[1] had had no impact on sport theory! It is disappointing, therefore, to find ourselves, two decades on, among so few female contributors to another academic reader. It is also interesting to ponder on what it might mean that women have been approached to write *this* chapter? Do women have nothing to say about the other topics in the book? Is it only women who are expected to consider and have something to say about the title question of this chapter? We know the answer to these two questions is 'no' but will this chapter by us, as women, imply that the answer is 'yes' and will it lead to continued marginalization of feminist and women's work? We hope, of course, that our readers will take note and help challenge existing practices that seem to reinforce the notion that SES is indeed a man's game.

However reluctantly, we do need to address the title question. In so doing, we will summarize some previous themes on gender and subject, retreading well-trod paths from the 1980s and 1990s in disciplines such as the biological sciences, psychology and sociology. We will attempt to locate these discussions specifically within the context of SES (interpreted here as including sport and exercise physiology, psychology, and biomechanics but not, as would be included in the continental European tradition, leisure studies). We take a mainly UK perspective. It is worth noting here, also, that exercise science is now embedded in the same professional structures as sport science. The influx of health promotion and fitness personnel into exercise science might have an impact on the gender order but this is unclear at the present time.

The chapter begins with a general discussion of gender and science and an exploration of the extent to which gender equity has permeated sport science organizations – both structures and cultures. It then proceeds to a consideration of why gender equity might be an ethical issue in sport science. Throughout the chapter, we provide boxed illustrative examples using both statistical and narrative data about the place of women in SES.[2] Many of these are drawn from our own collective experience of life as academic and applied scientists working in sport or exercise. That we attempt to offer an account that is descriptive, analytic *and* personal is important because the 'facts' of sport and exercise science, as reflected in, for example, publication rates and grant funding, can never fully reflect the experience of being a sport or exercise scientist. We argue that the lived experience of the sport or exercise scientist (whether as consultant, teacher, researcher or manager/leader) is a significant component in the practice of SES and that the associated subjectivities should be both acknowledged and celebrated in any account of the subject field. Finally, in returning to the question of whether sport and exercise science (in all its manifestations) is a man's game, we affirm our strong suspicions by reaching the inescapable conclusion that the answer is 'yes'. Moreover, we argue that there are serious, negative ethical implications of this state of affairs for the future of the field that sport and exercise scientists themselves should address.

## Gender and science

Gender[3] has been systematically linked with epistemology by several generations of feminist scholars such as Spender (1980, 1981), Acker (1990, 1993, 1994) and Harding (1986). Building on work in the 1970s on the sociology of knowledge, feminist scholars in many disciplines have shown how knowledge hierarchies are gendered and how scientific power is closely associated with the gendering process. Indeed, the very choice of the terms 'hard' and 'soft' to privilege the natural over the social sciences is a reflection of male bias. These critiques point to the androcentricism[4] inherent in research question formulation, research methods, interpretations of data and publication (e.g. Bleir 1984; Burman 1990; Fausto-Sterling 1992; Weisstein 1993; Choi 1999). Men determine what counts as scientific knowledge, they judge scientific merit and accord recognition on the basis of their own parameters. Thus, gender determines not only *how* we research but what we see as research-worthy. If a gender perspective is defined only as addressing 'individual differences', or if gender itself is ignored altogether, then it is little wonder that the discriminatory gender order of SES remains intact (see Boxes 9.1 and 9.2). Rather, a gender perspective goes beyond mere description of difference and problematizes both gendered structures *and* gender–power relations.

---

**Box 9.1 Harding's five research programmes**

Talbot (1999) reports Harding's (1986) five research programmes for addressing gender equity:

1 equity studies – to show gender composition;
2 the uses/abuses of biology, the social sciences and their technologies and how science is used in the service of racist, sexist, homophobic and classist social projects – to show that science is not value free;
3 critique – to illustrate bias in the selection and definition of acceptable research projects;
4 reading science as 'text' – to reveal its socially structured meanings and hidden agendas;
5 epistemological enquiry – to show how beliefs are grounded in social experience and how this influences what counts as science.

She challenges sport scientists to use them as a critical agenda for research in order to challenge the dominant paradigms of science.

---

**Box 9.2 Gender and knowledge**

Rejection by sport science journal editors of articles employing qualitative or reflexive methods.

Gender blindness/institutional discrimination in scientific awards schemes and committee representation.

Rejection of research into child abuse as 'political' rather than 'scientific'.

Exclusion of social science disciplines (e.g. sociology and history) from the sport and exercise science divisions within BASES.

---

Male scientists occupy the privileged spaces of the scientific world, mainly because of historical precedence rather than scientific ability. Illusions of political neutrality and value freedom have served this male hegemony. The next section will examine how this is maintained through the structure and culture of SES organizations.

---

**Box 9.3 Gender and structural power**

*Journal of Sports Sciences*

Editorial Board representation by women: 1 out of 7 (14%) in 2001, 1 out of 8 (13%) in 2002.

Advisory Board representation by women: 5 out of 51 (10%) in 2001, 5 out of 55 (9%) in 2002.

---

## Gender equity and equal opportunities

The term 'equity' carries multiple meanings. It is, first and foremost, associated with someone having a stake (usually financial) in some asset (usually business). However, it has also come to be associated with having a chance to achieve social goods (framed by such categories as race or class), including scientific and professional. The equity agenda is one shared by, and the responsibility of, both those in power and those without it. 'Equity' does not imply 'sameness' but, rather, a fair chance to pursue the rewards of social/academic/professional success. Having 'procedural equity' (i.e. in rules and regulations) does not necessarily guarantee 'distributive equity' (i.e. that all members have equal access).

The term 'equal opportunities' grew out of an analysis of social structures in the 1970s that exposed inequality and a lack of social diversity within most major social organizations. The term itself recognized that individuals who wished to join such structures in order to improve their lot could do so only when given appropriate opportunities. This understanding of equal opportunities implies that fairness is located in *individual* rather than *societal* responsibility. It also implies that those seeking to overcome disadvantage (whether this is socially, economically or academically based) can do so only when a common starting point provides an equal chance for them to achieve parity with others. In practice, this approach to equity has often absolved those in positions of power from doing anything more than simply 'offering opportunities'. This permissive approach has sometimes led to a 'blame-the-victim' culture, whereby those least equipped to challenge their own disadvantage carry the greatest responsibility for doing so. A conscious effort is needed, therefore, in order for resources to be shifted or redistributed to achieve greater equity. Equity is also often confused with diversity but it is possible to have diversity (across a range of social and other characteristics) without equity because power relations or gender cultures mediate the gender structure of an organization. Ideally, scientific organizations should seek to value and achieve both diversity and equity. An example of this might be the deliberate rotation and sharing of decision-making roles in an SES organization.

Equality and 'equity' are frequently interchangeable in the language of social democracy. Most recently they have become supplanted by the term social exclusion/inclusion through the UK government's own liberal welfare discourse and the establishment of its Social Inclusion Unit. The terms 'social inclusion' and 'exclusion' imply a greater degree of consciousness on behalf of those doing either the including or the excluding than did the earlier, associated terms. Even with this change of emphasis, the business case for social diversity is compelling (Mavin and Ryans 1999; Wilkinson 1995); socially diverse organizations are demonstrably stronger, more responsive, more creative and ultimately more resilient when faced with threats, than organizations characterized by rigid hierarchies and homogeneous memberships.

'Institutional sexism' is widespread in many large public, commercial and voluntary organizations (Pemberton 1995). It is important to stress that the term 'institutional' does not necessarily imply a conscious act on the part of any single individual. Instead, it refers to the net effect, usually over a protracted period of time, of taken-for-granted practices and conditions that lead to certain people and groups being privileged over others in their membership of that organization; an example would be the debate about institutional racism in London's Metropolitan Police sparked by enquiry into the murder of Stephen Lawrence. Institutional sexism is exhibited in, for example, the differential representation of women in positions of power in an organization, their lower rates of pay for the same work as men, and their reduced access to opportunities for promotion (see Box 9.4 in which, interestingly, the Exercise Science Committee of the British Association of Sport and Exercise Sciences [BASES], unlike many of its counterpart committees, shows a gender balance.)

In addition to the surface elements of organizational structures that can be identified to describe institutional sexism, there are powerful and embedded *cultural* features of organizations that can act as a brake on gender transformation. These normative features of organizations include the customs, habits and traditions that grow over time and that usually pass from one generation to the next through rituals, inherited statuses and expectations (see Box 9.5). In the quest for modernization of UK politics, for example, New Labour is seeking to change the working practices of Members of Parliament to make their 'office hours' more amenable to those with child care, elder care or other family responsibilities. In the legal profession, the custom of 'dining' on a fixed number of evenings in order to qualify as a barrister is a form of indirect discrimination against aspiring lawyers, especially women.

Hearn (in Hearn *et al.* 1989) has coined the term 'organization sexuality' to describe how organizations and not just individuals display sexuality in the way they function and how this acts to oppress those from excluded identities. The organization sexuality of sport science is a good example of hegemonic masculine heterosexuality in which occupational fitness is often associated with sporting fitness and prowess. This is frequently reflected in the clothing and athletic self-presentation of male sport scientists at conferences whose macho image management appears to be almost a badge of honour. As happens with athletes themselves (Griffin 1998), women sport scientists who adopt such practices are labelled as lesbian (regardless of their own sexual identity) and demeaned in the workplace. The cultural traditions and mores of sport science conferences and banquets, often overtly heterosexual and fuelled by alcohol, also reinforce a particular kind of rugged masculine heterosexual hegemony which marginalizes

**Box 9.4 Institutional sexism in the British Association of Sport and Exercise Sciences, at 2000 (Source: Choi *et al.* 2000a, 2000b)**

Overall membership by gender at July 2000 (Head office data)

|        | No.  | %   |
|--------|------|-----|
| Male   | 1487 | 62  |
| Female | 923  | 38  |
| *Total* | 2410 | 100 |

With the membership ratio at roughly 60/40 men to women we might expect a higher representation of women in committees, but almost half have no women members at all . . .

Committee membership

|                                            | Male | Female         |
|--------------------------------------------|------|----------------|
| Executive                                  | 7    | 3              |
| Elected committees:                        |      |                |
| Psychology                                 | 3    | 1              |
| Physiology                                 | 4    | 0              |
| Biomechanics                               | 4    | 0              |
| Interdisciplinary                          | 2    | 2              |
| Accreditation and Fellowships Committee    | 4    | 1              |
| Education and Training Committee           | 6    | 0              |
| Exercise Science Special Committee         | 3    | 3              |
| Sport Science Special Committee            | 5    | 1              |
| SES Special Research Committee             | 10   | 0 [now defunct] |
| Physiology Section                         | 7    | 0              |
| Biomechanics Section                       | 5    | 0              |
| Interdisciplinary Section                  | 2    | 2              |

Section membership by gender (survey response $n = 223$)

| Section           | Male | | | Female | | |
|-------------------|------|------------------|----------------------|--------|------------------|----------------------|
|                   | No.  | % of section | % of total membership | No.    | % of section | % of total membership |
| Biomechanics      | 7    | 78               | 2.6                  | 2      | 22               | 0.7                  |
| Physiology        | 57   | 64               | 20.8                 | 32     | 36               | 11.7                 |
| Psychology        | 46   | 60               | 16.8                 | 30     | 40               | 10.9                 |
| Interdisciplinary | 24   | 49               | 8.8                  | 25     | 51               | 9.1                  |
| *Total*           | 134  | 60               | 60.6                 | 89     | 40               | 39.4                 |

**Box 9.5 Gender and the experience of cultures**

'I went to a workshop on women in sport and sport science . . .. People walked out when the convenor highlighted the inequities and discrimination faced by women! One bloke thought she was being too feminist or something. We eventually got into small groups for discussion and I remember one quite senior bloke raised the point that he supervises lots of women students, PhDs, postdocs and all that but they all seem to disappear – "Where do they all go?" he asked. The lack of understanding seemed to me to be just amazing.' (Author's reflections.)

Presumptions of 'subjects' (that is, participants) in exhibited posters being all-male.

Selection of all-white, all-male keynote lists for conference programmes.

Use in debates of gender-exclusive language when non-sex-referent alternatives are available, e.g. chairman rather than chair or convenor.

**Box 9.6 Gendered perceptions**

On attempting to do interdisciplinary research: 'I just feel I live in another world, and not only that, but it is very much denied. They can't (or won't) understand it so it mustn't exist or something.'

On attending a conference dinner: '[O]ne after dinner speaker who made sexist jokes was applauded by some while others left the room in disgust. Really he should have publicly apologised.'

On discussing equity issues at a sport and exercise science committee meeting: 'I am sitting here looking at a sea of male faces – bored, hostile, indifferent. They can't understand why I am here. They don't understand what I am saying. They can't see the issue. I am wasting their time. Am I wasting mine?'

On the perceived importance of positivism: 'Why can't they understand that their "truth" is just a hand-me-down? Why do I have to confirm to their norm?'

On arguing for blind review in conference submissions: 'There was the usual blah, blah about how, while it was a good thing in theory, in practice is was going to be hard to implement. Then some senior bloke spoke against it on the grounds that one needed to know because submissions from some labs/people are going to be better than others . . ..'

not only women but also many men who prefer to adopt more diverse and socially sensitive identities (see Box 9.6).

## Gender equality and sport science

Sport itself is a masculine domain so it is hardly surprising that sport science follows suit. Indeed, Kolnes (1995) argues that gender is an 'organizing principle' in sport and that, historically, sport grew up as a public arrangement for the recreation of privileged males. Both modern sport and modern science have developed as public activities, the one associated with leisure spaces and the other with work spaces, so it is not surprising that women's traditional relegation to the private/domestic world has disadvantaged their skill development in both spheres. Despite the historically avowed status of science as 'value-free', we argue that the sciences, and the sport sciences more than most, adopt this claim as a mask that conceals their collusion with both the masculine heterosexual hegemony and the benefits that this accrues for men. An example of this is that the 1999 European Congress of Sport Psychology chose all male keynote speakers despite the fact that female scientists with expertise in relevant areas were available. Those who organized the keynote speakers were clearly 'blind' to the gender issue.

In a recent dictionary of sport psychology terms, Cashmore (2002) includes both 'gay' and 'gender' in his glossary but his entry for 'equality' talks only about equal performance outcomes in sporting events and does not mention equity, let alone its gender, race, religious or other dimensions, as a social or ethical imperative. We believe that it is precisely this failure to contextualize equity as a professional and not just a performance issue that has reinforced gender inequity in the sport and exercise sciences.

'[T]he concept of gender relations has been conspicuously absent from most sport psychology scholarship' (Plaisted, in Morris and Summers 1995: 538). Plaisted reports that, in 1982, two-thirds of research in the parent discipline of psychology was by men. On this basis it is not surprising that women have faced an extreme challenge in seeking equality in their sub-discipline. Adopting the male standard (norms) as the default position in sport or exercise science research leads to the reinforcement of the deficit model, whereby women athletes or exercisers are viewed as inferior versions of male athletes. In other words, research participants are falsely assumed to be homogeneous. This deficit approach is implicit in many examples of published sport and exercise science research which exhibit a lack of awareness of the female, otherwise known as 'gender blindness' (see Box 9.7). Not all journals, however, follow this trend. Indeed, Aitchison (1999: 255) praises the *Journal of Sport and Exercise Psychology* for being 'gender-aware'.

The attempt to widen participation and to make sport and exercise science organizations more equitable is advantageous for *all* their members, both from a principled and from a pragmatic standpoint. Gender and other forms of diversity among its membership affords SES the widest possible opportunity for creativity, for seeing new research questions and finding new solutions. The practice of SES consultancy raises particularly interesting questions about gender relations and professional advancement. For example, should male sport science consultants always or only work with male athletes or does this restrict the occupational opportunities for female sport scientists? Do invasive scientific practices pose gender dilemmas for sport and exercise scientists, such as taking skinfold measures, putting on electrodes, checking genital development as an indicator of maturity, or conducting massage for relaxation?

---

**Box 9.7 Gender blindness in published work**

In 51 per cent of the 126 articles reporting studies using empirical data with human subjects in the *Journal of Sports Sciences* (JSS) (Volumes 19 and 20) only male subjects were used. In 36 per cent both male and female subjects were used and in 10 per cent only female subjects were used. In 3 per cent of these articles the sex of the participants was not specified.

The titles of some articles revealed gender blindness:

'Exercise . . . in healthy humans' – this study incorporated 17 males but generalizes to *all* humans in its title.
'Human perceptions' – this study used only male golfers and yet again generalizes to all humans in the title.

In 18 of the 144 studies analysed from *JSS* the authors did not describe the sex of their participants, but left the reader to assume that they were male by dint of the sport or activity under scrutiny, for example Greco-Roman wrestling, county cricket, professional baseball, and international soccer refereeing. However, it is clearly not beyond the bounds of possibility that women could be involved in these activities.

At a recent conference presentation on a study that involved only males the answer to the question of why there were no female participants was as follows: 'Women provide too much variation in the data and add complexity to the lab timetable.' If this is acceptable then of course we will only have a science of *men* in sport. There are clearly issues that must be studied in each gender such as the lactate threshold, the benefits of creatine, and responses to consultations about sport and exercise.

---

Equity issues are often addressed by organizations only after some catastrophic breakdown in professional relationships, perhaps leading to industrial tribunals, civil or even criminal proceedings. Such crises can destabilize the very fabric of an organization. No such catastrophe is known to have had afflicted SES organizations but they are not immune to examples of demeaning or embarrassing incidents and exclusionary practices that damage the reputations of all involved.

A number of SES organizations, such as BASES (Graydon and Choi 1998; Choi and Brackenridge 2001; Choi 2002) have established equal opportunities, equity or diversity initiatives. But without formal structures for promoting gender equity (such as committees, statutes and full representation), women members have little opportunity to impact upon the development of the organization. Even where such structures exist, there is often slow progress towards gender equity (for example, women in the boardrooms of the UK's top 100 companies have been steady at 2 per cent representation for the past 10 years: *The Guardian*, 5 Oct 2002: 5). One reason for this slow progress is that, historically, sport and exercise science professionals have advanced the view that *individual* solutions should be sought to what have been considered *individual* problems. It is, therefore, unsurprising that there has been an apparent lack of *collective* analysis or *corporate* responsibility for changing what is, in organizational development terms, a fairly conservative and static community. In addition, traditional male sport scientists have prized apparent 'political neutrality' and apparent 'scientific objectivity' very highly and have therefore struggled to accept the relevance or validity of research and researchers whom they consider to challenge these tenets or initiatives, like equal opportunities, that appear to them to have no scientific relevance (see Box 9.8).

---

**Box 9.8 Conflation of gender and misogyny**

An Equal Opportunities Policy was adopted by the 1997 Annual General Meeting of BASES, with 56 votes for, 5 against and 22 abstentions. The large number of abstentions reflected, at best, ambivalence or misunderstanding and perhaps even hostility towards the issue by the male-dominated culture of the organization.

---

Whereas the case for social diversity in business was well-established and accepted by the 1990s (Mavin and Ryans 1999; Wilkinson 1995), the case for social diversity in academia is not yet won. Along with the leaders of most other scholarly organizations, those scientists who run our major SES associations may believe that they operate academic meritocracies where scientific ability and applied/practice achievements are the only criteria for acceptance and promotion. However, in reality, this utopian and gender blind view of professional science may be politically naïve and damaging to the professional development of sport and exercise science.

Choices and judgements made about sport and exercise scientists are shaped by historical traditions, received 'wisdom', the forces of the self-fulfilling prophecy, and not just by scientific capabilities. As a result it is often the case that some scientific topics, research methods, areas of application, modes of writing and individuals are more accepted than others (see Box 9.9). Put bluntly, just like those in any other professions, 'science' and 'scientists' are as much socio-politically as intellectually constructed.

---

**Box 9.9 Gender and authorship**

From 122 articles reporting empirical data in *Journal of Sport Sciences* Volumes 19 (2001) and 20 (2002) (excluding conference communication issues) the following pattern of authorship was found:

Male authors = [260/417] 62%
Female authors = [42/417] 10%
Author sex not known or identified = [115/417] 28%
Male first author = [81/122] 66%
Female first author = [14/122] 11%
First author sex not known or identified = [27/122] 22%

---

## Gender inequity and discrimination

All of the examples of gender-based exclusion or bias in sport and exercise sciences constitute forms of discrimination, some more severe than others. Personal discriminatory behaviour, harassment or abuse operates within a social and cultural context. Where personal prejudice goes *unchallenged*, then it does so within a context of institutionally discrimination. In other words, silence towards, ignorance of, or failure to challenge, personal acts of discrimination represent collusion and acceptance. Tolerance of such behaviour from individual members reflects an organization that lacks corporate awareness and responsibility, and has no commitment to social justice.

Gender *inequity* is manifested in discrimination, harassment and/or abuse, but there is no universally accepted set of definitions for these practices (Brackenridge 2001). Even though these behaviours may be defined *objectively* it is important to recognize that they are experienced *subjectively*. Thus, the personal and psychological impact of the same behaviour may be vastly different depending on the individual person's background and perceptions. Researchers from different disciplines also adopt different definitions.

As a result, it is more helpful to think of discrimination, harassment and abuse as representing different kinds of sequentially more serious behaviours. In Figure 9.1, harassment and abuse are represented as the middle and extreme points along a continuum of exploitation whereby abuse is a subset of harassment and harassment is a subset of discrimination.

Discrimination is rooted in institutional practices that undermine the confidence, performance and advancement prospects of an individual (usually but not exclusively affecting females, non-white, the aged, disabled or gay

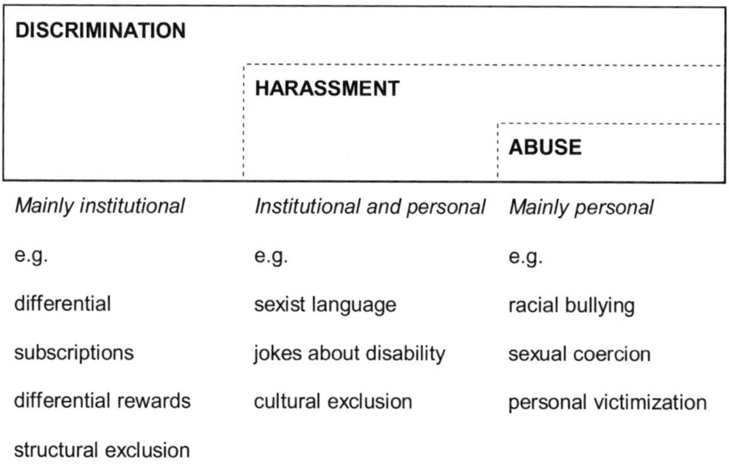

| DISCRIMINATION | | |
| --- | --- | --- |
| | HARASSMENT | |
| | | ABUSE |
| Mainly institutional | Institutional and personal | Mainly personal |
| e.g. | e.g. | e.g. |
| differential | sexist language | racial bullying |
| subscriptions | jokes about disability | sexual coercion |
| differential rewards | cultural exclusion | personal victimization |
| structural exclusion | | |

*Figure 9.1* Links between discrimination, harassment and abuse. (Source: Choi *et al.* 2000a: 8.)

people). Discrimination itself derives from the division of individuals on the basis of personal attributes or 'what people are' (age, sex, race, physical ability) or acquired characteristics or 'what people become' (sexual preference, scientific discipline, theoretical or methodological preferences). These differences are differently valued, leading to hierarchies that include some and exclude others.

Sex discrimination, one of the most prominent aspects of discrimination, is associated mainly with public organizations characterized by 'occupational sex segregation' (OSS) (Witz 1992). In other words, men and women in the organization occupy not only different levels (*vertical segregation*), with males usually at the top and females at the bottom, but also different types of work (*horizontal segregation*), where jobs occupied by males afford more power and rewards than those occupied by females. Vertical segregation in British sport and exercise science is illustrated in Box 9.3, which shows male dominance in the prestigious roles of editorial board and advisory board member for the *Journal of Sports Sciences*, which has the highest impact rating of the British SES journals.

Horizontal segregation is often based on stereotypical accounts of male and female capacities. It tends to lead to occupational cultures that are not only split along gender lines but also perpetuate the belief that male work is more valuable than female work. With reference to SES, for example, implicit and legitimate vertical segregation that privileges male professors over female research students may lead to *illegitimate* differential treatment of male and female research students. Examples include the allocation of greater resources to the 'harder' sciences, which are occupied by more males than females, and the false equation of academic budgets with academic merit. A million-pound research budget is always seen as more important than a thousand-pound budget even if publications of equal merit emerged. Similarly, implicit horizontal segregation separates biomechanics, exercise physiology and psychology from interdisciplinary studies: these are legitimate organizational differentiations yet can lead to *illegitimate* intellectual and personal valuations. Box 9.4 depicts horizontal segregation in BASES with the gender/subject hierarchy privileging biomechanics, physiology, then psychology and lastly interdisciplinary scientists. Vertical and horizontal separations frequently merge and are compounded in intricate hierarchies reflecting issues of gender, race, disability and subject (and many other factors including research institution, reputation, country of origin and so on).

Ann Witz's account of OSS (see Figure 9.2), originally based on the labour market, offers us a useful framework with which to analyse and understand the activities of voluntary and professional associations, including particular groups within BASES. For example, it can help us to map whether and how gendered strategies of occupational closure are used to maintain power and what strategies are possible to challenge or resist this.

With respect to vertical segregation, the dominant group (hypothetically, for example, those with sport or exercise science research accreditation) adopts *exclusionary strategies* to keep subordinates out (such as raising the threshold qualifications required to achieve accreditation 'bringing up the drawbridge behind them'), whilst the subordinate groups (for example, aspiring student or

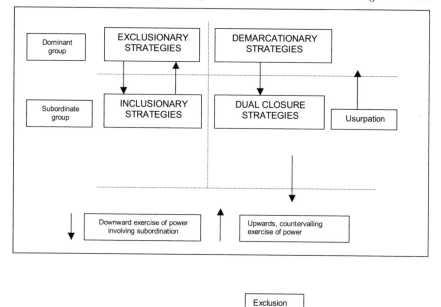

*Figure 9.2* Conceptual framework of gendered occupational closure strategies. (Adapted from Witz 1992: 45.)

women members) pursue *inclusionary strategies* to try to achieve parity. An example of an exclusionary strategy would be the exclusion of a qualitative research article from recognized sport and exercise journals on the grounds that it was 'not appropriate' for publication. An example of an inclusionary strategy would be the perpetuation of a theme or topic in the literature despite its theoretical redundancy, in order to sustain the intellectual and career interests of researchers in that field.

With respect to horizontal segregation, the dominant group adopts *demarcationary strategies* to maintain power within a realm defined as appropriate for them only (hypothetically, psychologists demanding evidence of a statistical or mathematical competence as a condition of acceptance into the group). Any attempt by a member of the subordinate group to enter this domain is seen by the power élite as *usurpation*. The subordinate group may also claim primacy over their domain by adopting *dual closure strategy* (vertical and horizontal), prohibiting all who do not share their interests or characteristics (for example, setting up their own exclusive sport or exercise science association). This has happened recently in Britain where a splinter group has separated from the British Association of Sport and Exercise Medicine (BASEM). Whereas BASEM is inclusive of any scientist or practitioner interested in sport and exercise medicine, the new group (United Kingdom Association of Doctors in Sport, UKADIS) insists that only those with medical qualifications may join.

Sex discrimination is based in the collective policies and practices endorsed by organizations but has individual consequences for women and other minorities. It is thus mainly institutionally based and institutionally manifested. As explained above, institutional discrimination is not, therefore, traceable to individual prejudice but reflects the cultural and historical accretion of attitudes, beliefs and working practices that serve to exclude and marginalize women and minority individuals. Discrimination usually creates an environment of discomfort for those who are excluded or unwelcome which has been aptly labelled 'the chilly climate'.

## Equity in sport science – an ethical issue?

In Nideffer's (1981) *The Ethics and Practice of Applied Sport Psychology* there is no mention of sex or gender in the contents table. This sport science text, like many of its time, is almost completely gender blind: bar its use of some examples of female athletes it does not problematize gender at all. There is, however, a whole chapter on ethical standards for sport psychologists which takes the reader through, among other topics, responsibility, competence, confidentiality and professional relationships.

In her exploration of feminist bioethics, Rosemarie Tong (1997:1) attempts to identify what is distinctive about feminist from nonfeminist ethics and says:

> Although feminists are eager to distinguish their approaches to ethics from those of non-feminists, they do not wish to reject all the moral principles, concepts, and virtues that have guided the Western tradition for centuries. Even if it were possible for feminists to interpret ethics entirely *de novo*, it would be very foolish for them to do so.

In looking at the ethical perspectives of gender and sport science, therefore, it makes sense to draw from established ethical analyses and feminist critiques of them. What is it about SES, then, that disadvantages women? If objectivity is the holy grail of traditional positivism then there ought to be no gender bias in sport or any other kind of science. But we have seen enough already to understand that gender bias affects the knowledge, research methods, management and practice of SES. To this extent, the gender-based unfairnesses in SES (discrimination, gender blindness, exclusion, discrimination, harassment and so on) *are* properly the focus of ethical scrutiny. Tong points out that feminist bioethicists have 'almost always faulted the dominant nonfeminist approaches to bioethics for emphasizing rules over relationships, norms over virtues, and justice over caring' (1997: 3).

One route to rectifying the unfairnesses, then, would be for those with authority in SES to place more emphasis on relationships, virtues and caring and less on the traditional and hierarchal practices of their disciplines. Successful transformation in the gender culture of SES may not depend on structural adjustments but is likely to be made easier if rules and structures themselves are made more inclusive (Box 9.10).

---

**Box 9.10 Examples of gender transformation in sport and exercise science**

*Committee restructuring* – such as appointing co-chairs – one male and one female, or including a place for novice female scientist in a shadowing/observation role.

*Mentoring schemes* – whereby young women scientists are helped by more experienced scientists, male or female, to learn the professional craft of sports science and scientific support. Women in science, engineering and technology have recognized the need for such support and advice from people who understand the challenges that women face, as well as the opportunities that we present to employers. They have set up a mentoring scheme that sport and exercise scientists could join. (Read more about the scheme at http://www.mentorset.org.uk.)

*Child protection and ethics policies and procedures* – which engage sport scientists in both the welfare of athletes and their own professional relationships and protection.

*Positive psychology* – which redresses the traditional emphasis of sport psychology on negative issues (e.g. anxiety, stress, performance breakdown) and values the internal goods of sport and exercise (e.g. flow, peak performance, optimal satisfaction).

*Equal opportunities initiatives* – that require the greatest efforts towards outreach and inclusion from those in the least diverse areas of science, e.g. biomechanics.

---

We have attempted to explain how, despite its claims to neutrality and objectivity, sport and exercise science is a 'man's game' in all its manifestations. Both the structures and the cultures of sport and exercise science render women, and often women's choices of research, invisible – once described as 'symbolic annihilation' – or inferior to men's. This is also a denial of women's moral agency.

In criticizing sport science as androcentric, Choi (1999: 38) argues that the continued failure of sport and exercise science to adopt a gender perspective is not just because of a benign commitment to positivism: '[S]exual divisiveness is very useful for the patriarchy who are the dominant social group and naturally wish to maintain their superiority.' Thus, despite Harding's five research programmes to challenge gender inequity in science, called for almost 20 years ago (Box 9.1), research of this nature continues to be marginalised and considered inferior by mainstream positivist science. In the experience of the authors of this chapter, when we write as feminists we are no longer sport or exercise scientists, and hear all-too-often the refrain that our work is politics, not science.

In a critique of sex differences research, Choi (2001) goes so far as to suggest that biological reductionism (which she considers to be endemic within sport science and medicine (see Choi 2000)), is a deliberate strategy by the patriarchy 'to ensure that a just society is *not* created' (Choi 2001: 282). Further, she notes that the popular and scientific revival of biological theories has coincided with both the feminist backlash and the crisis of masculinity. It does seem ironic that, in books like this, SES is beginning to ask questions about sex and gender, when gender theorists have been moving *away* from these divisions for the past 10 years or so into much more fluid interpretations of sexuality and identity (Butler 1990; Charles and Hughes-Freeland 1996). This is perhaps a reflection of a social and political time lag in the sciences. However, it could also be a sign of more active resistance by men to the successful incursion of women into SES in the same way that the incursion of female athletes in sport has been resisted (Choi 2000). Arguably, being so new, SES has had to strive for respectability and has thus adopted unwittingly all the wrongs of its parent disciplines in relation to gender equity. Perhaps with increasing maturity it might be able to relax and diversify into a more socially diverse and just enterprise.

## Bibliography

Acker, S. (1990) 'Hierarchies, job, bodies: A theory of gendered organizations', *Gender and Society*, 4(2).

Acker, S. (1993) 'Contradiction in terms: women academics in British universities', in M. Arnot and K. Weiler (eds) *Feminism and Social Justice in Education*, London: Falmer Press, 146–66.

Acker, S. (1994) *Gendered Education*, Milton Keynes: Open University.

Aitchison, C. (1999) 'Leisure studies: Gender, power and knowledge', Unpublished doctoral thesis, University of Bristol.

Bleir, R. (1984) *Science and Gender: A Critique of Biology and Its Theories of Women*, New York: Pergamon Press.

Brackenridge, C.H. (2001) *Spoilsports: Understanding and Preventing Sexual Exploitation in Sport*, London: Routledge.

Burkitt, I. (1999) *Bodies of Thought: Embodiment. Identity and Modernity*, London: Sage.

Burman, E. (1990) *Feminists and Psychological Practice*, London: Sage.

Butler, J. (1990) *Gender Trouble: Feminism and the Subversion of Identity*, London: Routledge.

Cashmore, E. (2002) *Sport Psychology: The Key Concepts*, London: Routledge.

Charles, N. and Hughes-Freeland, F. (eds) (1996) *Practising Feminism: Identity, Difference, Power*, London: Routledge.

Choi, P.Y.L. (1999) 'Masculine domains of hunting and sport: Androcentrism in theories of evolution and sport,' *Psychology, Evolution and Gender*, 1(1), 33–43.

Choi, P.Y.L. (2000) *Femininity and the Physically Active Woman*, London: Routledge.

Choi, P.Y.L. (2001) 'Genes and gender roles. Why is the nature argument so appealing?', *Psychology, Evolution and Gender*, 3(3), 279–85.

Choi, P.Y.L (2002) 'Awards remit reflects range of excellence', *BASES World*, March issue. Leeds: BASES.

Choi, P.Y.L., Brackenridge, C.H. and Hardman, A. (2000a) 'Equal or Opposite? Aspects of social equity and exclusion in BASES', Unpublished report of BASES Equity Audity, Leeds: BASES.

Choi, P.Y.L., Brackenridge, C.H. and Hardman, A. (2000b) 'Equal or Opposite? Aspects of social equity and exclusion in BASES', *BASES Newsletter*, December.

Choi, P.Y.L. and Brackenridge, C.H. (2001) 'Equity audit's sparked change', *BASES World*, September issue, Leeds: BASES.

Connell, R.W. (1987) *Gender and Power*, Oxford: Polity Press.

Dewar, A. and Horn, T. (1992) 'A critical analysis of knowledge construction in sport psychology', in T. Horn (ed.) *Advances in Sport Psychology*, Champaign, IL: Human Kinetics, 13–22.

Fausto-Sterling, A. (1992) *Myths of Gender: Biological Theories about Women and Men*, New York: Basic Books.

Featherstone, M., Hepworth, M. and Turner, B.S. (eds) (1991) *The Body: Social Process and Cultural Theory*, London: Sage.

Graydon, J. and Choi, P.Y.L. (1998) *British Association of Sport and Exercise Sciences Equal Opportunities Policy*, Leeds: BASES.

Griffin, P. (1998) *Strong Women, Deep Closets: Lesbians and Homophobia in Sport*, Champaign, IL: Human Kinetics.

Hall, M.A., Cullen, D. and Slack, T. (1989) 'Organizational elites recreating themselves: The gender structure of national sport organizations', *Quest*, (41), 28–45.

Harding, S. (1986) *The Science Question in Feminism*, Milton Keynes: Open University Press.

Hearn, J., Sheppard, D., Tancred-Sheriff, P. and Burrell, G. (eds) (1989) *The Sexuality of Organization*, London: Sage.

Kolnes, L. (1995) 'Heterosexuality as an organising principle in women's sports', *International Review for the Sociology of Sport*, 30, 61–80.

Mavin, P. and Ryans, S. (1999) 'Gender on the agenda in management education?', *Women in Management Review*, (3), 136–45.

Morris, T. and Summers, J. (1995) *Sport Psychology: Theory, Applications and Issues*, Brisbane: John Wiley & Sons.

Nideffer, R.M. (1981) *The Ethics and Practice of Applied Sport Psychology*, Ithaca, NY: Mouvement Publications.

Pemberton, C. (1995) 'Organizational culture and equalities work', in J. Shaw and D. Perrons (eds) *Making Gender Work: Managing Equal Opportunities*, Milton Keynes: Open University Press.

Shilling, C. (1993) *The Body and Social Theory*, London: Sage.

Spender, D. (1980) *Man Made Language*, London: Routledge Kegan Paul.

Spender, D. (ed.) (1981) *Men's Studies Modified: The Impact of Feminism on the Academic Disciplines*, Oxford: Pergamon Press.

*The Guardian* (2002) 'Women struggle to shatter glass ceiling', 5 October, 5.

Talbot, M. (1999) 'Working together towards more inclusive sport and exercise science', keynote speech to the Annual BASES Conference, Leeds, 7 September.

Tong, R. (1997) *Feminist Approaches to Bioethics: Theoretical Reflections and Practical Applications*, Oxford: Westview Press.

Weisstein, N. (1993) 'Psychology constructs the female; or, the fantasy life of the male psychologist (with some attention to the fantasies of his friends the male biologist and the male anthropologist)', *Feminism and Psychology*, 3(2), 195–210.

Wilkinson, H. (1995) *No Turning Back: Generations and the Genderquake*, London: Demos.

Wilkinson, S. (1977) 'Still seeking transformation: Feminist challenges in Psychology', in L. Stanley (ed.) *Knowing Feminisms*, London: Sage.

Witz, A. (1992) *Professions and Patriarchy*, London: Routledge.

## Notes

1   First-wave feminism was the era of the suffragettes (1920s and 30s); second-wave feminism grew out of the Civil Rights movement in the southern United States in the late 1960s and early 1970s.

2   These data are taken from sport science journals, BASES publications and from the career reflections of the authors.

3   Sex and gender identities have never been so much a source of discussion, debate and deconstruction as now (Connell 1987; Butler 1990; Featherstone *et al.* 1991; Shilling 1993; Burkitt 1999). There is broad acceptance in the scientific literature, however, of sex as a biologically ascribed status and gender a socially constructed one. In order to avoid the convolutions of this complex debate we will work here with these relatively simple interpretations in order to allow for social and ethical discussion rather than biological reductionism or theoretical kite-flying.

4   'Androcentric theory is the view that the male sex is primary and the female secondary in the organic scheme, that all things centre, as it were, about the male.' (Definition taken from the *Oxford English Dictionary*, http://athens.oed.com/entrance.dtl, accessed online 15 September 2003.)

# 10 Autoethnography: self-indulgence or rigorous methodology?

*Jacquelyn Allen Collinson and John Hockey*

## Introduction

Sport and exercise are particularly embodied activities, and as a consequence perhaps, have generated a great deal of research on their *physiological* aspects. In common with large amounts of the psychological research on sport and exercise, physiological studies primarily employ a positivistic framework, which constructs as 'objective' the observation, recording and measurement of phenomena (whether physiological, psychological or social) using quantitatively based research techniques or tools such as surveys, scales and structured interviews. This chapter will consider an alternative and very different mode of examining sporting and other activity, namely, autoethnography, where the focus centres upon the meaning of the activity to the researcher/participant herself or himself, and upon the cultural and social context. At this juncture, in congruence with the spirit of the autoethnographic enterprise, it is necessary to make visible some relevant 'accountable knowledge' (Stanley 1990), in order to explain our interest and involvement in the autoethnographic approach. In brief, collectively we have an athletic background of distance running and racing which has required a commitment to training 6 or 7 days a week, sometimes twice a day, for 18 years and 37 years respectively. In addition, we have trained together on a regular basis for 17 years. By a strange coincidence, we both suffered severe running injuries almost simultaneously, and decided to undertake a collective autoethnographic study of the subsequent rehabilitative process. In this sense, it was one of those unhappy accidents of current biography which provided access, physical and psychological, to the research setting (Lofland and Lofland 1985: 11) and stimulated our interest in autoethnography.

Before describing and discussing autoethnography itself, it is first necessary to situate this particular methodological approach within its ethnographic heritage. With its intellectual roots in anthropology and sociology, ethnography utilizes a spectrum of qualitative methods to gain access to particular kinds of human phenomena. While not enjoying the more established tradition of its positivistic counterparts in the study of sport (Sparkes 2002), sports ethnography now has a developing body of literature. This principally comprises ethnographic accounts based upon in-depth interviewing, or constructed via intensive participant observation (see for example, Donnelly 2000; Sands 2002). The latter method involves deep researcher participation in the lives of those under study for extended periods of time, and can generate detailed, rich, analytical descriptions of sporting activity which do not rely on, nor indeed valorize, quantitative data. Autoethnography is an innovative variation of this ethnographic approach and has in many ways challenged the epistemological foundations of much social scientific investigation, as will be discussed. As a result, it remains a somewhat contentious methodological form and is still regarded with suspicion and scepticism in many social science quarters.

## Ethnography and autoethnography

Traditionally, ethnographers have sought to acknowledge reflexivity, and to subject to analysis their own experiences of the social worlds of those under study; as a result, as Van Maanen (1988: ix) notes: 'Ethnography is therefore highly particular and hauntingly personal'. Accounts of such involvement of the self in the research field have largely been confined to publications independent of the actual ethnographic texts, often in the form of 'confessional' tales about the difficulties of undertaking participant observation (see for example, Lareau and Schultz 1996) or occasional accounts of revisiting former fieldwork locations (Ellis 1995). Participant observation, more than other methods, requires that the researcher be the prime and direct instrument of data collection, and this inevitably involves the immersion of the researcher's self or subjectivity in the fieldwork process. The turn towards autoethnography by some researchers has resulted in their experiences of the research process being 'written in' as narratives central to the research endeavour, rather than subsidiary or second-order texts.

In recent decades, the term autoethnography has begun to gain more widespread usage and acceptance within the sociological and anthropological communities (see for example Hayano 1979; Ellis 1997; Hayano 1982; Young 1991; Reed-Danahay 1997; Okley and Callaway 1992; Van Maanen 1995; Coffey 1999; Sparkes 2000), and David Hayano (1979) is typically credited with coining the current usage of the term. There is still, however, some debate about the appropriateness of the terminology, and a whole panoply of other terms co-exists, for example, self-narratives, *récits de soi/moi*, personal narratives, ethnographic autobiography (see Ellis and Bochner 2000: 739 for a comprehensive listing). Whilst bearing in mind the problematic nature of labels, for the purposes of this chapter, the term 'autoethnography' will be used. This has been defined as an autobiographical genre of writing and research (Ellis and Bochner 2000: 739), which examines the dialectics of subjectivity and culture. Autoethnographers constitute a heterogeneous group and vary widely in their focus, whether on the research process (graphy), culture (ethnos) or self (auto) (Ellis and Bochner 2000). Autoethnography in general entails the detailed analysis of oneself *qua* member of a social group or category as, for example, a distance runner (Denison 2002; Allen Collinson and Hockey 2001) or an Olympic rower (Tsang 2000). It is usually distinguished from autobiography by its particular forms of analysis and its emphasis on experiences within the writer's life that aim to illuminate wider cultural or subcultural aspects. The distinctiveness of autoethnography as an investigative process lies in its efforts to combine detailed fieldnotes, analysing the research 'field' (for example, a soccer match), with 'headnotes' (Sanjek 1990), the researcher's actual experience of engaging with the phenomenon at hand (for example, playing soccer). The self and the ethnographic field are then symbiotic, and in effect this combination forms the pivot of analysis (Coffey 1999).

As indicated, autoethnographers have sought to 'write themselves in' to their accounts of fieldwork (Tedlock 1991), in a rigorous, analytic fashion, and by so doing are engaged in writing about aspects of their identities (Coffey 1999) as an *integral* part of the research process. The reasons for this are explored in the section below on *representation*. Some ethnographic researchers in sport and dance have seized upon this challenging development and begun to utlize their own embodied sporting experiences to produce a range of detailed autoethnographies or 'narratives of the self' (Sparkes 2000) relating to various sporting and physical activities, and also to health problems such as sports injuries (see for example Denison 1999; Allen Collinson 2003; Allen Collinson and Hockey 2001; Duncan 2000; Fernandez-Balboa 1998; Kaskisaari 1994; Messner and Sabo 1994; Rinehart 1995; Silvennoinen 1999a, 1999b; Sparkes 1996, 2003; Sudwell 1999; Swan 1999; Tiihonen 1994; Tinning 1998).

## Methodology

Autoethnography, in common with its ethnographic parent, is a particular *methodology*; a research strategy which underpins the use and selection of specific methods in order to approach certain research questions. There exists a plurality of autoethnographic methods to gather and analyse research data, including: personal diaries, video and audio recordings, logs, and fieldnotes gathered by participant observation. Linked to autoethnographic methodology and methods are numerous *theoretical* perspectives (e.g. symbolic interactionism, phenomenology, feminism and so on), which constitute particular ways of seeing, understanding and explaining social life. For example, researchers of a symbolic interactionist persuasion view the social world as constructed interactionally, via language, communication, interrelationships, and social groups (see for example Crossett (1995) on golf; Fine (1987) on children's baseball; and Chambliss (1989) on swimming). Symbolic interactionism emphasizes the fluidity and mutability of meanings, and their context-dependency. The processual character of interaction can thus be best explored and charted by particular methods of investigation, and participant observation has traditionally been granted pride of place in the pantheon of methods.

The sets of assumptions underpinning symbolic interactionism and other theoretical perspectives sit within a wider theory of knowledge or epistemology which has become known as *constructionism*. As Crotty (1998: 43) explains: 'What constructionism claims is that meanings are constructed by human beings as they engage with the world they are interpreting.' Hence there is no 'objective' truth independent of actors' consciousness and experience; meaning has to be constructed by actors, within social situations. Researchers working within this paradigm, who assert that there exists no fact-like, 'objective' truth out there, independent of our consciousness and waiting to be discovered, contend that an objectivist epistemology and positivisitic perspectives are either logically impossible (taking the strong position) or (at the weaker end of the continuum) at the very least inappropriate for researching social phenomena. Constructionism, as Crotty (1998: 4) also notes, 'is the epistemology found, or at least claimed in most perspectives other than those representing positivistic and post-positivistic paradigms'. So, whilst specific theories may develop key concepts particular to themselves, for example *social worlds*, *social objects*, and the *self* (Blumer 1969) in the case of symbolic interactionism, their epistemological foundations are shared by a number of other theories which are situated intellectually within constructionism. This, in brief, is the intellectual 'baggage' contextualizing the ethnographic and autoethnographic enterprises.

In general, autoethnogaphers have tended to concentrate upon the phenomenological and interactional dimensions of sporting experience. On one level, they have sought to reveal their own place in the interactional milieux of sporting settings, as researchers and participants, where the researcher also becomes the subject of research, thus blurring the boundaries between the social and the personal, between self and other, as illustrated for example in Rinehart's (1998) analysis of swimming lessons. Autoethnographic researchers have also been concerned to reveal not only the interactional elements of the sporting self, but also the emotional dimension. Of particular interest has been a focus on feelings as an embodied form of consciousness (Denzin 1984) when participating in sport or indeed when deprived of that participation (Sparkes 2002) and a concern to portray self-consciousness; to 'open up the realm of the interior and the personal' (Fiske 1990: 90).

Given the focus on these concerns, other kinds of research questions and aims such as, for example, attempts at the quantification of sporting activity, the assessment of fitness levels, and so on, have not formed the target of autoethnographic attention. This is due to a number of features. First, attempts at measurement and quantification, with a heavy emphasis on statistical generalizability, have generally been rejected as a goal by auto/ethnographic researchers. Of greater relevance to the latter are case studies, each of which harbours its own sets of meaning, structure and normative order (Denzin 1983: 133–4), and requires in-depth analytic dénouement in order to develop the knowledge base of the topic or group under investigation. Second, whilst one of the primary autoethnographic objectives is to reveal information about the researcher's membership of social groups, categories (e.g. injured athletes) and social processes, a strong biographical imperative to reflect upon the researcher's own life experiences in a highly self-reflexive fashion is also apparent. This objective of making sense of sporting and other kinds of experience (cf. Spry 2001) fuels the involvement of many researchers in this particular methodological form. In addition, autoethnographers are often committed to uncovering their own motives for undertaking this form of research, and making visible the 'accidents of current biography' (Lofland and Lofland 1985: 11) which stimulate the researcher/author to embark upon the study. The processes, problems and questions which autoethnographers examine tend to be relatively focused in scope and range, and typically link directly to biography, subjectivity and interaction.

## Representation

As indicated, autoethnography has been employed as a research approach for over two decades (Hayano 1979) and some of the early literature focuses upon sports and games, such as Hayano's (1982) study of poker players. The development of the genre was given considerable impetus during the 1980s by the engagement of some ethnographers in a fundamental questioning of the ways in which ethnographic accounts were constructed, and whether these constructions could be deemed 'objective'. One of the consequences of this questioning, termed the 'crisis of representation and legitimation' (Denzin and Lincoln 2000) has been the flourishing of autoethnography, where researchers explore different ways of undertaking and writing ethnography, and as a corollary seek alternative ways of legitimating this particular methodological and narrative form.

One of the fundamental tenets of ethnographic research had previously been that researchers could directly capture the lived experience of those they were researching. This precept was subsequently rendered highly problematic when it was argued that such experience was formed within the text crafted by the researcher. Consequently, some of the focus shifted to an examination of the ways in which ethnographic texts were constructed (cf. Van Maanen 1995). Traditional modes of writing in the natural and social sciences, in which the author is construed as 'silent', other than being credited as the author, were deemed highly problematic (Van Maanen 1995). The embodied self of the researcher has become recognized as a crucial component of the research process, having a fundamental impact upon the way in which (s)he chooses to construct the ethnographic text and to represent reality. Indeed some would contend (for example, Behar 1997: 6) that there needs to be clarification and exposition of what occurs *within* the observer if we are to understand fully what has been observed and in turn written. The traditional way of writing ethnographic texts, such as the 'classic' ethnographies of, for example, Whyte (1943), Becker *et al.* (1961) and Atkinson (1981), has also come under sustained criticism from some quarters, although it should be borne in mind that these texts are inevitably products of their time. The criticism has been levelled not just at the 'silent' author approach taken, but also because the voices of those under study in these so-called 'realist' works may seem 'orchestrated to serve the theoretical needs of an absent, disembodied author' (Sparkes 1995: 164). In this instance, 'disembodied' can be taken to mean that the author, as a physical entity, does not feature in the analysis. The result, critics maintain, is a somewhat narrow account of what happened, a limited, very partial version of reality, which apparently precludes other interpretations of what has been observed (Van

Maanen 1988: 53), but does not 'come clean' about this partiality. One response to this critical onslaught has been the development of new ways of writing, for as Richardson (1994: 516) notes: 'Writing is also a way of "knowing" – a method of discovery and analysis. By writing in different ways, we discover new aspects of our topic and our relationship to it.' Some of the elements of this new form of writing will now be examined before issues of legitimation are explored further.

## New writing

Richardson (1994) describes the narrative of self as an evocative textual form which produces highly personalized and revealing accounts. Ellis (1999: 669) has described her autoethnographic goal as being 'to extend ethnography to include the heart, the autobiographical, and the artistic text'. Particular language forms are often used, for example the first person singular and plural, metaphor, 'colourful' language, dramatic or unusual turns of phrase, juxtaposition of ideas, and so on, in an attempt to convey an immediacy, to make a connection, to *show* the reader the feelings and emotions of the experience, rather than merely *telling* what these things mean or meant (see Sparkes 2003: 65). Autoethnographers invite the reader not only to analyse, but to *share* the feelings and the sensations, to connect with the experience. The reasons for this are many and varied, but Simpson (2003: 115) captures something of the quest in his discussion of mountaineers and their willingness to encounter great risk:

> Why? Perhaps it all boils down to sensation – what we feel is all we really know; all we can accurately say we are. Yet others may not feel the same way. This isolates us. We hope that others also experience the same things because it keeps us sane and allows us to build a construct within which to live.

Describing autoethnography in the abstract cannot really capture its distinctiveness. In order to convey some of the flavour of autoethnographic research accounts, it is necessary to consider some examples of the genre, and it is hoped that the following small selection will provide some indication. For example, the use of imagery and colour is well illustrated in the following account from Jim Denison (2002: 132) in which he contrasts the activities of writing and running, inviting the reader to visualize and feel, vicariously, the experience:

> Writing and running are both visual. For instance, I may shape a scene with words, but images still appear in my mind. And out running I used to picture a radiant blue beam emanating from my waist that pulled me forwards mile after mile, lap after lap. When I write my arms become light, turn to wings almost, and I feel weightless in my chair. Exactly how running at night used to feel, when shrouded in blackness I became an apparition floating above the road ... somehow the process of moving in and through language, like moving in and through water, puts me inside myself and I trust the words that appear. Running's vital elements always felt cerebral too, with a touch

of aquamarine. I realize now that I should have trusted myself more. After all, it was my body, no one else's.

As Greenhalgh (2001: 55) has noted, there is still a degree of risk involved in this genre of 'vulnerable writing', particularly when it focuses upon the emotion and pain experienced by the author(s). Two extracts from different autoethnographic accounts, both in relation to the pain of injury, may serve to illustrate authors' attempts to convey accurately and vividly the problematic physicality, the intense feelings and emotion of the experience:

> Deeper now in my left buttock I feel it. Sharper, tugging, less playful now. With each left step I wait for the brief cut of pain . . . Left step – *stab*. Right step – fine. Left step – *stab*. Right step – fine. Left step – *stab*. Left, left, left – *stab, stab, stab* . . . (Sparkes 2003: 57).

> At the initial point of injury, each of us came to a juddering halt, in a state of shock, the pain stabbing the knee, jangling through the body, standing then sitting in fear, drenched with anxiety, asking the same question over and over: 'Will I be able to run again?' (Allen Collinson 2003).

Autoethnographers often seek to communicate not only the immediacy, the physicality and emotionality of the experience, but also its psychological and social elements, the internal dialogue of the writer with her/himself, and also to situate the experience within its wider structural context. Tsang (2000), for example, a competitive rower with the Canadian national team, recounts an instance where one of her teammates asked: 'So are you going to shave your legs before the Olympics?' The account continues:

> 'Maybe Rebecca and I will have to tie you down and Neet[1] your legs for you,' Chris quips. A few of my crewmates laugh at this. It's a joke. Or is it? . . . A flitter of fear or panic scampers across my consciousness as I picture the scene she has suggested, and then it is gone. These are my friends. The panic in my mind is replaced by a multitude of different thoughts and emotions surrounding the subject of my legs. I feel a slight resentment at being pressured to change something about myself that has been a choice characterized by struggle. The struggle of knowingly going against cultural standards of beauty and thereby risking the acceptance of friends, or potential lovers, and of employers. Not to mention my own internal struggle with myself and my choices: deep down I actually prefer the aesthetics and sensation of smooth, soft legs, yet intellectually and politically I feel it important enough to act against these impulses. (48–9.)

Writing in this personal and emotional style seeks to challenge the orthodoxy of the researcher/author as neutral, distanced, absent, silent, and this may leave the autoethnographer vulnerable to charges of being 'irrational, particularistic,

private, and subjective, rather than reasonable, universal, public, and objective'
(Greenhalgh 2001: 55). Writing in this way can also be therapeutic, even
cathartic, a learning experience, as described by Ellis (1999) who asked one of
her students if she had learned anything new from writing her autoethnographic
account of surviving breast cancer:

> Yes, that cancer is more than a medical story; it's a feeling story. I learned
> how scared I am even though I've been a survivor now for 7 years. And that's
> the interesting thing – there's little about long-term survivors in stories or in
> social science research . . .. I try so hard to pretend that I'm an upbeat,
> optimistic person with no worries, a warrior who has learned from her
> experiences. But what I had to face as I wrote my story is that I'm scared all
> the time that the cancer will come back . . .. Maybe I can write myself as a
> survivor in a deeper, more meaningful way. (678–9.)

## Issues of legitimation

Contemporaneous with this 'new writing' came the search for its legitimation,
given the prevalent view that all academic writing needs to be based upon a set
of scrutinized principles. In the domains of sport, exercise and health research,
the crisis of representation and in turn of legitimation appears to have had a
differential impact upon the various disciplines and sub-disciplines which make
up the field. Some researchers have argued that the questioning of traditional
criteria appears to be stronger amongst sociologists of sport than amongst social
psychologists for example (Sparkes 2002: 7), and by no means all sociologists
accept the arguments for a radical overhaul. Critics, including many who work
within the qualitative tradition, regard autoethnography as failing to meet
'appropriate' academic criteria, such as validity and generalizability. Some of the
dangers of the approach are perceived to be its narcissism, 'navel-gazing' and self-
indulgence (Coffey 1999), and it has even been likened to the confessional tales
of 'reality TV'. As one of Ellis and Bochner's (2000: 749) participants questions
in relation to personal narratives:

> How do you react to critics who say that personal narratives simulate reality
> TV? Aren't these narratives reflective of the culture of confession and
> victimization and don't they end up as spectacles that sentimentalise,
> humiliate, and take pleasure in revealing anguish and pain? Personal
> narratives remind me of victim art. They play on your sympathies and
> manipulate your emotions.

Autoethnographers have responded to such critiques in a variety of ways, one
response being: if personal narratives 'play upon' or better still, evoke, the reader's
sympathies, then they have clearly achieved one of their purposes. This leads us
to discussions regarding the kinds of criteria to be employed in evaluating

autoethnographic accounts. If an account of a research project is acknowledged to be just one perspective, one interpretation of what has occurred, constructed via the author's craft of writing rather than any supposedly 'objective' description, then the conventional criteria for evaluation are undermined. Writing, it is now recognized by many, is an integral feature of the research enterprise, and 'there can be no such thing as a neutral, innocent report since the conventions of the text and the language forms used are actively involved in the construction of various realities' (Sparkes 2002: 12). In such cases the research output cannot be checked against the reality it supposedly represents. Therefore, it is argued, the traditional criteria used to evaluate much qualitative research cannot legitimately be applied to autoethnographic research.

### Traditional criteria: validity, reliability and generalizability

Before proceeding to consider some of the fallout from this crisis of legitimation, a brief recap of the 'holy trinity' (Sparkes 1998: 365) of traditional criteria for evaluating research may be necessary at this juncture.

Questions of *validity* pertain to whether a measure or operational definition actually relates to the concept that it is claimed to examine. A classic case would be whether the IQ test actually measures levels of intelligence, or whether it is measuring something quite different. Various forms of validity have been proposed, including for example, face validity: whether there *appears* to be a correspondence between the measure and the concept; construct validity: whether one can hypothesize a connection between the concept of interest and another related concept (Bryman 1995: 59). *Reliability* refers to the consistency of a measure and is usually taken to comprise two elements: external and internal reliability. External reliability relates to the degree of consistency over time, often gauged by testing and retesting the measure on subsequent occasions. Internal reliability refers to the degree of internal consistency of a measure (for a detailed explanation, see Bryman 1995: 57). *Generalizability* relates to the degree to which the data from one research study can be extended or generalized beyond the specific population or settings of that piece of research to the general population, other populations or other contexts. In many forms of qualitative research, which are not based upon statistical samples, generalizability usually relates to whether the findings of one study can be replicated in other similar circumstances, or to what extent the findings can be extrapolated to the theory which the research was designed to test (Brannen 1992: 9).

### Alternative criteria for evaluation

Under the critical challenges of postmodernism, poststructuralism and feminism, these traditional criteria for the evaluation of qualitative research have been problematized and treated with suspicion, particularly by autoethnographers, so that widely taken-for-granted terms like 'validity', 'generalizability', and 'reliability', have been subjected to serious rethinking within certain disciplines and sub-disciplines.

The evocative narratives of autoethnographic accounts often contrast starkly with the more traditional conventions of much social scientific writing, on a whole series of dimensions (see Ellis and Bochner 2000: 744), including, for example: the blurring of the roles of researcher and researched (with their potential connotations of hierarchy); the attempt to write evocatively, in emotional and emotive language, which presents a direct challenge to the notion of the researcher/author as a neutral, 'objective', distanced observer, in control of her or his research setting. Given the very distinctive methodological foundations of autoethnographic research, the question arises as to how we should approach its evaluation, and what criteria should be employed to judge qualitative work, and more specifically autoethnographic research accounts.

In relation to qualitative inquiry in general, researchers such as Sparkes (1998) have emphasized that subjecting qualitative research to the kinds of criteria usually employed to evaluate positivistic or postpositivistic social science research is highly problematic, even nonsensical. Given their different paradigmatic foundations, it seems pointless, indeed imperialistic, to apply inappropriate criteria derived from other traditions. It is argued that different criteria are therefore required to evaluate qualitative research; so for example, the conventional criteria of validity, reliability and generalizability might be replaced with criteria such as credibility, transferability, dependability, and confirmability (Lincoln and Guba 1985: 42–3). These 'substitute' criteria may, however, themselves be deemed problematic, as Sparkes has pointed out:

> [E]ven though the criteria used in conventional research were defined as inappropriate for qualitative inquiry, attempts were made to develop their *parallels* under a different guise. Thus, an essentially parallel perspective developed in response to the legitimisation problem in qualitative inquiry. (1998: 366, emphasis added.)

The philosophical contradictions of this 'parallel position' have been revealed and trenchantly critiqued (see for example, Smith 1990, 1993), leading some to argue for the abandonment of concepts such as validity altogether, in order to seek alternative, more appropriate criteria for the evaluation of ethnographic and autoethnographic research. Consequently, radically different, more open-ended, flexible criteria have been proposed, such as authenticity, fidelity, believability, congruence, resonance, aesthetic appeal, to name but a few. Believability, resonance and congruence with the reader's experience were certainly key criteria which we sought to meet in our own autoethnographic research accounts (Allen Collinson and Hockey 2001; Allen Collinson 2003). As ethnographers it was therefore important for us to convey as accurately, vividly, analytically and evocatively as possible the subjective experience of the injury and rehabilitative processes that we underwent, so that the reader could form a judgement as to whether our account was believable. Such believability would, we considered, be based upon a close congruence or resonance with the reader's own similar life experiences, or the experiences of someone whom they knew well.

As a consequence of the emergence of this plurality of criteria, 'there can be no canonical approach to this form of inquiry, no recipes or rigid formulas . . .' (Sparkes 1998: 380). Judgements regarding the most appropriate criteria to employ will always be context-dependent. We would hasten to add, however, this does not imply a position of total relativism of a particular form, where anything and everything is acceptable. It is argued, rather, that qualitative researchers, including autoethnographers, must seek to reach agreement on appropriate criteria via rigorous, free, open and ongoing dialogue and debate. Reaching agreement and passing judgement may then become practical and moral tasks rather than epistemological ones (Sparkes 1998: 381), for the very criteria we use to evaluate research are themselves of course historically and culturally situated, and therefore subject to review, interpretation and reinterpretation over time and epoch (see Smith 1993: 139), and across cultures.

## Why use autoethnography?

Having portrayed something of the complexity of the autoethnographic enterprise, it remains to contemplate why this particular methodology should be seriously considered as a legitimate means of enquiry into sport, physical activity and health. Sport after all involves action, either based on individual or collective participation, and is a thoroughly embodied and practically accomplished activity. Ultimately what makes that activity possible is that it is meaningful to participants. In order to grasp fully that meaning, the actor's subjective point of view needs to be examined in depth. This leads to the problem of subjectivity and the inaccessibility of mind. Researchers working within the ethnographic tradition have long tried to gain access to participants' subjective experiences by employing techniques such as in-depth interviewing and participant observation. The 'sporting mind' in particular has largely been accessed imperfectly, for as Bain (1995) indicates, there is scant research into and within sport which comprehensively recognizes subjective knowledge. Even when the study is conducted via qualitative methods, ultimately an objectivist interpretation of the data is often all too evident. The result can be a failure to provide 'an in-depth analysis of meaning as constructed by the participants themselves' (Bain 1995:243).

A more fruitful approach may well be that of phenomenology, with its greater emphasis on the consciousness of individuals as the focus of study. In addition, phenomenologists view the organization of everyday life as 'centred around the here and now of bodily existence and presence' (Münch 1994: 151), acknowledging the centrality of the body in the relationship between self-consciousness and the self. As Crossley (1995: 47) has noted, the mind is inseparable from the body; they remain 'reversible aspects of a single fabric'. It is perhaps ironic that in such a thoroughly embodied activity as sport, there appears to be relatively little written from a phenomenological perspective, in terms of material rooted in the actual embodied sporting activity of participants (Kerry and Armour 2000: 10) and their thoughts and feelings during that process. As Kerry and Armour (2000: 3) indicate in relation to endurance athletes who suffer glycogen depletion: 'An embodied phenomenological approach would endeavour to capture the lived meaning of marathon running and hitting the wall. What is it actually like to hit the wall?' The body as 'objectively' measured and assessed, and the body lived and experienced subjectively, are in essence dissimilar (Rintala 1991: 274); for example, as Luijpen (1966: 50) explains, our hands are not any old hands, but rather are 'I-myself-grasping-things'; our feet are not just an item in some anatomy discussion, but rather 'I-myself-walking'. As Rintala (1991: 271–2) perceptively notes:

> The runner may not know her or his percent body fat and may have no data on hand to assert that the running mechanics are efficient. The computer printout that lists all of the known variables about that individual may be meaningless to the runner, but she or he can discuss what it is like to run . . . feeling one's feet strike the ground, or knowing the experience of one's heart pounding.

There is consequently a need for research on sport, physical activity and health to render visible and knowable this kind of experience, for example: I-myself-cross-country-running, or the feeling of being hit in a heavy rugby tackle, or undergoing a medical procedure. As Kerry and Armour (2000: 9) contend, the purpose of writing within the phenomenological approach is 'to bring the essence of such lived experiences into being', and achieving this may well require a vivid, evocative style, rich in narrative (Smith 1992). Autoethnography, with its unorthodox narrative forms and strong emphasis on embodiment, emotions and feelings, is a methodology which offers fertile possibilities for the development of very distinctive forms of phenomenological sporting and medical accounts, which are presently in a state of underdevelopment. This would also begin to remedy an imbalance in the relationship between theory and practice in the study of sport, for it is interesting to note that readers can access considerable theoretical resources (cf. Maguire and Young 2002), and abundant physiological data, but little in the way of systematic phenomenological depictions and analysis of actual, lived sporting experience. Autoethnographic accounts of sport and physical activity offer the promise, over time, of insight not only into the individual's meaningful sporting subjectivity but also into the ways in which certain categories of sports participants share the experiences of their own particular sport(s) and physical activity. In addition, autoethnography continues the work of poststructuralist and deconstructionist writers such as Derrida (1978) and Foucault (1970) in challenging and altering the very ways in which we understand the connections between author, text and reader (Ellis and Bochner 2000). All this is not to say, however, that autoethnographic accounts should in any way supersede other kinds of research tradition, but rather to highlight the potential complementarity of this methodological approach.

Autoethnography and, for example, experimental methods might complement each other by examining phenomena from different perspectives, as in the above example of 'hitting the wall' in an endurance event.

## Concluding remarks

To conclude on a more personal note, our involvement in a collective autoethnographic project (Allen Collinson and Hockey 2001; Allen Collinson 2003) provided an opportunity to undertake a systematic analysis of a traumatic sporting-injury event and its aftermath; a very difficult period in both our biographies, which posed a serious threat to our running careers and subjectivities. The research helped us psychologically to come to terms with an intensely negative and highly emotional period, and also to sustain the momentum of recovery. One of the aims of our autoethnographic study was to convey, as accurately and evocatively as possible, the lived experience of this emotionally charged journey, to share with the reader the feelings and emotions, and hopefully to make an empathic connection with the audience. In addition, we were concerned to present, analytically *and* experientially, the ways in which we managed to sustain rehabilitative momentum, in the hope that this might help others suffering from injury. For us, our own small autoethnographic enterprise was validated by the words of one journal reviewer who wrote in some detail about the high degree of empathic resonance (s)he had felt in reading the account. To have achieved such a writer–text–reader connection meant that one of our own principal criteria for evaluating an autoethnographic account had been satisfied in full.

## Bibliography

Allen Collinson, J. (2003) 'Running into injury time: distance running and temporality', *Sociology of Sport Journal*, 20(4), 331–350.

Allen Collinson, J. and Hockey, J. (2001) 'Runners' tales: Autoethnography, injury and narrative', *Auto/Biography*, IX(1 and 2), 95–106.

Atkinson, P. (1981) *The Clinical Experience*, Farnborough: Gower.

Bain, L.L. (1995) 'Mindfulness and subjective knowledge', *Quest*, 47, 238–53.

Becker, H.S., Geer, B., Hughes, E.L. and Strauss, A.L. (1961) *Boys in White*, Chicago: Chicago University Press.

Behar, R. (1997) *The Vulnerable Observer: Anthropology that Breaks Your Heart*, Boston: Beacon.

Blumer, H. (1969) *Symbolic Interactionism: Perspective and Method*, Englewood Cliffs, NJ: Prentice-Hall.

Brannen, J. (1992) 'Combining qualitative and quantitative approaches: an overview', in J. Brannen (ed.), *Mixing Methods: Qualitative and Quantitative Research*, Aldershot: Avebury, 3–37.

Bryman, A. (1995) *Research Methods and Organization Studies*, London: Routledge.

Chambliss, D. (1989) 'The mundanity of excellence', *Sociological Theory*, 7, 70–86.

Coffey, A. (1999) *The Ethnographic Self: Fieldwork and the Representation of Identity*, London: Sage.

Crossett, T. (1995) *Outsiders in the Clubhouse: The World of Women's Professional Golf*, Albany, NY: State University of New York Press.

Crossley, N. (1995) Merleau-Ponty, the elusive body and carnal sociology, *Body and Society*, 1(1), 43–63.

Crotty, M. (1998) *The Foundations of Social Research*, London: Sage.

Denison, J. (1999) 'Boxed in', in A. Sparkes and M. Silvennoinen (eds) *Talking Bodies*, Jyvaskyla, Finland: SoPhi, 29–36.

Denison, J. (2002) Writing a 'true' sports story, *Auto/Biography*, X(1 and 2), 131–7.

Denzin, N.K. (1983) 'Interpretative interactionism', in G. Morgan (ed.) *Beyond Method: Strategies for Social Research*, Beverley Hills, CA: Sage, 129–46.

Denzin, N.K. (1984) *On Understanding Emotion*, San Francisco: Jossey Bass.

Denzin, N.K. and Lincoln, Y.S. (2000) 'The policies and practices of interpretation', in N.K. Denzin and Y.S. Lincoln (eds) *Handbook of Qualitative Research*, 2nd edn, Thousand Oaks, CA: Sage, 897–992.

Derrida, J. (1978) *Writing and Difference* (trans. A. Bass), Chicago: University of Chicago Press.

Donnelly, P. (2000) 'Interpretive approaches to the sociology of sport,' in J. Coakley and E. Dunning (eds) *Handbook of Sports Studies*, London: Sage, 77–92.

Duncan, M.C. (2000) Reflex, *Sociology of Sport Journal*, 17(10), 60–8.

Ellis, C. (1995) Emotional and ethical quagmires in returning to the field, *Journal of Contemporary Ethnography*, 24, 68–98.

Ellis, C. (1997) 'Evocative autoethnography', in W. Tierney and Y. Lincoln (eds) *Representation and the Text*, New York: State University of New York Press, 115–39.

Ellis, C. (1999) 'Heartful autoethnography', *Qualitative Health Research*, 9(5), 669–83.

Ellis, C. and Bochner, A. (2000) 'Autoethnography, personal narrative, reflexivity. Researcher as subject', in N.K. Denzin and Y. Lincoln (eds) *Handbook of Qualitative Research*, 2nd edn, London: Sage, 733–68.

Fernandez-Balboa, J.-M. (1998) 'Transcending masculinities', in C. Hickey, L. Fitzclarence and R. Matthews (eds) *Where the Boys Are*, Geelong, Australia: Deakin University Press, 121–39.

Fine, G.A. (1987) *With the Boys: Little League Baseball and Preadolescent Culture*, Chicago: University of Chicago Press.

Fiske, J. (1990) 'Ethnosemiotics: Some personal and theoretical reflections', *Cultural Studies*, 4, 85–99.

Foucault, M. (1970) *The Order of Things: An Archaeology of the Human Sciences*, New York: Random House.

Greenhalgh, S. (2001) *Under the Medical Gaze: Facts and Fictions of Chronic Pain*, Berkeley: University of California Press.

Hayano, D.M. (1979) 'Auto-ethnography: Paradigms, problems and prospects,' *Human Organization*, 38(1), 99–104.

Hayano, D.M. (1982) *Poker Faces: The Life and Work of Professional Card Players*, Berkeley: University of California Press.

Kaskisaari, M. (1994) 'The rhythmbody', *International Review for the Sociology of Sport*, 29(1), 15–23.

Kerry, D.S. and Armour, K.M. (2000) 'Sport sciences and the promise of phenomenology: Philosophy, method, and insight,' *Quest*, 52(1), 1–17.

Lareau, A. and Schultz, J. (1996) *Journeys Through Ethnography: Realistic Accounts of Fieldwork*, Boulder, CO: Westview.

Lincoln, Y. and Gubba, E. (1985) *Naturalistic Inquiry*, Thousand Oaks, CA: Sage.

Lofland, J. and Lofland, L.H. (1985) *Analyzing Social Settings: A Guide to Qualitative Observation and Analysis*, 3rd edn, Belmont, CA: Wadsworth Publishing Company.

Luijpen, W.A. (1966) *Phenomenology and Humanism – Primer in Existential Phenomenology*, Pittsburgh: Duquesne University Press.

Maguire, J. and Young, K. (eds) (2002) *Theory, Sport and Society*, London: JAI.

Messner, M.A. and Sabo, D.F. (1994) *Sex, Violence and Power in Sports: Rethinking Masculinity*, Freedom, CA: Crossing Press.

Münch, R. (1994) *Sociological Theory: From the 1920s to the 1960s*, Chicago: Nelson Hall.

Okley, J. and Callaway, H. (1992) *Anthropology and Autobiography*, London: Routledge.

Reed-Danahay, D. (ed.) (1997) *Auto/Ethnography*, Oxford: Berg.

Richardson, L. (1994) 'Writing: a method of inquiry', in N.K. Denzin and Y. Lincoln (eds) *Handbook of Qualitative Research*, London: Sage, 516–29.

Rinehart, R. (1995) 'Pentecostal aquatics', *Studies in Symbolic Interactionism*, 19, 109–21.

Rinehart, R. (1998) 'Born-again sport: Ethics in biographical research', in G. Rail (ed.) *Sport and Postmodern Times*, Albany, NY: State University of New York Press, 33–46.

Rintala, J. (1991) 'The mind-body revisited', *Quest*, 43, 260–79.

Sands, R.R. (2002) *Sport Ethnography*, Champaign, IL: Human Kinetics.

Sanjek, R. (ed.) (1990) *Fieldnotes: The Making of Anthropology*, Ithaca, NY: Cornell University Press.

Silvennoinen, M. (1999a) 'Anguish of the body', in A. Sparkes and M. Silvennoinen (eds) *Talking Bodies*, Jyvaskyla, Finland: SoPhi, 93–8.

Silvennoinen, M. (1999b) 'My body as metaphor', in A. Sparkes and M. Silvennoinen (eds) *Talking Bodies*, Jyvaskyla, Finland: SoPhi, 163–75.

Simpson, J. (2003) *The Beckoning Silence*, London: Vintage.

Smith, J.K. (1990) 'Goodness criteria: alternative research paradigms and the problem of criteria', in E. Guba (ed.) *The Paradigm Dialog*, London: Sage, 167–87.

Smith, J.K. (1993) *After the Demise of Empiricism: The Problem of Judging Social and Educational Inquiry*, Norwood, NJ: Ablex.

Smith, S.J. (1992) 'Studying the lifeworld of physical education: a phenomenological orientation', in A.C. Sparkes (ed.) *Research in Physical Education and Sport: Exploring Alternative Visions*, London: Falmer, 61–89.

Sparkes, A. (1995) 'Writing people: Reflections on the dual crises of representation and legitimation in qualitative inquiry', *Quest*, 47, 158–95.

Sparkes, A. (1996) 'The fatal flaw', *Qualitative Inquiry*, 2(4), 463–94.

Sparkes, A. (1998) 'Validity in qualitative inquiry and the problem of criteria: implications for sport psychology', *The Sport Psychologist*, 12, 363–86.

Sparkes, A. (2000) 'Autoethnography and narratives of the self: Reflections on criteria in action', *Sociology of Sport Journal*, 17, 21–43.

Sparkes, A. (2002) *Telling Tales in Sport and Physical Activity: A Qualitative Journey*, Champaign, IL: Human Kinetics.

Sparkes, A. (2003) 'Bodies, identities, selves: autoethnographic fragments and reflections', in J. Denison and P. Markula (eds) *Moving Writing: Crafting Movement in Sport and Research*, New York: Peter Lang, 51–76.

Spry, T. (2001) 'Performing autoethnography: An embodied methodological praxis', *Qualitative Inquiry*, 7(6), 706–32.

Stanley, L. (1990) 'Feminist auto/biography and feminist epistemology', in A. Jane and S. Walby (eds) *Out of the Margins: Women's Studies in the Nineties*, London: Falmer Press, 204–19.

Sudwell, M. (1999) 'The body bridge', in A. Sparkes, and M. Silvennoinen (eds), *Talking Bodies*, Jyvaskyla, Finland: SoPhi, 13–28.

Swan, P. (1999) 'Three ages of changing', in: A. Sparkes, and M. Silvennoinen (eds) *Talking Bodies*, Jyvaskyla, Finland: SoPhi, 37–47.

Tedlock, B. (1991) 'From participant observation to the observation of participation: the emergence of narrative ethnography', *Journal of Anthropological Research*, 41, 69–94.

Tiihonen, A. (1994) 'Asthma', *International Review for the Sociology of Sport*, 29(1), 51–62.

Tinning, R. (1998) 'What position do you play?', in C. Hickey, L. Fitzclarence and R. Matthews (eds), *Where the Boys Are*, Geelong, Australia: Deakin University Press, 109–20.

Tsang, T. (2000) 'Let me tell you a story: a narrative exploration of identity in high-performance sport', *Sociology of Sport Journal*, 17(1), 44–59.

Van Maanen, J. (1988) *Tales of the Field: On Writing Ethnography*, Chicago: University of Chicago Press.

Van Maanen, J. (ed.) (1995) *Representation in Ethnography*, London: Sage.

Whyte, S.F. (1943) *Street Corner Society*, Chicago: Chicago University Press.

Young, K. (1991) 'Perspectives on embodiment', *Journal of Narrative and Life History*, 1(2 and 3), 213–43.

## Note

1 Brand name of depilatory product.

# 11 Is investigative sociology just investigative journalism?

*John Sugden*

## Introduction

In a leading article for the BSA's (British Sociological Association) Newsletter, Ivor Gaber (2003), freelance journalist and Emeritus Professor of Broadcast Journalism at Goldsmiths College, University of London, suggested that sociologists might improve their skills of interpretation and communication by developing closer relations with journalism. In this chapter I will explore some of the broader implications of this position. In particular I will be reflecting upon and exemplifying issues that have emerged through my own field work and that of colleagues, researching the governing body of world football, FIFA (Sugden and Tomlinson 1998, 1999, 2003), and investigating the underground economy that has grown up around the same game in the UK (Sugden and Tomlinson 2002). Much of this output inhabits a grey area between investigative journalism and investigative sociology. Trying to make sense of the differences and similarities between the two professions raises a series of epistemological and ethical issues. The remainder of this chapter explores these and related methodological concerns.[1] In doing so I raise more questions than provide answers, but I hope what follows at least provides the impetus for lively debate.

## Finding and telling the truth

What, then, are investigative journalists and how do they differ from their sociological counterparts? According to Hugo De Burgh, investigative journalists are usually driven people whose mission it is to probe into and uncover corruption, malpractice and abuse of power usually in corporate, government and/or criminal settings:

> Investigative journalists attempt to get at the truth where the truth is obscure because it suits others that it be so; they choose their topics from a sense of right and wrong which we can only call a moral sense, but in the manner of their research they attempt to be dispassionately evidential. They are doing more than disagreeing with how society runs; they are pointing out that it is failing by its own standards. They expose, but they expose in the

public interest, which they define. Their efforts, if successful, alert us to failures in the system and lead to politicians, lawyers and policemen taking action, even as they fulminate, action that may result in legislation or regulation. (2000: 23.)

Simon Jenkins, columnist for *The Times*, makes the same point, but a little more pithily than De Burgh, when he suggests that, for more than 200 years, the investigative journalist's imperative has been, 'find out what the bastards are up to and tell the world!' (Sanders 2003: 8). In this formulation one is immediately struck by the unproblematic notion of truth that apparently fires the investigative journalists' imaginations. For them the truth is a taken-for-granted fact that is unquestionably out there: the journalist's essential task under this description is one of finding truth and simply revealing it.

We sociologists, on the other hand, in a post-postmodern moment, are so hung up on the philosophical questions of what is truth and who can legitimately seek it, that we are sometimes reluctant to take to the field in the first place. The central tenet of positivism and the driving force for the development of most sociology in the twentieth century, that explanation and theorization should be based on inductive and empirically grounded reasoning, has become increasingly questioned. Some important critiques of positivism privilege a standpoint epistemology which holds that only those who embody and live through the identities and experiences under scrutiny can have sufficient empathetic understanding to construct adequate interpretations. Such a view can, for instance, be found in the writings of Wacquant: 'that women's subjugation puts them in a privileged position to produce true knowledge' of women's subjugation (1993: 497). Logically, therefore, only women can study and interpret women: and presumably men men; blacks blacks; native Americans native Americans; football hooligans football hooligans and so on. To adopt such a position takes away the overviewing and interpretative role of the sociologist. It makes of sociological work a series of generated accounts in which, say, experiential narratives are not necessarily related to any transcending social structural and cultural contexts.

Observing this trend, the sociologist Steven Ward has argued that realist (positivistic) epistemology has become unfashionable in much of contemporary sociology, some of which views the concept of positive science as itself ideologically constructed:

This attack (on realist epistemology) has been instigated, at least in part, by a loose confederation of deconstructionists, feminist theorists, science studies practitioners and cultural studies theorists. These theorists, who are often grouped under the convenient label of postmodernists, question the possibility of ever grounding scientific knowledge in any firm absolutes.... They reject the notion that scientific truth can ever transcend the local semantic practices, power dynamics, social hierarchies or cultural forms which shape it. Truth, therefore, is not a result of the unearthing and reporting of the already there, but always and forever a product of rhetoric, power and persuasion. (1997: 773.)

Ward refers to the relativist position in the theory of method as 'standpoint epistemology' whereby, 'all knowledge is localised perspective and all interpretations are mediated by and can be reduced to the linguistic or social characteristics of the groups which produce them' (Ward 1997: 774). He goes on to reveal the ontological weaknesses in the standpoint position, emphasizing that it encourages cultural relativism and results in the anarchy of opinion rather than the cultivation of shared understanding. Positivistic sociology, in this scenario, is displaced by something resembling an entirely theoretical sociology of knowledge wherein theoretical reasoning and positioning take precedent over the observation and interpretation of everyday life (Bridges 2002). Ward concludes his attack on postmodernist and culturally relativistic thinking by attempting to stake out a middle ground between standpoint epistemology and scientific realism. He calls for an 'associational epistemology': a theory of method based on the moral commitment of a community of scholars objectively, rigorously and systematically to seek out shared truths (Ward 1997: 83–5).

It has been argued elsewhere that Ward's case is both overstated and oversimplified (Sugden and Tomlinson 2002). By grouping together under the heading of 'standpoint epistemology' a wide and diverse body of scholarship, particularly in feminist and postcolonial theory, he fails to notice that it is not so much the standpoint of the researcher that is important, but what she or he says about this in relation to the observations and interpretations made and theories constructed. Gouldner has a radically different use for the notion of standpoint-based social research. In his hands, one meaning of sociological objectivity is the ability of the sociologist to

> take the standpoint of someone outside of those most immediately engaged in a specific conflict, or outside of the group being investigated . . .. It is only when we have a standpoint somewhat different from the participants' that it becomes possible to do justice to their standpoints. (Gouldner 1973: 56–7.)

For Gouldner such a position is absolutely essential for any empirical work that aims to avoid the pitfalls of cultural relativism. It is possible to research and theorize power relations in ways that are honest about the perspective that frames the gaze of the researcher, while at the same time, through self-reflection and dialogue with existing theory and research, contributing to the accumulation of 'associational' sociological knowledge. Belinda Wheaton's account of her experiences being a woman researching a male-dominated windsurfing subculture provides an excellent example of how to achieve this through interrogating the insider–outsider relationship (Wheaton 2002).

By singling out a narrowly defined positive-realism as the only standpoint from which to embark on research Ward could also leave himself open to the charge of academic elitism. Yes, sociologists should talk to one another in a shared language that is also accessible to a wider audience, but the development of this code of communication is a democratic project. In other words it cannot be a white, middle class, western and male-dominated code, but one that is inclusive across all social categories (race, class, gender, religion and so forth). Ward is right to suggest, however, that neither can it simply be a melting pot or battlefield of ideologies and local perspectives. On the contrary, the code of communication becomes the metalanguage, a kind of exchange rate system, through which interpretations of and debates about distinctive spheres of social life are conducted on common ground. Without such a language, relativism prevails and the 'disenchantment of the world' cannot be achieved. Sociologists should not be against the empowerment of the marginalized and oppressed through the authentic reporting of local perspectives. If local voices are to make a contribution to shared understanding, however, such perspectives must themselves be re-evaluated through a metalanguage of social science. The task is always to relate different accounts to each other, and to construct the bigger picture.

There will always be problems with any epistemological position that privileges the assumed authenticity of any single voice. Objective critique and healthy scepticism are necessary for the defence of an associational realism upon which any metalanguage of the critical social science community must surely be based. Willis, for instance, in his seminal ethnographic work, *Learning to Labour* (1977), never left the voices of his subjects to speak merely for themselves. His ethnography of 'the lads' is mediated by his interpretative conceptualizing, and then separately and densely theorized in the metalanguage of social science. By doing so Willis avoids falling into any reductionist relativism or romantic celebration of the voices of the less powerful.

Investigative sociologists, then, should have a commitment to the objective, rigorous and systematic quest for a socially constructed truth. This, however, can never be the absolute truth that Ward seems to be talking about or the uncritical notion of truth which works for journalists. Rather it is a sociological truth. Clegg argues that, whereas the former asks what is truth (a question that Foucault believed unanswerable), sociological truth is 'what passes for truth' (Clegg 2000: 141), in other words what people believe to be true in the context of the social worlds within which they abide. Given this formulation, and given that there are multiple vantage points, there are multiple truths. Getting at, and spelling out, such multiple truths and, detached from any particular standpoint among them, constructing a model of the social whole, is what sociological research and scholarship should be about. Thus, in the context of particular social hierarchies and networks of power, it is the task of the researcher to identify, gain access to, and share as many vantage points as possible. On this basis it is possible to construct an overall interpretation that may not be true to any single vantage point, but which, by taking account of them all including that of the researcher, is the most honest representation of a given milieu's shared truth about itself at a given point in history. It is also the most balanced way to build towards appropriate interpretation and theorization. This approach can be explained through an artistic metaphor:

To clarify this, think of the difference between a photograph and an impressionist painter's canvas. The photograph captures a moment of reality (or truth) that is immediately transient, and dependent on prevailing and instantly passing conditions of light, shade, expression and so forth. And remember, just like respondents in interviews, the camera can lie. The impressionist painting, on the other hand, is constructed over time and incorporates the various dimensions of the artist's gaze and what is known about the places and people that are painted. It also leaves room for interpretation by those who view the work in the gallery. Thus, what is produced is not reality *per se*, but an informed *impression* of that reality. The artist then offers the painting for public appraisal, acclaim or ridicule, implicitly challenging other artists to depict the chosen scene differently. In this way we regard ourselves as rigorous social scientists and as *social impressionists* (Sugden and Tomlinson 2002: 18).

McDonald makes a further and useful distinction between radical and moralistic epistemological positions. According to him 'moralistic social research collapses the boundaries between research and activism' (2002: 114). People working in this way not only privilege the voices of the oppressed but manipulate those voices to serve their own activist agendas. 'Little attention is paid to the conventions of sound scholarly habits, which are dismissed anyway as elitist and bogus, as the aim of research is to support the attainment of immediate political goals' (ibid.). The radical approach, on the other hand, with its explicit political agenda, incorporates this as one perspective amongst many and accounts for it as part of a multilayered process of getting at the sociological truth.

Underpinning this approach is a view that there is no special virtue in those that lack power and authority, and more than in those who possess them. In particular, there is no reason to believe that the perspective of those placed at the bottom of society is more likely to be true than those at the top (McDonald 2002: 109).

Taking a leaf out of Dunning's (and he after Elias's) book (Dunning 1999: 215), McDonald argues that we can be permissive with regard to politic matters set out in the sociological agenda and be encouraging of others (and ourselves as activists if necessary) to use the yield of sociological enquiry to promote equitable social change. We should not, however, allow this to influence the methods through which we gather and present the evidence and argument.

## The investigative imperative

How does one get at sociological truth if those who embody it do not want to give it up? Observing a swan swimming gracefully across a placid lake tells us little about the energy and turbulence generated by the bird's powerful legs and wide webbed feet below the surface. Social life is like this. What is visible at street level is only ever a part of the story. Investigative sociology is an important methodological tradition because passive forms of ethnography – that is, fieldwork in which the researcher's role is dictated and constrained by the flow of events presented to him or her as 'natural' – rarely allows for the full story to be told.

In the 1960s and 1970s, Jack Douglas, a sociologist at the University of California, retrieved this tradition, arguing that any valid critique of what is really going on must go beyond passive observation and embrace the investigative. His investigative mission combined a quest for truth with the recognition that observation is essential: 'Direct observation of things in their natural state (uncontrolled) is the primary basis of all truth ... this bedrock facticity of concrete experience and observation pervades our everyday lives' (Douglas 1976: 12). To get at the truth, direct observation, for Douglas, necessarily goes beyond gazing at the surface. His research strategy is based upon the assumption that everyday social life has a tendency to be duplicitous: that individuals and groups construct and present images of who they are and what they do that can mask underpinning social realities:

> The investigative paradigm is based upon the assumption that profound conflicts of interest, values, feelings and actions pervade social life. It is taken for granted that many of the people one deals with, perhaps all people to some extent, have good reason to hide from others what they are doing and even lie to them. Instead of trusting people and expecting trust in return, one suspects others and expects others to suspect him. Conflict is the reality of life; suspicion is the guiding principle. (Ibid.: 55.)

Douglas's view of the nature of social life is framed by his experience of researching relatively microscopic (albeit 'deviant') subcultures. His basic principles, however, can be taken to apply to all walks of life. He does not believe that all people are fraudulent all of the time, but he does maintain that even the most trivial areas of social interaction can be distorted through combinations of misinformation; evasions; outright lies; and stage management or 'front' as Goffman (1969) would have put it. Douglas argues that social research must account for this and advocates mixed methodologies that are simultaneously 'co-operative and investigative' (1976: 56) – that is, methodologies that take note of self-generated and freely given legends, but that also subject such 'official histories' to scrutiny from a multitude of vantage points.

## Investigative sociology and the fourth estate

Investigative sociology is not a new sub-discipline. It has for some years lain dormant within the social scientist's methodological repertoire. Classic sub-cultural studies by Robert Park and his contemporaries in the Chicago School in the 1920s and 1930s were in part dependent upon the methods of investigative and 'muck-raking' journalism, a tradition that can be traced back to Charles

Dickens and beyond (De Burgh 2000). This overtly politicized sociological cum journalistic tradition made an important contribution to the democratic process in the early twentieth-century United States, in particular in the legendary figure of Lincoln Steffens (Kaplan 1975).

Investigative journalists schooled in this tradition tend to view themselves, then, as keepers of the public conscience. Matthew Kieran has argued that

> journalism can usefully be characterised, in part, as an official Fourth Estate which has the function of pursuing and covering stories that concern the political legal or social interests of the public as citizens . . ... The basic Lockean thought is that citizens must be made aware of the nature, workings, and character of those in government so they are in a position to exercise their will as citizens and judge those to whom power is entrusted on their behalf. (2000: 156.)

In its role as a 'Fourth Estate', according to Curran and Seaton,

> the press scrutinises the actions of the executive (government), and relays public opinion to the law makers. The press also keeps people informed about what is happening in the world, and provides a forum of public debate. It thus lubricates the workings of democracy by facilitating the formation of public opinion. (2003: 346.)

In this vein, *The Washington Post*'s Watergate investigations that brought about the downfall of US President Nixon in the 1970s is clear example of this kind of work (Woodward and Bernstein 1981).

The aim to penetrate, interpret and, where relevant, make transparent the inner workings of public and private corporate organizations is too important a task to be left to journalists alone. Today global media are dominated by fewer and fewer self-interested and self-censoring conglomerates (Said 1993). According to John Pilger, investigative journalists are a threatened species. They are being crowded out, to be replaced by

> a new kind of 'multiskilled' journalist, who is not multiskilled at all, but a sad Protean figure required to work for a range of very different publications in the group but be loyal to none. There is no time to investigate (1999: 535).

The freedom of the press is likewise under threat as ideology and spin replace factual news and critical analysis. The more that the independence of the press and its role as the Fourth Estate is threatened, the more important it is that sociologists, at least occasionally, leave the relative sanctuary of the academy and reinvigorate the investigative tradition. Sociology has, indeed, made a significant contribution to this Fourth Estate. Some of my own work, particularly that with Alan Tomlinson, on power, politics and corruption within the governing body of world football, FIFA, for instance, is justified and driven by such Lockean principles:

> This book is not an epitaph for the people's game. We have written it because we believe that information is power. Pointing out who is doing what to your game, we believe that we can make a valuable contribution to the growing resistance and reaction against the total commodification of football. (Sugden and Tomlinson 1999: 8.)

## Themes and audiences

Unlike investigative sociologists, however, investigative journalists do not usually target the ordinary in everyday life. Sociologists' interests may include high-level corporate malpractice, but they also may embrace much less spectacular, but nonetheless interesting, spheres of social life. For instance, the social construction of status, identity and meaning among groups of volunteer charity workers may hold some fascination for certain sociologists and may lend itself to an investigative approach, but it is unlikely to fire the imagination of an investigative reporter because outside a relatively small, specialist, professional audience such questions seem trivial. Neither are investigative journalists so much concerned with the broader concerns of social structure and social process that frame and help to account for the kind of corruption and injustice that they choose to expose. In other words their commentaries lack any theoretical gravity. They are committed to getting below the surface of social and political life, but only just, and not to the extent that they are impelled to make more fundamental and connected interpretations and theorizations.

It would be a brave (and soon to be unemployed) newspaper reporter of even the most respected and highbrow broadsheet that attempted to invoke Bourdieu and Foucault in their feature on power and corruption in local government. In this context, in some of my own work I have felt the wrath of sceptical editors and publishers. I once submitted a book proposal to a publisher in the popular market. The idea for a book on football and the underground economy was warmly embraced apart from the last chapter in which I proposed to flesh out first-level narratives, characterizations and interpretations with broader theoretical issues and social–structural connections. The publisher in question agreed to publish the book (Sugden 2002), and even offered me a modest advance, provided that I omitted the final chapter. Of course, this has as much to do with target audiences and sales volume as it does with the substance of enquiry and mode of analysis. Usually, therefore, sociologists and journalists can be distinguished by what they write about, how they write, and for whom they write. Nevertheless, there is little point of aspiring to make a contribution to framing public opinion if the public cannot understand what is being written. If from time to time a sociologist (like me) becomes committed to delivering aspects of his work to a bigger and by definition popular audience, this raises another series of important issues and problems.

## The glass bead game

There is, in my view, a regrettable distinction between journalists and sociologists: the former are usually much better communicators. Journalists write for the general public, whereas sociologists usually write for more specialist and sociologically sensitized audiences. The latter, however, can have no excuse for the amount of impenetrable jargon that characterizes some contemporary sociology and even more in the genre of post-1980s cultural studies. It would be rude to name names, but go to any university library and try to pick one's way through volumes in the tradition of, for instance, the Frankfurt School and certain relatives from neo-Marxism, structuralism, post-structuralism, post-post-structuralism and beyond and the reader will soon understand what I mean. If sociologists are to make a contribution to the preservation and development of democracy they need to find voices that can be heard and understood.

For some, sociology has developed into a kind of *glass bead game*, whereby primacy is given to the apparent demonstration of general theoretical sophistication over the empirical analysis of social phenomena. The glass bead game is the fictional creation of German novelist and philosopher, Herman Hesse, who describes it thus:

> The only way to learn the rules of this Game of games is to take the usual prescribed course, which requires many years, and none of the initiates could ever possibly have any interest in making those rules easier to learn. These rules, the sign language and grammar of the Game, constitute a kind of highly developed secret language (1970: 18).

As Orwell argued vigorously, assumed technical sophistication is no excuse for bad English (1994). Orwell's tirade was directed towards political commentaries of his day. Surely, however, of all the academic disciplines, with the possible exception of English itself, sociology – the study of society – should be the most accessible of subjects. That it is not is nothing short of shameful. This view was endorsed by C. Wright Mills, who, in a searing critique of his fellow academics, said:

> To overcome academic prose, you must first overcome academic pose . . .. To be called a 'mere journalist' makes him feel undignified and shallow. It is this situation, I think, that is often at the bottom of the elaborate vocabulary and involved manner of speaking and writing . . ... It may be that it is the result of an academic closing of ranks on the part of the mediocre, who understandably wish to exclude those who win the attention of intelligent people, intelligent or otherwise (1970: 240).

As Mills demonstrates amply through his own research and writing, there is no good reason why the possession of a sociological imagination and the capacity to write clearly and succinctly should be mutually exclusive talents.

By comparison, journalism itself is by no means all virtue. On the contrary, driven by headline-hungry editors, journalists, unlike sociologists, can become overdependent upon sensationalist exposé and juicy stories. The danger here is that, too often, the journalist is tempted to use sources that are either too narrowly focused and/or require degrees of anonymity that make verification impossible. It may also encourage a resort to tactics that are not normally associated with the sociologists' method. This would include such things as 'cheque book journalism', 'faction' (dramatic reconstruction of events that are alleged to have taken place), 'stings' (entrapment operations) and a wide range of techniques based on deception. At worst it can lead journalists to fabrication – captured elegantly in the phrase that one should never let the truth get in the way of a good story.

Verification and reliability are much more important principles for sociologists who are required to present in full the context that lies behind the headlines. We must demonstrate in detail how we gather our data, and who our sources were in order that those who come after us can replicate our studies or at least test our findings and interpretations. Necessarily, however, this must go beyond a reliance on official sources and self-generated biographies/hagiographies and glossy institutional histories: sources that are notoriously unreliable. In order to cover all of the angles sometimes it is necessary to resort to or at least take advantage of forms of deception. I must confess that more than once while on the FIFA and football black market trails I have pretended to be other than I am in order to get inside and/or to get insider information. I have also used the yield of a newspaper 'sting' to inform my work on football's black economy.

## Ethical issues for sociologists and journalists

This raises another important set of issues that requires some thought and discussion. What, if anything, are, or should be, the differences in the ethical principles that underpin the regulation of investigative journalists' method compared with those of sociology? This is a very grey area. Sociologists, in the UK at least, are advised rather than regulated through the BSA's *Statement of Ethical Practice* (BSA 2002). This is, to say the least, an ambiguous document that has not been written with the investigative sociologist in mind. The overriding emphasis is on the protection of those studied and their empowerment in terms of the way data collected from and about them is interpreted, communicated and disseminated. Consider clause 24 which states, 'Clarification should also be given to research participants regarding the degree to which they will be consulted prior to publication. Where possible, participants should be offered feedback on findings . . .' (ibid.: 6). The spirit of this clause is hard to square with some of the underlying assumptions of investigative sociology outlined herein. If, even in relatively mundane spheres of social activity, individuals and groups hold views of themselves that are underpinned by self-interest, it is difficult to imagine how those same individuals and groups could be allowed to influence the researcher's interpretation of findings without undermining the search for sociological truth. This problem is magnified one hundred-fold when researching large official groups and organizations (like FIFA or Manchester United) that have public relations departments headed by communications directors (spin doctors), whose sole purpose is to promote squeaky-clean official histories that deflect attention from corruption and malpractice. Likewise, the veracity of investigations into so-called deviant and/ or criminal subcultures is unlikely to be enhanced by ongoing consultations with subjects with regard to the images of their worlds that we are constructing.

There is also the related issue of how a researcher is supposed to proceed in gathering insider information. Wherever possible we are advised to be candid with our research hosts about the nature of our research and our role as researchers. Usually access to a research setting is gained via a 'gatekeeper'. In these situations, the BSA reminds us, 'members should adhere to the principle of gaining informed consent directly from the research participants to whom access is required, while at the same time taking account of the gatekeepers' interest' (ibid.). This consent, we are told, should be 'regarded, not as a once and for all prior event, but as a process subject to renegotiation over time. In addition, particular care may need to be taken during periods of prolonged fieldwork where it is easy for research participants to forget that they are being studied' (ibid.).

Much of my own research experience has led me to take the opposite view. Wherever possible I have avoided fully covert work. Not only, as the BSA makes clear, is this ethically problematic, but it is also very risky, especially when working in potentially dangerous settings involving people who are suspicious of those who would study them. I have reached the conclusion that the most productive and certainly the most secure *modus operandi* for investigative sociology is to let the subject(s) know up-front, without going into too much detail, that you are a researcher. Then, as the fieldwork progresses, make it easy for them to forget by fading into the background and becoming part of the furniture. This allows for a greater sense of sociological naturalism to pervade the fieldwork.

Equally, though, I have occasionally found it useful to be less than fully honest about what my research interests are and where the product of my research will be disseminated. When embarking on our FIFA work, for instance, Alan Tomlinson and I told potential gatekeepers that we were social historians, not sociologists, the latter being regarded with some suspicion in the corporate world. The idea of academics producing a social history of some institution or other is far less threatening than the prospect of a potentially revealing and acerbic sociological analysis and critique, which our various FIFA publications tended to be.[2] In addition, in circumstances such as this, it proved useful to encourage a belief that the yield of our studies was targeted for a strictly academic clientele. Similarly, in my research into the black economy of football, my key gatekeeper assumed that the product of my fieldwork would end up gathering dust on a university library shelf. I did little to discourage that view as it helped me with ongoing insider access. That it ended up in paperback and sold thousands of copies on the high street was a very unpleasant surprise for my hosts.

One thing that investigative sociologists and journalists have in common is the resort to interpersonal treachery. In my experience, in order to gain full empathetic access to the world of the other, it is useful to develop a positive rapport with them. To achieve this it is important to find and focus upon an aspect of their character that you can at least pretend to like. Some of the subjects of my research have been pretty reprehensible, but I have almost always discovered in them something to which I can relate. By cutting out the bad and the ugly and homing in on the good the researcher can develop a line of communication through which the required information can flow more freely. This is the stock-in-trade of most 'fly-on-the-wall' television documentary makers, but it can also be a useful strategy for investigative sociologists. For both the researcher and the researched, however, this is an uncomfortable manipulation of the natural human desire for facilitation and friendship. In the end, because the subjects of investigative sociology can be exposed to public scrutiny in ways that either make them look foolish, bad, or both, such intimate research relationships can end with a deep sense of betrayal. I am absolutely certain that key gatekeepers in FIFA and in the football black market felt betrayed once they read what had been written about them and the networks of which they were guardians. According to Tomlinson, this is something that comes with the turf:

> In the messy world of social research at least, the integrity of the project should be at the forefront of the researcher's consideration. The social researcher, despite an argot of methodological reflexivity behind which moral issues might be veiled, faces the same moral issues as the investigative reporter ... to sense that the subject or respondent has been flattered and betrayed is sensitively to recognise the strengths of oral sources and use them critically. Merely to produce an oral account, or to over-anonymise it, would be a greater betrayal of the very task of interpretation. (Tomlinson 1997: 262.)

Using deceit in the service of sociology, however, requires ethical justification that goes beyond that required 'for integrity of the project'. Once more the BSA's guidelines are ambiguous. On the one hand, we are told, 'research relationships should be characterised by trust and integrity ... although sociologists, like other researchers, are committed to the advancement of knowledge, that goal does not, of itself, provide an entitlement to override the rights of others' (2002: 16). In the same code of practice sociologists are offered the following get-out clause: '[I]n some cases, where the public interest dictates otherwise and particularly where power is being abused, obligations of trust and protection may weigh less heavily. Nevertheless, these obligations should not be discarded lightly' (ibid.: 4). This is hardly a ringing endorsement of the methods of investigative sociology.

# In the public interest

Journalists, who are regulated through a variety of codes of conduct/practice, are subject to similar ethical considerations. There is some ambiguity, however, when it comes to the question of matters deemed to be in the public interest. The public interest as defined by the PCC (Press Complaints Commission) includes: 'detecting or exposing crime or serious misdemeanour; protecting public health and safety; preventing the public from being misled by some statement or action of an individual or organization' (1997: 1). Once, it seems, journalists have established that the focus of their inquiries is 'in the public interest' then, to a large extent, the end – i.e. publication and exposure – justifies the means. As Kieran puts it:

> If investigative journalists were required to be morally good they would be unable to penetrate the murky world they need to investigate and thus would be unable to do their job. It is something like this that underlies the presumption of many journalists that at a certain point ethical considerations are excluded from the sphere of investigative journalism. (Kieran 2000: 158.)

Kieran goes on to argue, however, that immoral actions used in the service of investigative journalism are only justifiable if the moral purpose for doing so is incontrovertible.

The problem remains, however, both for journalists and for sociologists, to discover some secure guidance as to precisely what constitutes 'the public interest'. Within journalism the answer to this question appears to be established through trial and error and the establishment of precedent thereafter. For instance the PCC makes the point that 'the public interest is not whatever happens to interest the public' (Sanders: 2003: 48). Thus they can rule that the use of subterfuge by *Sun* journalists to investigate 'Sex in the Suburbs' cannot be justified on the grounds of the public interest, but that the work of *Sunday Times* investigators exposing the practice of MPs accepting cash for questions can (ibid.: 48–9).

It is clearly in the public's interest to know about the results of in-depth sociological investigations into the affairs of individuals, groups and organizations in the world of sport. It is also my contention that the same flexible approach should be taken. I have argued elsewhere that 'getting one's hands dirty' does not mean that the investigator has become morally corrupt (Sugden and Tomlinson 1999). As is the case with journalism, however, such strategies should only be deployed as a last resort when they are the only way through which to establish proof of neglect, corruption and/or criminal practice that has resulted or may result in significant harm to others or the undermining of the commonwealth. Without such licence the sociologists' capacity to make meaningful contributions to social policy and social change in the world of sport is undermined.

## Concluding remarks

I have argued that the ethical context for investigative research is a very grey area that, in my experience, is a question of principle and balance that can only be worked out in practice. I have in the past, for instance, turned down the opportunity to misappropriate important documents, even though they might have shed important light on the subject of my inquiry, largely because of the consequences that might befall the person who left them unguarded. In other situations I have participated in black market activities (for no personal gain) when I judged that this would get me deeper inside the subcultural world that I was investigating without resulting in any substantial harm to others. In this case I believed that the story was worth, in public interest terms, the immorality and the risk.

It is with a brief discussion of risk that I close this chapter. If we are to follow Gidden's (1976) wisdom (somewhat ironically meted out from his armchair), researchers must 'immerse' themselves and live out the experiences where structure and agency collide. I have argued elsewhere that ethnography is inherently perilous (Sugden 1996). The risks multiply when the (under)worlds that you set out to access and share are at the margins of society and those that you research have something to hide. The level of risk can, however, be minimized. The most important thing is for the researcher to be acutely aware that, once in the field, he or she is always at risk. In order to maximize understanding, fieldworkers should be ever alert to what is going on around them.

To achieve this they need to develop sensitively tuned sociological antennae. This is required for the generation of data, but it is also essential for self-preservation. For the purpose of generating open and fluid lines of communication, the researcher should work hard to engender trust, but trust nobody. In the field one is required to make decisions about who one can be up-front with regarding the role and who not to tell; what is safe to do and who it is safe to be with.

An escape route is also necessary. One of the main reasons why I do not favour fully covert research is that it offers no protection. There may come a time when the researcher may need to invoke the protection of his or her identity through a well-placed insider. Once you have let key gatekeepers know that you are doing research this can act as an amnesty – a kind of 'get out of jail free' card – later in the investigation, should you find yourself compromised. For instance, while studying football's black economy, on different occasions, I was accused of being an undercover police officer, invited to take part in a variety of illegal scams, and threatened with arrest as 'one of them'. At such times it was valuable for me to reaffirm my researcher's role and make for the exit.

Getting under the surface-soil of social life, digging deeply into and making coherent sense of the social experience of others, and translating those findings and interpretations into a universal language for widespread consumption, are hugely challenging tasks. Taking account of the checks and balances outlined herein, to help us meet these challenges I believe we do have much to learn from the traditions and techniques of investigative journalism. Kieran's view of investigative journalism, that 'getting one's hands dirty is something that comes with the territory' (2000: 158) should not discourage sociologists from using similar approaches. Yes, it may mean occasionally getting our hands dirty, but, so long as the grime is only skin deep, the product is clean and the story is in the public interest in the first place, it is usually worth the dig. What is needed is further debate on the ethical frameworks that guide us through – rather than inhibit – this important style of fieldwork.

## Bibliography

British Sociological Association (2002) *Statement of Ethical Practice*, British Sociological Association. Available online at http://www.britsoc.org.uk/about/ethic.htm.

Clegg, S. (2000) 'Theories of power', *Theory, Culture and Society*, 17(6), 139–47.

Curran, J. and Seaton, J. (2003) *Power Without Responsibility. The Press, Broadcasting and the New Media in Britain*, 6th edn, London: Routledge.

De Burgh, H. (2000) *Investigative Journalism. Context and Practice*, London: Routledge.

Douglas, J. (1976) *Investigative Social Research: Individual and Team Field Research*, Beverly Hills: Sage.

Dunning, E. (1999) *Sport Matters. Sociological Studies of Sport, Violence and Civilization*, London: Routledge.

Gaber, I. (2003) 'Taming the daily beast', *Network*, 84, February, 2–3.

Goffman, E. (1969) *The Presentation of Self in Everyday Life*, Harmondsworth: Penguin.

Gouldner, A. (1973) *For Sociology. Renewal and Critique for Sociology Today*, London: Allen Lane.

Hesse, H. (1970) *The Glass Bead Game* (Magister Ludi), London: Cape.

Kaplan, J. (1975) *Lincoln Steffens: A Biography*, London: Jonathan Cape.

Kieran, M. (2000) 'The regulatory and ethical framework', in H. De Burgh (ed.) *Investigative Journalism. Context and Practice*, London: Routledge, 156–76.

McDonald, I. (2002) 'Critical social research and political intervention: Moralistic versus radical approaches', in J. Sugden and A. Tomlinson (eds) *Power Games. A Critical Sociology of Sport*, London: Routledge, 100–16.

Mills, C.W. (1970) *The Sociological Imagination*, Harmondsworth: Pelican.

Orwell, G. (1994) 'Politics and the English Language', in *The Penguin Essays of George Orwell*, London: Penguin, 348–59.

Pilger, J. (1999) *Hidden Agendas*, London: Vantage.

Said, E. (1993) *Culture and Imperialism*, London: Chatto and Windus.

Sanders, K. (2003) *Ethics and Journalism*, London: Sage.

Sugden, J. (1996) *Boxing and Society. An International Analysis*, Manchester: Manchester University Press.

Sugden, J. (2002) *Scum Airways. Inside Football's Underground Economy*, London: Mainstream.

Sugden, J. and Tomlinson, A. (1998) *FIFA and the Contest for World Football. Who Rules the People's Game?* London: Polity.

Sugden, J. and Tomlinson, A. (1999) *Great Balls of Fire. How Big Money is Hi-Jacking World Football*, London: Mainstream.

Sugden, J. and Tomlinson, A. (2002) 'Critical sociology of sport: theory and method', in J. Sugden and A. Tomlinson (eds) *Power Games. A Critical Sociology of Sport*, London: Routledge, 3–21.

Sugden, J. and Tomlinson, A. (2003) *Badfellas. FIFA Family at War*, London: Mainstream.

Tomlinson, A. (1997) 'Flattery and betrayal: observations on qualitative and oral sources', in A. Tomlinson and S. Fleming (eds) *Ethics, Sport and Leisure*, Aachen: Meyer and Meyer, 223–44.

Wacquant, L. (1993) 'Positivism', in W. Outhwaite and T. Bottomore (eds) *The Blackwell Dictionary of Twentieth Century Social Thought*, Oxford: Blackwell.

Ward, S. (1997) 'Being objective about objectivity: the ironies of standpoint epistemological critiques of science', *Sociology* 31(4), 773–91.

Willis, P. (1977) *Learning to Labour. How Working Class Kids Get Working Class Jobs*, Farnborough: Saxon House.

Woodward, B. and Bernstein, C. (1981) *All The President's Men*, London: Hodder and Stoughton.

## Notes

1   Some of the material in this chapter builds upon work with Alan Tomlinson previously published by us in *Power Games: A Critical Sociology of Sport* (2002).
2   At the time of writing, the author and co-writer of the FIFA corpus were the subject of litigation initiated in Swiss courts by FIFA and its President Joseph 'Sepp' Blatter.

# 12 Is research with and on students ethically defensible?

*Roger Homan*

## Preamble

The author of this chapter is an offender and a moralizer.

He is an offender because he conducted and published field work in which he deceived the subjects he observed into thinking he shared their religious beliefs and affiliation. His doctoral thesis (Homan 1979) was a study of pentecostal behaviour conducted in over 80 assemblies in England and Wales, Canada and the United States. Most of these were visited only once or twice; in some cases the research role was explicit, consent was obtained from a gatekeeper and he wielded the standard apparatus of an observer in the field, the clipboard. In other cases, especially where such devices might have been intrusive or reactive, observation was covert. In one case, an assembly was visited and observed two or three times a week over a period of 15 months without the research interest being declared. When this was first reported in the *Sociological Review* (Homan 1978) fellow sociologists were outraged. One of them asked, 'How are the next legitimate researchers into Pentecostalism going to be received when the deceit of one of their colleagues becomes known?' (Dingwall 1979: 7).

The author's view of covertness (Homan 1980) is a position that he continues to defend (Homan 1992a: 113–19; Homan forthcoming). It is recognized to be unethical but, he has maintained, it has been in many ways the more moral. For example, an overt investigator may commence an interview by reminding the respondent that participation is voluntary and then go on so to sequence questions and develop rapport as to break down the defences of the interviewee. Again, they may ask interviewees to report transactions with third parties whose consent was not sought but who become the effective subjects of the research. A covert observer may well have a more genuine regard for the privacy and dignity of participants. It is therefore possible that those who in certain respects contravene the ethical codes honour the higher moral principles which they are designed to safeguard. So in his writings on research ethics the author of this chapter has claimed to occupy the moral high ground and assign 'ethics' – as distinct from 'morality' – to the low ground (Homan 1992a: 119–26, 178–83; 1992b).

Thus he is a moralizer. He dares now to suggest virtues and vices in the treatment of human participants, their entitlements and the moral obligations of researchers.

It may be thought that one who has flouted the rules of his own profession has no authority to proclaim the rights and wrongs of professional and moral practice. Not so. The codes and guidelines are frequently incompatible with the principles that underlie them; a fundamentalist adherence to them will sometimes disfavour the research subjects. The reverse is equally true: taking a moral stance may involve transcending codified habits. As the apostle Paul warned, the letter killeth but the spirit giveth life (2 Corinthians 3. 6).

The approach which is adopted in this chapter and in other writings by its author (Homan 1992a, 1992b; forthcoming) is therefore to identify moral obligations that are over and above what the codes prescribe. We recognize a moral position in the established professional guidelines, not by looking at them but by looking through them.

The pentecostals observed in prayer meetings had a right to know that they were participating in a research act. They were also entitled not to be interrupted in their worship or rendered self-conscious. In collaboration with the pastor of a neighbouring congregation it was decided that their prayer behaviour would have been devalued had they known they were being observed. Again, they were entitled to some kind of protection. The subjects of open research have the opportunity to control what data are collected from them; as the consent of pentecostal subjects was not sought, the investigator felt a duty of protection on their behalf. Private or potentially embarrassing data were not reported. This procedure is arguably more moral than the practice of open researchers who secure consent at the outset and then use skills to break down the defences of subjects and invade their private domains (Homan 1992b). The power relationship of a skilled investigator and a naïve or partially informed respondent belies the morality of securing initial consent: the interviewer is more competent to invade privacy than the respondent to defend it. Further, it may be that a researcher wanting to be noticed by fellow professionals has more to gain than an anonymous interviewee has to lose.

This chapter, however, is not about how social researchers deceive their subjects but, in a sense, about how they deceive themselves. It is an invitation to approach research in a particular way, not by starting with the formal rules and seeking how to apply them but identifying the principles or moral values that we might want to honour – things like respect for others and respect for truth. The focus of this chapter is upon one or two instances in which the letter of the law may contradict its spirit.

## Codes and other controls

In order to protect the human subjects of research and to respect their interests, to maintain as good a reputation as possible for the research community and – let us face it – to minimize the prospect of litigation, several kinds of safeguard are in operation in universities.

First, we may rely on the good judgement of the practitioner. Those involved in research will not want to deploy methods that cause their subjects discomfort or distress or inflict pain. For example, they would not want to stick pins in their subjects gratuitously. Second, we may trust the wisdom and discretion of experienced supervisors and mentors who will foresee and forestall the worst effects of clinical experiments. They have, after all, accumulated knowledge and understanding, and will design and advise tests accordingly.

It is, however, naïve to trust in either of these safeguards. The infamous work of Stanley Milgram (1974) has demonstrated the willingness of a research supervisor to direct experiments that cause apparently excruciating pain in the laboratory setting and certain distress in the longer term, as well as the passive willingness of assistants to conduct and persist with these. Milgram's assistants were prepared to inflict severe electric shocks on other participants and he has been held responsible for the adverse after-effects in their emotional lives.

Milgram's study received critical attention outside the research profession from, for example, the playwright Dannie Abse (1973). It is one of a number of scandals that have prompted the various professional groups researching human and social behaviour to draw up codes and guidelines. There was already in the form of the Nuremberg Code of 1947 a role of principles governing medical research; this followed the involuntary freezing of internees in prison camps in order to discover the effects of frostbite. The principle of informed consent is the mechanism by which it is ensured that a procedure be voluntary on the part of any competent patient who should be aware of its purpose, risks and consequences. The Nuremberg Code was emphatically concerned with human dignity:

> The voluntary consent of the human subject is absolutely essential. This means that the person involved should have legal capacity to give consent, should be so situated as to be able to exercise free power of choice without the intervention of any element of force, fraud, deceit, duress, over-reaching or any other form of constraint or coercion; and should have sufficient knowledge and comprehension of the elements of the subject matter involved as to enable him to make an understanding and enlightened decision (reprinted in Reynolds 1982: 143).

The content of codes in social research varies according to the discipline of the professional group. For example, the Code of Conduct of the British Association of Sport and Exercise Sciences (BASES) stresses aspects of safety, whereas the British Sociological Association's Statement dwells more upon issues of consent, subjects' rights, publication and sponsor control.

The code of conduct of the British Association of Sport and Exercise Sciences (n.d.) rests on a foundation of three moral principles, the first of which draws particularly heavily on the Nuremberg Code:

> All clients have the right to expect the highest standards of professionalism, consideration and respect.
>
> The pursuit of scientific knowledge requires that research and testing is [sic] carried out in a safe and ethical manner.

The law requires that working practices are safe and that the welfare of the client is paramount.

BASES is constituted of four sections – Biomechanics, Physiology, Psychology and the Open Section. Its code offers an indicative list of the procedures likely to be undertaken by members including the administration of ergogenic aids, the employment of biopsy or venipuncture, the imposition of unusual or severe physical or psychological stress, the taking of capillary blood and the involvement of children and persons with disabilities. Ethical clearance for these procedures calls for specialist knowledge by the committee and an assessment of the skills of the investigator. The issue of competence, both to use equipment and to analyse and report results, is a peculiar and important feature of the BASES code.

The BASES code is comprehensive in respect of other ethical principles such as informed consent, confidentiality, data protection and disciplinary procedures for members who fall short of the standards of their profession. Some details, though held in common with other professional codes, are worth highlighting at this stage as they will be challenged later in this chapter:

> Informed consent is the knowing consent of a client ... who is in a position to exercise free power or choice without any undue inducement ...
>
> It is of paramount importance that all BASES members must preserve the confidentiality of the information acquired in their work
>
> Members should seek to maximise the accessibility of research findings and, where possible, to publish them ...
>
> Publication of data must not disclose the identity of any individual ... (sections 4a–4d).

Though at times feeble as means of control, professional and institutional codes and guidelines have the potential of providing a useful basis of ethical education. Even if their prescriptions are crude, their agenda is a good starting-point. Too often they purport to provide answers by way of cut-and-dried taboos, whereas books like this raise the questions in all their complexity.

In recent years the 'ethical screening' of research at the proposal stage has become standard in British universities. This development follows the practice of Institutional Review Boards (IRBs) in North America and the local and multicentre research ethics committees (LRECs and MRECs) operated within the National Health Service in Britain. Each university has a research ethics committee to which students are advised to submit forms or 'protocols' detailing the nature of research and the information given to participants, together with a copy of the consent form and details of funding and of any identified hazards. Inevitably, some disciplines are more sensitive of the need for peer review and screening than others. For those working in medicine and health, ethical screening is now mandatory but elsewhere the urgency of screening has yet to be appreciated. One of the conclusions submitted below is that ethics committees serve an important protective function, not only for participants but also for those conducting research. Ethical issues are so complex that individual students and their supervisors cannot always be expected to recognize them or address them adequately.

## Case studies

What follows is a series of four fictional but typical case studies that reflect the kinds of research undertaken at a range of levels. Each raises different issues that are then discussed. The basic facts of each case are set out as a preface to the respective discussion: it is suggested that some readers may wish to use the narratives for teaching purposes and to conduct their own discussion, as though acting in the role of an ethics committee.

### Case Study One: Eating, drinking and sleeping

Dr Early had a bright idea for a longitudinal research project. He wanted to look at the effects of alcohol, smoking, hours of sleep and certain diets on the improvement of physical performance. He teaches undergraduates and therefore had a handy population in which to conduct his tests. By approaching them early in their first year he was able to track them over a period of almost 3 years. He knew that some would drop off the course and be lost but the expectation was that early in the course most members of a cohort would be willing to take part and would not subsequently wish to withdraw from the project.

Before the end of October, Dr Early introduced the project to his first year class and most of the students were willing to take part. It involved keeping a record of units of alcohol consumed, numbers of cigarettes smoked, hours of sleep and basic descriptions of diet. This did not need to be done every day of the 3 years but in a sample of weeks which Dr Early had chosen. He had been careful to avoid intruding into the private domain of his subjects by testing some variables that might have a bearing on performance, such as the use of drugs and the frequency of sexual activity.

Each participating student nominated one or two sports and Dr Early found an indicative measure respectively. These were kept simple: for example, if a student nominated golf the measure would be the average length of five drives taken on each of four occasions in each year, always from the same tee. In other cases it was possible to exercise greater control over variables such as climate: some jumping, throwing and sprinting could be measured in a local indoor stadium.

From the first cohort, he recruited 22 students in the first year of which 15 survived the project until graduation. In accordance with the statement of good practice set out in the BASES code, students were given copies of their own data and several of them made use of these in their final year dissertations.

## Discussion of Case One

The project was more or less naturalistic: that is to say, it did not ask participants to adopt a daily behaviour that they would not otherwise have chosen. It involved measurement but not experimentation. Safety considerations were minimal. Participation was voluntary. Those conducting the investigation were interested in measurements not in persons and so anonymity was assured.

The reason for enlisting students early in their course is to maximize the period over which the study could be conducted. Coincidentally, they are less resistant to claims upon their commitments in the early stages than they are once they have a clearer view of their schedule. This is one of the reasons why there are so many invitations to sign up for student societies during freshers' week. Concern over competence to give consent is the subject of great debate in the medical world and in a milder way it applies to those who are disoriented by transitions in their lives. Researchers who are always intent upon securing a high rate of response are apt to choose their moments on the basis of strategic rather than ethical considerations. The extent of information given to subjects and the rate of their response often vary inversely; Dr Early, it may be thought, was strategically approaching his subjects before they were realistically informed or aware.

It is well established that information given at the outset of a project should include all foreseeable risks. However, the project did not and – because of an omission in planning or a lack of experience – could not feature the benefits of participation, such as the accumulation of data that students could use at a later stage in connection with their dissertations. No one foresaw that some students in the year group would be advantaged in that throughout their 3 years they had one of their tutors operating as a research assistant. While the investigator may have been careful to identify any known risks to participants, he might also have signalled the cost of non-participation; his failure to do so means that students of the course who were not participants in the study reckon themselves to have been deprived of what turned out to be a beneficial element of the course.

There is a further and less tangible benefit that raises a still more serious issue. We have to consider the possibility that long-term cooperation in such a project, like being a teacher's helper at school, may predispose a tutor to a positive assessment and favourable expectations of students. They have done him a long-term favour. What is at issue is no more than the hope of participants and the suspicion of those who decline to take part that they will be reciprocally favoured or disadvantaged in assessment. In the context of what are termed 'consensual relationships' between tutors and students, there would be recognizable grounds for concern. The possibility that participation may weigh with assessors in the same way is discussed further in the commentary at the end of this chapter. If no payment is offered we are bound to ask what are the motivations of those who continue to cooperate.

A distinction is sometimes made between the technical and the ethical aspects of research as though one can be good without the other. Indeed, those who seek ethical clearance are often irritated when an ethics committee gives feedback on operational elements of method. The principle adopted by such ethics committees may be expressed thus: that which is technically flawed cannot be ethically sound. A bad research design wastes people's time and resources and may misinform policy-makers. This is undesirable: among other reasons, it gets research a bad name. It is therefore important to question the reliability of Dr Early's results. It is out of concern that research be well designed that, for instance, many ethics committees include a statistician in their membership. The novelty of recording diet, counting drinks and timing sleep may soon wear off in the lives of young undergraduates. Maybe the first week they will keep records meticulously but the project will soon become a burdensome chore and respondents will be likely to forget, invent and rely on fallible capacities of recall. If the results are suspect, the research and others of its kind will be discredited. It is therefore not unreasonable of research ethics committees to give attention to issues of design.

### Case Study Two: Telling the truth

Two years ago there was a vacancy for a lecturing post in the PE and Dance department of a teacher education faculty. Candida Smart had trained there only 3 years previously. She had enjoyed her short time teaching in schools but was an ambitious person and decided to apply. One of the criteria on the job specifications was that applicants should hold a postgraduate degree. However, this was given as 'desirable' rather than 'required'. The interview went well. They remembered her favourably and would be pleased to have her back in the department but were concerned that her appointment may be a lost opportunity to raise its academic profile. It was informally agreed that after a year settling in she would register for a master's degree. Such a course was available in the faculty and staff members did not have to pay fees.

In due time Candida started the course on a part-time basis. The first year was given to taught courses with short assignments. The second was given to a dissertation, in the guidance for which there was much commendation of action research. Candida was allotted a supervisor who was head of the department in which she taught. There loomed an inspection by the government agents OFSTED; this provided many opportunities to observe forms of administrative activity and there were more meetings than usual, which Candida would naturally attend. The inspectors would visit students on practice in schools and Candida's supervisor had the idea that she could monitor the briefing and special support given to these students by the university tutors.

As a piece of action research the assignment worked well. Candida was able to identify a number of ways in which the partnership between the university and PE departments in schools could be improved. A number of those acting as mentors had not received formal training; some of them had a friendly relationship with university tutors because they had played team games together. Candida suggested that this was not necessarily a good starting-point for a professional relationship in which they needed sometimes to draw attention to inadequacies in the schools' provisions. Though heavily committed to the OFSTED inspection, Candida's supervisor was able to spare her time for regular tutorials; they both felt that she was collecting rich and valuable data. When it came to writing up the dissertation, her supervisor was particularly helpful in identifying conclusions and recommendations that were 'constructive'.

### Discussion of Case Two

From a purely pragmatic point of view this kind of arrangement has considerable benefits. Two or more birds are killed with one stone. The head of department maintains his focus upon his responsibilities in respect of the OFSTED visitation even when he turns to his role as supervisor. Perhaps Candida's research provides him with a fuller picture of what is going on than he could otherwise achieve: in effect, he gets regular briefings without cost to his department. And at the end of the day Candida gets a master's degree and the academic profile of the department is improved.

A university board, however, might be concerned with a number of issues that Candida would be advised to consider.

There are problems arising from the fact that her supervisor is the head of those whom she will observe or interview. So-called 'raw' data are often seen by supervisors when they advise on options for analysis. But Candida's supervisor will not have an impartial interest in data that reflect upon the efficiency of his colleagues or their views about the management of his department. If Candida keeps her data to herself she may lose some of the benefit of her supervisor's guidance: but if he sees them, she may be betraying the implicit trust of her respondents.

Candida's relationships in her workplace are in jeopardy. Insider research has the potential of estranging its practitioners from their colleagues. Researchers come to possess a great deal of local information that they will not reveal or discuss; this can be disconcerting and alienating. Because Candida reports to the head of department in her role as a tutor, there is also the possibility that she will be suspected of betraying those she has engaged as research subjects; she may find that colleagues are reluctant to speak off the record or sit next to her at the staff party.

The relationship of student and supervisor in this case may affect the quality of data collected. Participants would be wise to be circumspect. The expectation is that Candida will be less cautious with her supervisor than they will be with her.

The possibility of inhibition affects not only the reliability of the findings that Candida reaches and hence the quality of her dissertation, but also the usefulness of such meetings as she attends. Reactivity is normally defined in terms of the effect that a researcher's role or style may have upon the nature of responses; in this case, there is a conflict of role on the part of the supervisor that is likely to inhibit the supply of data. The relationship of power lends an unusual dimension to the meaning of reactivity.

Candida must ask how candid she will be when it comes to writing up. Certain conclusions may be unpalatable to the one who has supervised and will mark the dissertation. If, for example, there were a consensus among colleagues in schools that the managers of the university department were aloof, inaccessible and out of touch, Candida would have to work this finding particularly carefully in order to avert a negative disposition to and low evaluation of her interpretation of data.

The supervisor's offer to help Candida formulate recommendations that are 'constructive' is very ominous. *Constructive* is a word that conveys a judgement likely to be based on self-interest and compatibility with predetermined intentions. What a manager may regard as constructive may not be helpful in terms of the intellectual development of the research. Internally supervised research that is intended to impact upon local practice ('action research') raises the problem of a vested interest in findings and thereby of the intellectual freedom of the investigator. If it is thinkable at the outset that certain conclusions will not be acceptable and/or will prejudice the student, careful consideration should be given to the integrity of the project.

It is in cases like this that research ethics committees come into their own. It may well be that all the conventional protections of subjects have been given, information has been comprehensive and an exemplary consent form has been devised. But Candida has not protected herself. Always supposing that the supervisor puts forward the proposal for ethical clearance, a good research ethics committee will pick up the prospect of estrangement and the reactive presence of the supervisor and suggest ways in which these hazards may be averted.

### Case Study Three: Buttock tone

Mark Thyme is a Ph.D. student whose master's degree was in sports physiology. His dissertation tutor had published many articles on aspects of enhancing athletic performance. When Mark was looking for ideas on what to do next he went back to his tutor who had an idea for an exciting new project on buttock tone as a factor in triple jumping. Mark registered for the degree and the project began. He used contacts in athletic clubs to recruit 25 healthy male volunteers who were active in high, long and triple jumping.

Participants were asked to keep a diary of exercise and diet over the period of a month during which they would need to attend the laboratory three times. Each of these visits was preceded by a period of controlled fasting and abstinence. Laboratory tests included short periods of vigorous exercise, the giving of blood and urine samples and the installation of a thermometer up what is technically known as the tradesmen's entrance. The opportunity was taken to test a new digital flabometer giving accurate readings on muscle–fat ratios for samples of tissue taken from each quadrant. Mark collected and analysed data from the diaries but all the surgical stuff was carried out by his supervisor. Mark and his supervisor agreed in advance that anything they were to publish would be jointly authored, their names appearing in alphabetical order.

### Discussion of Case Three

Mark, the research ethics committee, and those who have his interests at heart would want to ask a number of questions before proceeding.

One of the standards required of medical research is that any risks or discomforts are justifiable. In medicine this normally takes the form of the hope or expectation of findings that will be beneficial for all sufferers of a particular condition. Beside this standard, the justification of invasive measures on the basis that people may be able to jump further is less convincing. On the other hand, those who are taking part are themselves athletes who will in their own way want access to research findings and the latest technology: it is arguable that they have a moral obligation to support research and that to refrain from it while enjoying its benefits is effectively 'free-riding'.

There is an issue of safety. It may well be that there is an impressive and reassuring quantity of guidelines in the institution. One would want to ask whether the supervisor is properly qualified to conduct invasions, incisions and insertions. Such a project as this would need the approval of a research ethics committee. Further, heeding the recommendations that followed the controversial work of Stanley Milgram, it would not be a bad thing to seek the view of an independent expert in the field.

Participants will of course be invited to give written consent to such research on the basis of informative notes. Sometimes the full facts of risks and sacrifices deter volunteers; there is consequently a temptation to understate the commitment that participants are making. A third party who is both neutral and familiar with this type of work should be asked whether the risks involved in any way exceed the statement issued to participants.

No mention is made above of payment to volunteers. Practice varies. Some participants in drug trials may earn thousands of pounds while others are offered nothing. If participants are travelling to the laboratory from distant clubs it is assumed they would be paid expenses. If they are paid any fee, we must be sure that they do not thereby surrender rights in the event of injury or adverse after-effects. If the fee is so high, there is a risk that volunteers may take risks themselves, for example failing to notify the investigator of a condition such as haemophilia that could disqualify them from taking part.

Mark may well be satisfied that the human subjects of this project are not being exploited. He must then question his own part and his relationship with the director of his research. Supervisors have often had crazy ideas and committed their graduate or research students to dubious designs. The Rosenhan (1979) study involved students faking the symptoms of insanity and having to stay some months in mental hospitals; Festinger's students posed as emissaries of outer space and greeted a group of spiritualists who were at that time expecting the end of the world (Festinger *et al.* 1964).

In due course Mark and his supervisor publish their epoch-making paper 'Breakthrough in buttock tone'. It was agreed at the outset that their names should appear in alphabetical order. At that time Mark did not know the conventions. As the name of Mark Thyme finds its way into journals and bibliographies he finds that he is sometimes represented as '*et al.*' as though he were a forgettable assistant. It is unlikely that a supervisor with a name like Zygmund would have made such a stipulation. Unless they have surnames like Abdullah, young researchers would be wise to check the principles and study the subtle difference between *with* and *and*: in the trade these nuances signal different levels of responsibility and initiative.

## Case Study Four: Taking a gamble

*Pilot study.* In an unlikely development the women's game of bowls has attracted from other sports an underworld of international betting rings and match-fixers. Cigar smoke now drifts across the greens and the hollow percussion of woods is accompanied by a symphony of mobile phones. Newspapers in the Far East devote whole pages to form guides on which gamblers are exclusively dependent. The players themselves are incorruptible but every game at county level begins to attract a marginal following. Off the green, tipsters and bookmakers meet to do business. Once in a while, it is agreed, tipsters will get their forecasts deliberately wrong, enabling particular big-time gamblers to place bets on longer odds.

This phenomenon lends itself to qualitative research. In the first phase of his research, Jack High decides to hang around bars and other places where deals are being struck. His purpose is not to blow the whistle on a criminal element but to develop a theory of the relations between sport and gambling. He hypothesized that the commercial exploitation of an amateur sport was the first of two or three stages of its transition to professional status. He sets out to write a book on the commercialization of sport and lets it be known among those he observes that this is what he is doing.

## Discussion of Case Four

This procedure barely conforms with the letter of the codes though it does to some extent with its spirit. Consent in this case takes no literate form. Jack's description of his research interest diverts subjects from the likely focus upon them as criminals or parasites. There is no negotiation of the research act: on the other hand, they are of such a type that they can look after themselves and at the fieldwork stage – albeit not upon publication – the subjects could be considered more powerful than the researcher.

Jack's statement of his interest reflects a true sense of his purpose as a researcher. He is not a journalist. He is not seeking a sensational story – although his subsequent book may be more attractive to publishers if he finds one. He has no intention of identifying or exposing individuals. But he has to recognize and live with the fears and suspicions that are engendered by the practice of investigative journalism. Sugden and Tomlinson (1999: 390; and Sugden *loc. cit.*) clarify the distinction between the investigative forms of journalism and research. The habit of the social scientist is distinguished by 'the pursuit of objective understanding; the generation of theory; and the value of interpretation and explanation rather than mere exposé'.

*Follow-up study.* Jack then moves to the second phase of his project which is altogether more explicit. He approaches some of the acquaintances he has made and asks whether they would be prepared to take part in in-depth interviews lasting not more than one hour. He assures them of absolute confidentiality. Records of interviews will be kept under lock and key and names will be changed, not only in the published account but even as labels on tape recordings and notes. Interviews will be conducted in a private place, ideally in Jack's apartment or in the home of the respondent. All these details are set out in an information sheet given to respondents; here he explains that his purpose is not to expose the marginal world of punters and fixers but to develop a grand theory on the demise of amateurism in sport; it is made clear that participants may withdraw at any time without giving a reason. Jack will give each respondent a transcript of the interview and later a copy of the text in which it is reported and interpreted; if at any time participants are unhappy with the way their responses are represented, he undertakes to delete them.

### Discussion of follow-up to Case Four

In terms of the codes that are generally observed in research of this kind, Jack is now behaving 'ethically'. He is punctilious in informing consent, in stressing that participation is voluntary and in making arrangements to ensure anonymity. He honours participants in assigning them rights of ownership or control over their own data. In all these respects this is a highly 'ethical' approach to research.

It is, however, deeply problematic and in many ways undesirable. It highlights the issue of whether ethical practice is necessarily good research practice.

By respecting the rights of subjects to control the account he gives of them, he denies the public the right to know. Research will be discredited if its reports convey only the interpretation that principal actors want to be heard. If subjects assert the rights he gives them, he abdicates his duty to report and interpret and becomes a mouthpiece for them, giving credence to their perspective by according it the name of research. The rights that subjects have do not include entitlement to secretarial services in the recording and reporting of their thoughts and sayings. A researcher is more than a reporter and should not surrender the responsibility to interpret.

The subjects' right of veto is unwise not merely because it denies the public the right to know but also because it denies the investigator the right to issue a report. For Jack this may be 2–3 years work wasted. In related circumstances, say, for registered research students, it may mean missing a vital deadline.

The degree of anonymity he offers is neither possible nor desirable. Social researchers do not enjoy the rights of priests and doctors to withhold evidence of criminal activity that is confided in them. In Britain, 'pleading the fifth' is not an option. Moreover, the use of pseudonyms or other anonymizing devices will not be sufficient to put other investigators like journalists or police off the scent. In the end, one has to change significant contextual details, even the identity of the sport or the level at which it is played. While Jack may claim an exclusive interest in generating theory, his publisher and his readers may have more worldly interests.

It may well be that Jack can look after himself when lurking in the underworld. Lesser mortals would be ill-advised, however, to go alone once they are in possession of sensitive data or are interviewing persons of a volatile disposition. Supervisors should be aware that safety is a consideration not only for subjects but also for those working in the field.

## Commentary

In the forms of research featured in this chapter, there are already in place detailed guidelines to ensure high standards of safety and dignity. In particular the Code of Conduct of the British Association of Sport and Exercise Sciences provides a model on which departments base their own codes of practice.

We may now make a number of general observations.

In medical and social science research the principle of informed consent is axiomatic. So it is in research in the sport and exercise sciences, in physiology, psychology and in biomechanics. However, there is in these fields a greater sense of acute risk than in, say, naturalistic methods such as the observation of routine human behaviour by anthropologists, sociologists, flies on the wall and other voyeurs. The concern with safety is much more technical than the concern with consent. The assessment of risks during strenuous exercise is a science in itself: it involves screening of participants to ensure that they are fit for the experimental procedure and the control of laboratory conditions including the provision of specialist staff in the event of accident or expiry. The effect of these factors is to shift the responsibility of whether to proceed from the participant to the researcher. Whereas an interviewer may secure consent and then leave the respondent to protect his or her own interests (Homan 1992b), the laboratory supervisor has a continuing responsibility.

While students' participation in the experimental research of peers or tutors may be in the technical sense voluntary, there may be an element of moral obligation and subtle coercion. Where students will in due time need to recruit peers for their own research, the feelings of guilt suffered by those who free-ride on the willingness of others will diminish the sense in which participation is entirely free and voluntary. In respect of medical research the Helsinki Declaration counsels: 'When obtaining informed consent for the research project the physician should be particularly cautious if the subject is in a dependent relationship with the physician or may consent under duress' (World Medical Association 2000: B23).

We have to question whether students who are invited to participate in experimental research conducted by their tutors are genuinely 'in a position to exercise free power or choice without any undue inducement . . .', as properly required by the code of BASES. We may consider the possibility of two students of comparable physical and intellectual capacity and with a similar personality, both taking the same course: throughout the 3 years one of these consistently declines to take part while the other always does so. At the end of the 3 years they both apply for the same job or for a master's course; the tutor is asked to complete an employer's reference request form and to grade the students on attributes such as cooperative disposition. Even if the tutor is so utterly professional as to make a judgement independently of the experience of recruiting participants, the probability is that students will perceive participation and refusal as factors in personal assessment. It is this very perception that academic judgement may be impaired by factors outside the formal tutorial context that is the basis of concern about so-called 'consensual relationships'. The prospect of an adverse reference may be held to constitute a measure of coercion. The principle of volition is compromised by the suspicion of sanction: Brackenridge (2001: 59) has observed that in sport 'sexual harassment becomes the price for reaching elite athlete status' and so those who research sport will want to be sure that some other favour does not become the price for academic distinction or an alternative to honest work.

Those screening research in the field of sport and exercise science need to be particularly sensitive of the hazards of vested interest. Where students act as participants in their own studies or where a supervisor has expectations of the outcome of a study there may be a temptation to take risks, to persevere on the treadmill a minute or two too long, to forget that a student was drinking heavily the previous evening.

The necessity of ethical screening by committees of experts cannot be stressed too heavily. Students and supervisors who decline to submit their proposals to a research ethics committee often believe that no hazards beset their designs. Such people need the benefit of a suspicious mind or two. Though perceived as a hurdle to be cleared, the purpose of ethical screening is to pre-empt embarrassment, humiliation or legal action. Until such time as the nuances of ethical principles are understood by all who propose and pursue research with human subjects, screening by peers is an important safeguard.

## Bibliography

Abse, D. (1973) *The Dogs of Pavlov*, Valentine: Mitchell.

Brackenridge, C.H. (2001) *Spoilsports: Understanding and Preventing Sexual Exploitation in Sport*, London: Routledge.

British Association of Sport and Exercise Sciences (n.d.) *Code of Conduct*.

Dingwall, R. (1979) 'Covert observation: a question of ethics', Correspondence with Ronald Frankenberg, *Network*, 14, 7.

Festinger, L., Riecken, H.W. and Schachter, S. (1964) *When Prophecy Fails: A Social and Psychological Study of a Modern Group that Predicted the Destruction of the World*, New York: Harper and Row.

Homan, R. (1978) 'Interpersonal communication in pentecostal meetings', *Sociological Review*, 26(3), 499–518.

Homan, R. (1979) 'A sociological analysis of the language-behaviour of old-time pentecostals', Ph.D. thesis, University of Lancaster.

Homan, R. (1980) 'The ethics of covert methods', *British Journal of Sociology*, 31, 46–59.

Homan, R. (1992a) *The Ethics of Social Research*, London: Longman.

Homan, R. (1992b) 'The ethics of open methods', *British Journal of Sociology*, 43(3), 321–32.

Homan, R. (forthcoming) 'Covert research' and 'Deception', in M. Lewis-Beck, A. Bryman and T. Futing Lao (eds) *Encyclopedia of Social Science Research Methods*, Thousand Oaks, CA: Sage.

Milgram, S. (1974) *Obedience to Authority*, London: Tavistock.

Reynolds, P.D. (1982) *Ethics and Social Science Research*, Englewood Cliffs, NJ: Prentice-Hall.

Rosenhan, D. (1979) 'On being sane in insane places', *Science*, 179 (19 January), 230–8.

Sugden, J. and Tomlinson, A. (1999) 'Digging the dirt and staying clean: retrieving the investigative tradition for a critical sociology of sport', *International Review for the Sociology of Sport*, 34(4), 385–98.

World Medical Association (2000) Declaration of Helsinki: Ethical Principles for Medical Research Involving Human Subjects.

# 13  Obesity, type 2 diabetes mellitus and the metabolic syndrome: What are the choices for prevention in the twenty-first century?

*Simon Williams and Rhys Williams*

### Hypokinetic disease and the risk factor concept

Many contemporary textbooks that discuss the connection between physical activity and health often begin by delineating how the principal infectious diseases of the past, for example cholera, tuberculosis, polio and diphtheria, have been replaced as the foremost causes of premature mortality (death) by non-infectious diseases associated with lifestyle changes. The most important lifestyle changes are those that have accompanied the 'modernization' of populations – a reduction in fruit and vegetable intake, an increase in the consumption of refined, 'fast' foods that tend be high in saturated fats, sugar and salt, an increase in psychosocial stress and a reduction in physical activity. The reduction in physical activity has been attributed to changes in occupational activity, i.e. fewer manual jobs, the introduction of labour-saving devices in the household and garden, the proliferation of the motor car and the sudden and dramatic increased availability of sedentary leisure-time activities such as computer games.

Of the various hypokinetic (lack of movement) diseases, probably the most well known and extensively studied has been cardiovascular disease (CVD). Atherosclerosis, colloquially referred to as 'furring of the arteries', is the underlying pathological process that leads to the major cardiovascular diseases – coronary artery disease, cerebrovascular disease and peripheral vascular disease. The potential and ultimate end-points of each of these – myocardial infarction, stroke and lower-limb amputation respectively – are devastating for the person affected.

The relationship between physical activity and exercise (exercise can be regarded as a more structured and planned form of physical activity) with CVD risk has been studied extensively using large-scale epidemiological examinations, cross-sectional comparisons of active and sedentary subjects and also randomized and non-randomized intervention studies. Overwhelmingly, the epidemiological evidence suggests that physically active people are at lower risk of CVD (Wannamethee and Shaper 2001). Both cross-sectional and intervention studies suggest that this reduced risk is a consequence of a more favourable 'risk factor' profile existing in active people (Hardman and Stensel 2003). The term risk factor is used to describe certain physiological (e.g. blood pressure), biochemical (e.g. lipoproteins and lipids), physical (e.g. weight-for-height), psychological (e.g. stress) and demographic (e.g. socio-economic status) factors that predispose individuals to a certain disease – in this case CVD. High blood pressure (hypertension), cigarette smoking and elevated serum total and/or low-density lipoprotein (LDL) – cholesterol – are often considered to be the most important or primary risk factors because they meet several criteria that can be used to distinguish causative from non-causative associations (Fletcher *et al.* 1996). These criteria include:

- *Temporality* – the cause precedes the outcome.
- *Strength* – there is a large relative risk.
- *Dose–response* – larger exposures to the cause are associated with higher rates of the disease.
- *Reversibility* – a reduction in exposure to the cause is associated with lower rates of the disease.
- *Consistency* – the observation is made repeatedly by different researchers in different places under different circumstances and times.
- *Biological plausibility* – the association makes sense according to the biologic knowledge of the time.
- *Specificity* – one factor leads to one effect.

In addition to hypertension, cigarette smoking and elevated cholesterol there are many more CVD risk factors that have been, and are being, studied in relation to the criteria outlined above. The intention of this chapter is not to examine the strengths and weaknesses of the research with respect to the numerous CVD risk factors and whether or not they are truly causative or simply associated with CVD. Rather, we wish to turn our attention to one particular risk factor – diabetes mellitus and specifically type 2 diabetes mellitus (T2DM) as distinct from type 1 diabetes mellitus, gestational diabetes mellitus or any of the other rarer forms of this condition. A glance at the extraordinary incidence and prevalence data presented in the next section will reveal one of the reasons for choosing to discuss T2DM. It is, without question, one of the most significant and contemporary health issues. A second reason for choosing to discuss T2DM is that recent studies have shown that T2DM can be prevented by both the introduction of lifestyle changes, specifically dietary change and moderate physical activity (Eriksson and Lindgarde 1991; Pan *et al.* 1997; Tuomilehto *et al.* 2001; Swinburn *et al.* 2001; Knowler *et al.* 2002), and pharmacotherapy (Knowler *et al.* 2002; Chiasson *et al.* 2002; Azen *et al.* 1998; Torgerson *et al.* 2004; Freeman *et al.* 2001) in people who are at high risk of this disease because they have impaired glucose tolerance (IGT) and/or obesity. As health professionals, we are quick to promote these important findings to the wider population in an attempt to reduce the personal and economic burden of T2DM. Exercise professionals, dieticians and other behavioural therapists will, no doubt, powerfully advocate lifestyle intervention as the key initiative for preventing T2DM. The pharmaceutical industry has introduced several drug types for the treatment of T2DM and now also has data to support their use as a preventative measure. The 'medicalization' of people described as having pre-diabetes, i.e. people at very high risk of developing T2DM in the future and for whom pharmacological intervention has been shown to be beneficial, is clearly something that is in the interests of pharmaceutical companies.

## Obesity, type 2 diabetes mellitus and the metabolic syndrome

Overweight and obesity are conditions associated with an excessive enlargement of the body's fat mass. This increased fat mass is frequently associated with a number of morbid conditions and premature mortality (Williams *et al.* 1997). Amongst the most prevalent obesity-related non-communicable diseases are diseases of the cardiovascular system (coronary artery disease, peripheral artery disease, stroke, hypertension) and T2DM. Type 2 diabetes is itself strongly related to CVD risk (Kannel and McGee 1979; Haffner *et al.* 1998). That T2DM is a powerful predictor of CVD risk is indisputable. However, there is now accumulating evidence that the risk of CVD begins below the thresholds of fasting and post-prandial glucose whereby diabetes is diagnosed (Coutinho *et al.* 1999).

At this point, a brief and simple explanation of the physiology of T2DM and elevated fasting and post-prandial blood glucose concentrations is probably worthwhile. In the normal healthy state, the $\beta$-cells of the pancreas respond to increases in blood glucose following meals by releasing insulin. The role of insulin is to stimulate glucose uptake in insulin-sensitive tissues, thereby lowering the blood glucose concentration to its pre-meal levels. The principal insulin-sensitive tissues in this context are skeletal muscle and adipose tissue. The liver is also sensitive to the presence of insulin, but rather than stimulating glucose uptake, the function of insulin in the liver is to suppress glucose production by a process known as gluconeogenesis. T2DM is a condition characterized by insulin resistance. In other words, the skeletal muscle, adipose tissue and liver become desensitized to insulin, leading to an overall disturbance of glucose regulation. In the early stages of insulin resistance, the pancreatic $\beta$-cells respond by producing more insulin. This is referred to as compensatory hyperinsulinaemia and is often sufficient to maintain the fasting and post-prandial glucose levels within the normal range. However, in some genetically susceptible individuals, the $\beta$-cells are unable to maintain this level of compensatory hyperinsulinaemia indefinitely and there is eventual $\beta$-cell failure. When the $\beta$-cells begin to fail, the fasting and post-prandial glucose concentrations spiral upwards towards the threshold points for T2DM. Thus, $\beta$-cell failure and T2DM can be regarded as the end-points of an underlying process (insulin resistance) that may have been present for many years.

Insulin resistance is regarded as the primary defect in this whole process and is associated not just with disturbances in glucose regulation but also with disturbances in lipid and lipoprotein metabolism, blood pressure and haemodynamic function, inflammation, coagulation and fibrinolysis. As the defining feature of this cluster is thought to be insulin resistance, the term 'insulin resistance syndrome' has been used to describe the situation where they exist together. Simplified diagnostic criteria for identifying individuals with the insulin resistance or 'metabolic' syndrome have been proposed by the World Health Organization (Alberti and Zimmet 1998) and the National Cholesterol Education Program (Adult Treatment Panel III) (NIH 2001). These criteria are given in Table 13.1. The association between blood glucose and CVD below the threshold points for diabetes is, therefore, likely to be a consequence of the presence of several atherogenic factors that cluster in these individuals. Indeed, the metabolic syndrome has been shown to be a significant predictor of CVD (Lakka *et al.* 2002; Ninomiya *et al.* 2004; Kip *et al.* 2004) and end-stage renal disease (Chen *et al.* 2004).

As it is not practicable to assess body fatness in large-scale epidemiological studies, the association between obesity and premature morbidity and mortality has been established using a well-established surrogate measurement known as body mass index (BMI). BMI, calculated from measurements of body weight in kilograms divided by height squared ($kg/m^2$), is highly correlated with body fatness but is independent of height. Thus, BMI is a

*Table 13.1* National Cholesterol Education Program (NCEP) Adult Treatment Panel III (ATP III) and World Health Organization (WHO) criteria for diagnosis of the metabolic syndrome

| Metabolic syndrome components according to: | Critical value or 'cut-off' point |
| --- | --- |
| NCEP ATP III criteria[1] | |
| Waist girth | > 102 cm in men and > 88 cm in women |
| Fasting plasma glucose | > 6.1 mmol/l |
| Fasting HDL-cholesterol | < 0.9 mmol/l in men and > 1.00 mmol/l in women |
| Fasting triglycerides | > 1.7 mmol/l |
| Blood pressure | > 130 mmHg systolic and/or 90 mmHg diastolic or antihypertensive medication |
| WHO criteria[2] | |
| Central obesity | BMI > 30.0 $kg/m^2$ and/or waist-to-hip circumference ratio > 0.90 in men and > 0.85 in women |
| Blood pressure | > 140/90 mmHg |
| Fasting triglycerides and/or low HDL-cholesterol | Triglycerides > 1.70 mmol/l and/or HDL-cholesterol < 0.9 mmol/l in men and < 1.0 mmol/l in women |
| Microalbuminuria | Urinary albumin excretion rate > 20.0 $\mu$g/min or albumin:creatinine ratio > 30.0 mg/g |

[1]Metabolic syndrome diagnosis relies on the presence of at least three of the components.
[2]Metabolic syndrome diagnosis relies on the presence of IGT, insulin resistance and/or diabetes mellitus and at least two of the components.

measurement of weight-for-height that is unrelated to height. Individuals with BMI values between 25 and 29.9 kg/m$^2$ and greater than 30 kg/m$^2$ are classified as overweight or obese, respectively (Expert Panel on the Identification, Evaluation and Treatment of Overweight Adults 1998). Prospective epidemiological studies have now firmly established a positive association between BMI and CVD that is mediated through the association between obesity and several well-known CVD risk factors, particularly T2DM, hypertension and an atherogenic blood lipid profile, as outlined earlier.

The last two decades have seen a well-publicized and documented increase in obesity (Mokdad 2003; Seidell 2003). Whilst virtually no part of the world has escaped this explosive increase, modernized countries and cultures have been under the most intense scrutiny. In some of these countries, for example the United States of America, as many as 7 out of 10 adults are now classified as overweight. Of equal or perhaps greater concern is the fact that childhood obesity rates have also increased at an alarming rate (Guillaume and Rolland-Cachera 2002).

Whilst the obesity epidemic has been well publicized, less well known amongst the wider general population is the fact that obesity, particularly visceral obesity, where fat accumulates in the intra-abdominal cavity, is probably the most powerful risk factor for insulin resistance and T2DM (Colditz *et al.* 1995; Chan *et al.* 1994; Hu *et al.* 2001). Therefore, the prevalence of T2DM has also increased dramatically in recent years. It has been estimated that the global prevalence of T2DM will increase from 151 million in the year 2000, to 221 million by the year 2010 and to 300 million by 2025 (Zimmet *et al.* 2001; Amos *et al.* 1997; King *et al.* 1998). Furthermore, the prevalence of the metabolic syndrome in the USA is 13.9 per cent, 20.8 per cent and 24.3 per cent in black, Mexican American, and white men, respectively (Park *et al.* 2003). Among females, these figures are 20.9 per cent, 27.2 per cent and 22.9 per cent respectively (Park *et al.* 2003). In relation to obesity, the prevalence of the metabolic syndrome increases in a linear fashion with increases in BMI. For example, the study by Park *et al.* (2003) found prevalence rates of 4.6 per cent, 22.4 per cent and 59.6 per cent in normal-weight, overweight and obese men respectively. In women, the corresponding rates were 6.2 per cent, 28.1 per cent and 50.0 per cent.

Type 2 diabetes mellitus was once considered to be exclusively a disease of older people. However, the consequence of the increased prevalence of childhood obesity is that T2DM is now emerging at an alarming rate in children and adolescents (Fagot-Campagna and Narayan 2001). It is likely that in the next decade or so, T2DM will take over from type 1 diabetes, which is an autoimmune disease of $\beta$-cell destruction and, therefore, insulin deficiency, as the predominant form of the disease in young people. As several reports of high rates of T2DM in children have recently been published (Fagot-Campagna and Narayan 2001; Rosenbloom *et al.* 1999), an increased future incidence of diabetic complications such as CVD, renal disease, retinopathy and neuropathy, is likely.

## The case for prevention

The considerable personal health costs of obesity, T2DM and the metabolic syndrome that have been outlined are coupled with the economic cost of treating these complications. The economic cost is enormous. In developed countries, 10 per cent or more of the total health budget is expended on the management of diabetes and its complications. In the USA, diabetes cost the health care system $20.4 billion in 1987, $90 billion in 1994 and has now risen to about $132 billion (Hogan *et al.* 2002). The case for prevention of obesity, the metabolic syndrome and T2DM from both the personal and economic perspectives is, therefore, very strong. Furthermore, the United Kingdom Prospective Diabetes Study (United Kingdom Prospective Diabetes Study Group 1998) further supports the case for prevention as this landmark study showed that aggressive treatment of hyperglycaemia with pharmacotherapy (sulfonylureas and insulin) significantly reduced blood pressure and the complications of diabetes. However, blood glucose homeostasis continued to decline. Thus, the treatment successfully affected some of the complications of diabetes without halting or reversing the underlying disease process, i.e. the diabetes itself.

There are two distinct options available for the primary prevention of the metabolic syndrome and T2DM. One possibility is the introduction of pharmacological intervention for high-risk individuals. Several familial, genetic and clinical factors can be used to screen populations for such high-risk individuals. Obese individuals, particularly those with a high level of intra-abdominal fat, are one group for whom preventive strategies should be introduced. First-degree relatives of those with T2DM, individuals with hypertension and other features of the metabolic syndrome, people with impaired glucose tolerance (IGT) or impaired fasting glucose (IFG) and women with a history of gestational diabetes or polycystic ovarian syndrome are others for whom preventive measures should be introduced.

There are a number of drugs that are licensed for the pharmacological treatment of T2DM. The thiazolidinediones (TZDs) are one class of drug that offers the possibility for the prevention of T2DM as they address the underlying pathophysiology, i.e. the insulin resistance that precedes T2DM. TZDs are agonists at the peroxisome proliferator-activated receptor gamma (PPARγ). Activation of this nuclear receptor alters glucose and lipid metabolism as well as increasing insulin sensitivity (Olefsky and Saltiel 2000). Evidence to date suggests that TZDs are effective at reducing the progression to T2DM from IGT. For instance, the TRIPOD study (TRoglitazone In the Prevention of Diabetes) found a 56 per cent relative reduction in diabetes incidence in a group of high-risk women who were studied for 2.5 years (Azen *et al.* 1998). Drugs such as acarbose, which slows the absorption of glucose in the intestine, and metformin, another insulin-sensitizing agent, also present possibilities for T2DM prevention. In the STOP-NIDDM trial (the Study TO Prevent Non-Insulin Dependent Diabetes Mellitus (non-insulin dependent diabetes mellitus was the former name of T2DM)), acarbose was responsible for a significant reduction in the incidence of T2DM in comparison with a placebo (Chiasson *et al.* 2002). The pharmacological treatment of obesity is also possible with several drug types, although there is no evidence or basis for the prescription of these drugs for obesity prevention. The recent results from the XENDOS study, however, show that the gastrointestinal lipase inhibitor Orlistat, a drug that restricts dietary fat absorption, reduced the incidence of T2DM in obese individuals by 37 per cent when combined with lifestyle counselling in comparison with lifestyle counselling alone (Torgerson *et al.* 2004). The pharmacological prevention of the metabolic syndrome also has no supportive evidence thus far. Whilst intuitively the use of pharmacological agents to reduce the premature morbidity and mortality associated with the metabolic syndrome seems attractive, no trial has yet been conducted that evaluates the costs and benefits (economic and clinical) of prescribing drugs for this purpose.

## Evidence in support of lifestyle interventions

Type 2 diabetes is clearly a multidimensional disorder that is influenced strongly by environmental factors. Among the most powerful environmental influences are a sedentary lifestyle (Manson *et al.* 1992; Hu *et al.* 2001), dietary factors such as excess intake of saturated fat (Hu *et al.* 2001) and obesity (Colditz *et al.* 1995; Chan *et al.* 1994; Hu *et al.* 2001). For some time, epidemiological evidence has suggested that a more active lifestyle and a 'healthier' or 'hunter-gatherer' style diet are associated with a significantly reduced risk of T2DM. However, large-scale, purely observational studies suffer from several methodological limitations. For example, they use relatively weak measurement instruments to assess very complex behavioural attributes such as dietary intake and physical activity. Furthermore, the primary end-point, which could be death from any cause, death from a specific cause, or the presence of some disease, is evaluated against a behavioural, biochemical or physiological factor that was measured several or many years previously. Thus, no consideration can be made for the possibility that these factors may have changed in the intervening period. In more recent times, however, three randomized controlled trials (RCTs) investigating the effect of a structured lifestyle intervention on the progression from IGT to T2DM have revealed promising, consistent and highly publicized findings (Pan *et al.* 1997; Knowler *et al.* 2002; Tuomilehto *et al.* 2001). These Chinese, US and Finnish studies, known as the Da Qing IGT and Diabetes Study, the USA Diabetes Prevention Program (DPP) and the Finnish Diabetes Prevention Study (DPS) respectively, are the first RCTs to show that an intervention programme that encourages a more active lifestyle, adherence to a modified, healthy diet and promotes weight loss has clear, beneficial effects for reducing the risk of T2DM in subjects at high risk of progressing to this disease because they already demonstrate IGT. These studies indicate that a fairly dramatic change in population lifestyle would result in a substantial reduction in T2DM. Indeed, the DPP actually found that those subjects randomized to the lifestyle arm of the study experienced a greater reduction (58 per cent) in T2DM incidence than those randomized to the metformin arm (31 per cent). Coincidentally, the DPS also found a 58 per cent reduction in T2DM incidence in their lifestyle-treated subjects. These reductions compare very favourably with the reported reductions of 25 per cent in the STOP-NIDDM trial of acarbose (Chiasson *et al.* 2002) and 56 per cent reduction in the TRIPOD study of troglitazone (Azen *et al.* 1998). Thus, there appears to be strong evidence that lifestyle interventions should be the primary means of reducing the incidence of T2DM in high-risk subjects. The Da Qing study differed to the DPP and DPS as it randomized clinics to a particular intervention rather than individuals.

The findings of the DPS and the DPP raise several interesting and important questions with regard to future governmental strategies for reducing T2DM incidence. In essence, as referred to above, we now have scientific evidence demonstrating that T2DM can be prevented by changing lifestyle habits or using pharmacological agents. As yet, no study has evaluated the effect of combining these approaches so it is unclear whether or not a greater reduction in T2DM incidence is possible. Thus, in order that people can make fully informed decisions about their choices for preventing this very debilitating disease, a comprehensive discussion needs to take place between scientists (exercise professionals, dieticians, psychologists and behavioural scientists, clinicians etc.), economists, health-care administrators, policy-makers and, importantly, patient groups.

## How strong is the strong case for lifestyle intervention?

The DPS, DPP and Da Qing study have all shown that T2DM can be prevented, or at least delayed, in subjects at high risk of T2DM. However, these high-risk populations represent only a small proportion of people who are at risk of T2DM. Furthermore, the DPP and DPS were conducted in developed westernized countries. In this respect, Zimmet *et al.* (2003) have posed two important questions. First, whether these results can be replicated in other populations who are underprivileged or disenfranchised, and second, if the intervention strategies are sustainable and affordable in the context of demographic, cultural and socio-economic factors.

Another important factor to consider is whether these studies are externally valid. In other words, can the findings be reproduced in the 'real-life' situation? In science, the randomized controlled trial is held in high esteem as it provides evidence of a 'cause-and-effect' relationship between two variables. In the case of the DPS, the DPP and the Da Qing study, the variables are intervention by a lifestyle approach (and by the use of metformin in the DPP) and the relative reduction in T2DM incidence. Several methodological issues that affect the ability of a study to establish a cause and effect relationship are provided in Table 13.2. These methodological issues are referred to as threats to internal validity by Thomas and Nelson (1996) and can be controlled by adopting the RCT model. Thus, both internal validity (the ability of a study to establish cause-and-effect) and external validity (the ability to generalize the results of a study to the wider population) are important. However, they are often at odds with one another. By controlling as many variables as possible a study gains in internal validity but loses external validity or generalizability.

Thus, despite their undoubted strengths, the DPS, DPP and Da Qing study demonstrate that it is possible to reduce the risk of type 2 diabetes in high-risk subjects participating in carefully controlled scientific trials. For those of us interested in the prevention of T2DM through lifestyle changes, the DPP and the DPS are held in great esteem and are used to convince people of the potential for the primary prevention of the condition, but much remains to be done before this potential can be realized in everyday public health and clinical practice. Apparently, the financial cost of the DPP has been estimated to be in excess of $174 million (The Diabetes Prevention Program Research Group 2003). For the lifestyle intervention group, the direct medical cost over 3 years

*Table 13.2* Potential threats to the internal validity of experimental studies that aim to establish a cause-and-effect relationship between independent and dependent variables

| *Threat to internal validity* | *Description and explanation* |
| --- | --- |
| History | Any event or intervention, other than that being studied, that occurs during the experimental period and that affects the outcome or dependent variable |
| Maturation | Processes that occur within the subjects as a result of time passing (e.g. ageing) |
| Experimental mortality | Subjects leaving the study for reasons that are not random. For example, leaving the study because the intervention is too difficult or not enjoyable |
| Selection bias | Identifying experimental groups for reasons that are not random. This means the groups may be different even before the intervention is applied |
| Testing | The effect that performing a test on one occasion has on the performance of the same test on a subsequent occasion. Performance on that test can change simply because the subject has performed the test before |
| Instrumentation | Changes of instrumentation or calibration of instruments that takes place during the study period |
| Statistical regression | When subjects are not randomly assigned to groups but are chosen on the basis of obtaining an extreme (high or low) score. On a subsequent occasion they are less likely to exhibit this extreme score |
| Selection–maturation interaction | When the passing of time might affect one group but not another |

Source: Thomas and Nelson (1996).

was $2780 per person. Economically, any intervention has to be cost-effective and it remains to be seen if a positive outcome such as that demonstrated by the DPP and DPS can be shown with a less expensive treatment. In the DPP, approximately 50 per cent of the lifestyle intervention participants achieved the target of a 7 per cent weight reduction goal and 74 per cent the goal of 150 minutes per week of moderate intensity physical activity. Amongst other things, the DPP intervention included frequent and intensive lifestyle coaching from trained and qualified instructors, a 16-session curriculum on behavioural self-management, supervised physical activity sessions and an extensive network of training, feedback and clinical support (The Diabetes Prevention Program Research Group 2002a). A 'toolbox' of strategies was employed for individual participants when they experienced barriers to adherence. For each participant, approximately $100 per year was available to assist participants who were having trouble achieving one of the goals. For example, subjects struggling to meet the physical activity target were enrolled in community exercise classes. Thus, despite the comprehensive and multidisciplinary lifestyle intervention, 50 per cent of the subjects were still unable to meet the weight loss target and about 25 per cent the physical activity goal. Subsequent analysis of the DPP data suggests that without weight loss, exercise was not effective at reducing the incidence of T2DM (The Diabetes Prevention Program Research Group 2002b).

The humility needed now by workers in the fields of epidemiology, public health and other disciplines interested in the accumulation of empirical evidence in this area is related to the practicalities of modifying behaviour and the environment to prevent T2DM and its related disorders if this is deemed to be ethical and appropriate by other members of society. The moral question all should answer for themselves is whether the ultimate aim is to prevent ill-health or to offer individuals the choice to prevent their own ill-health if they so wish.

## Bibliography

Alberti, K.G. and Zimmet, P.Z. (1998) 'Definition, diagnosis, and classification of diabetes mellitus and its complications. Part 1: diagnosis and classification of diabetes mellitus: provisional report of a WHO consultation', *Diabetic Med*, 15, 539–53.

Amos, A., McCarty, D. and Zimmet, P. (1997) 'The rising global burden of diabetes and its complications: estimates and projections to the year 2010', *Diabetic Med*, 14, S1–S85.

Azen, S.P., Peters, R.K., Berkowitz, K., Kjos, S., Xiang, A. and Buchanan, T.A. (1998) 'TRIPOD (TRoglitazone In the Prevention of Diabetes): a randomized, placebo-controlled trial of troglitazone in women with prior gestational diabetes mellitus', *Control Clin Trials*, 19, 217–31.

Chan, J.M., Rimm, E.B., Colditz, G.A., Stampfer, M.J. and Willett, W.C. (1994) 'Obesity, fat distribution and weight gain as risk factors for clinical diabetes in men', *Diabetes Care*, 17, 961–9.

Chen, J., Muntner, P., Hamm, L., Jones, D.W., Batuman, V., Fonseca, V., Whelton, P.K. and He, J. (2004) 'The metabolic syndrome and chronic kidney disease in U.S. adults', *Ann Intern Med*, 140, 167–74.

Chiasson, J-L., Josse, R.G., Gomis, R., Hanefeld, M., Karasik, A. and Laakso, M. for the STOP-NIDDM Trial Research Group (2002) 'Acarbose for prevention of type 2 diabetes mellitus: the STOP-NIDDM randomised trial', *Lancet*, 359, 2072–7.

Colditz, G.A., Willett, W.C., Rotnitzky, A. and Manson, J.E. (1995) 'Weight gain as a risk factor for clinical diabetes mellitus in women', *Ann Intern Med*, 122, 481–6.

Coutinho, M., Gerstein, H.C., Wang, Y. and Yusuf, S. (1999) 'The relationship between glucose and incident cardiovascular events: a metaregression analysis of published data from 20 studies of 95,783 individuals followed for 124 years', *Diabetes Care*, 22, 233–40.

Eriksson, K.F. and Lindgarde, F. (1991) 'Prevention of Type 2 diabetes mellitus by diet and physical exercise. The 6-year Malmo feasibility study', *Diabetologia*, 41, 1010–16.

Expert Panel on the Identification, Evaluation and Treatment of Overweight in Adults (1998) 'The identification, evaluation and treatment of overweight and obesity in adults: executive summary', *Am J Clin Nutr*, 68, 899–917.

Fagot-Campagna, A. and Narayan, K. (2001) 'Type 2 diabetes in children', *BMJ*, 322, 377–87.

Fletcher, RH., Fletcher, S. and Wagner, EH. (1996) *Clinical Epidemiology. The Essentials*, 3rd edn, Baltimore: Williams and Wilkins, 228–48.

Freeman, D.J., Norrie, J., Sattar, N. *et al.* (2001) 'Pravastatin and the development of diabetes mellitus: evidence for a protective treatment effect in the West of Scotland Coronary Prevention Study', *Circulation*, 103, 357–62.

Guillaume, M. and Rolland-Cachera, M.F. (2002) 'Epidemiology', in W. Burniat *et al.* (eds) *Child and Adolescent Obesity. Causes and Consequences, Prevention and Management*, Cambridge: Cambridge University Press.

Haffner, S.M., Lehto, S., Ronnemma, T. *et al.* (1998) 'Mortality from coronary heart disease in subjects with type 2 diabetes and in nondiabetic subjects with and without myocardial infarction', *N Engl J Med*, 339, 229–34.

Hardman, A.E. and Stensel, D.J. (2003) *Physical Activity and Health. The Evidence Explained*, London: Routledge, 76–92.

Hogan, P., Dall, T. and Nikolov, P. (2003) 'Economic costs of diabetes in the US in 2002', *Diabetes Care*, 26, 917–32.

Hu, F.B., Manson, J.E. and Stampfer, M.J. *et al.* (2001) 'Diet, lifestyle, and the risk of type 2 diabetes mellitus in women', *N Engl J Med*, 345, 790–7.

Kannel, W.B. and McGee, D.L. (1979) 'Diabetes and cardiovascular disease: the Framingham Study', *JAMA*, 241, 2035–8.

King, H., Aubert, R. and Herman, W. (1998) 'Global burden of diabetes, 1995–2025, prevalence, numerical estimates and projections', *Diabetes Care*, 21, 1414–31.

Kip, K.E., Marroquin, O.C., Kelley, D.E., Johnson, D., Kelsey, S.F., Shaw, L.J., Rogers, W.J. and Reis, S.E. (2004) 'Clinical importance of obesity versus the metabolic syndrome in cardiovascular risk in women. A report from the Women's Ischemia Syndrome Evaluation (WISE) Study', *Circulation*, 109, 706–13.

Knowler, W.C., Barrett-Connor, E., Fowler, S.E. *et al.* (2002) 'Reduction in the incidence of type 2 diabetes with lifestyle intervention or metformin', *N Engl J Med*, 346, 393–403.

Lakka, H.M., Laaksonen, D.E., Lakka, T.A. *et al.* (2002) 'The metabolic syndrome and total and cardiovascular disease mortality in middle-aged men', *JAMA*, 288, 2709-.

Manson, J.E., Nathan, D.M., Krolewski, A.S., Stampfer, M.J., Willett, W.C. and Hennekens, C.H. (1992) 'A prospective study of exercise and incidence of diabetes among US male physicians', *JAMA*, 268, 63–7.

Mokdad, A.H. (2003) 'Obesity in the United States', in G. Medieros-Neto, A. Halpern and C. Bouchard (eds) *Progress in Obesity Research: 9. Proceedings of the Ninth International Congress on Obesity*, Sao Paulo, Brazil: John Libbey, 561–3.

National Institutes of Health (2001) Third report of the National Cholesterol Education Program Expert Panel on Detection, Evaluation, and Treatment of High Blood Cholesterol in Adults (Adult Treatment Panel III), Bethesda, MD, NIH publication no. 01-3670.

Ninomiya, J.K., L'Italien, G., Criqui, M.H., Whyte, J.L., Gamst, A. and Chen, R.S. (2004) 'Association of the metabolic syndrome with history of myocardial infarction and stroke in the Third National Health and Nutrition Examination Survey', *Circulation*, 109, 42–6.

Olefsky, J.M. and Saltiel, A.R. (2000) 'PPAR-γ and the treatment of insulin resistance', *Trends Endocrinol Metab*, 11, 362–8.

Pan, X.R., Li, G.W., Hu, Y.H. *et al.* (1997) 'The Da Qing IGT Diabetes Study. Effects of diet and exercise in preventing NIDDM in people with impaired glucose tolerance', *Diabetes Care*, 20, 537–44.

Park, Y-W., Zhu, S., Palaniappan, L., Heshka, S., Carnethon, M.R. and Heymsfield, S.B. (2003) 'The Metabolic Syndrome: Prevalence and associated risk factor findings in the US population from the third National Health and Nutrition Examination Survey, 1988–1994', *Arch Intern Med*, 163, 427.

Rosenbloom, A., Joe, J., Young, R. and Winter, W. (1999) 'Emerging epidemic of Type 2 diabetes in youth', *Diabetes Care*, 22, 345–54.

Seidell, J.C. (2003) 'Prevalence and time trends of obesity in Europe', in G. Medieros-Neto, A. Halpern and C. Bouchard (eds) *Progress in Obesity Research: 9. Proceedings of the Ninth International Congress on Obesity*, Sao Paulo, Brazil: John Libbey, 571–8.

Swinburn, B.A., Metcalf, P.A. and Ley, S.J. (2001) 'Long-term (5 year) effects of a reduced-fat diet intervention in individuals with glucose intolerance', *Diabetes Care*, 24, 619–24.

The Diabetes Prevention Program (DPP) Research Group (2002a) 'The Diabetes Prevention Program (DPP). Description of lifestyle intervention', *Diabetes Care*, 25, 2165–71.

The Diabetes Prevention Program (DPP) Research Group (2002b) 'Effects of change in weight, diet and physical activity on risk of diabetes with intensive lifestyle (ILS) intervention in the Diabetes Prevention Program (DPP)', *Diabetes (Suppl)*, 2, A115.

The Diabetes Prevention Program Research Group (2003) 'Costs associated with the primary prevention of Type 2 diabetes mellitus in the Diabetes Prevention Program', *Diabetes Care*, 26, 36–47.

Thomas, J.R. and Nelson, J.K. (1996) *Research Methods in Physical Activity*, 3rd edn, Champaign, IL: Human Kinetics, 344–63.

Torgerson, J.S., Hauptman, J., Boldrin, M. and Sjostrom, L. (2004) 'XENical in the prevention of diabetes in obese subjects (XENDOS) Study. A randomized study of orlistat as an adjunct to lifestyle changes for the prevention of type 2 diabetes in obese patients', *Diabetes Care*, 27, 155–161.

Tuomilehto, J., Lindstrom, J., Erikkson, J.G. *et al.* (2001) 'Prevention of type 2 diabetes by changes in lifestyle among subjects with impaired glucose tolerance', *N Engl J Med*, 344, 1343–50.

United Kingdom Prospective Diabetes Study Group (1998) 'Intensive blood-glucose control with sulfonylureas or insulin compared with conventional treatment and risk of complications in patients with Type 2 diabetes (UKPDS 33)', *Lancet*, 353, 837–53.

Wannamethee, G.S. and Shaper, A.G. (2001) 'Physical activity in the prevention of cardiovascular disease: an epidemiological perspective', *Sports Med*, 31, 101–14.

Williams, S.R.P., Jones, E., Bell, W., Davies, B. and Bourne, M.W. (1997) 'Body habitus and coronary heart disease in men. A review with reference to methods of body habitus assessment', *Eur Heart J*, 18, 376–93.

Zimmet, P., Alberti, K.G. and Shaw, J. (2001) 'Global and societal implications of the diabetic epidemic', *Nature*, 414, 782–7.

Zimmet, P., Shaw, J. and Alberti, K.G.M.M. (2003) 'Preventing type 2 diabetes and the dysmetabolic syndrome in the real world: a realistic view', *Diabetic Med*, 20, 693–702.

# Index

# eBooks

eBooks – at www.eBookstore.tandf.co.uk

## A library at your fingertips!

eBooks are electronic versions of printed books. You can store them on your PC/laptop or browse them online.

They have advantages for anyone needing rapid access to a wide variety of published, copyright information.

eBooks can help your research by enabling you to bookmark chapters, annotate text and use instant searches to find specific words or phrases. Several eBook files would fit on even a small laptop or PDA.

**NEW:** Save money by eSubscribing: cheap, online access to any eBook for as long as you need it.

### Annual subscription packages

We now offer special low-cost bulk subscriptions to packages of eBooks in certain subject areas. These are available to libraries or to individuals.

For more information please contact webmaster.ebooks@tandf.co.uk

We're continually developing the eBook concept, so keep up to date by visiting the website.

## www.eBookstore.tandf.co.uk